Second
Edition

Social Work
in Health Care

SAGE SOURCEBOOKS FOR
THE HUMAN SERVICES SERIES

Series Editors: ARMAND LAUFFER and CHARLES GARVIN

Second
Edition

Social Work
in Health Care

Its Past and Future

Surjit Singh Dhooper

University of Kentucky

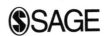

Los Angeles | London | New Delhi
Singapore | Washington DC

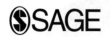

Los Angeles | London | New Delhi
Singapore | Washington DC

FOR INFORMATION:

SAGE Publications, Inc.
2455 Teller Road
Thousand Oaks, California 91320
E-mail: order@sagepub.com

SAGE Publications Ltd.
1 Oliver's Yard
55 City Road
London EC1Y 1SP
United Kingdom

SAGE Publications India Pvt. Ltd.
B 1/I 1 Mohan Cooperative Industrial Area
Mathura Road, New Delhi 110 044
India

SAGE Publications Asia-Pacific Pte. Ltd.
33 Pekin Street #02-01
Far East Square
Singapore 048763

Acquisitions Editor: Kassie Graves
Editorial Assistant: Courtney Munz
Production Editor: Karen Wiley
Copy Editor: Megan Granger
Typesetter: C&M Digitals (P) Ltd.
Proofreader: Caryne Brown
Indexer: Kathy Paparchontis
Cover Designer: Anupama Krishnan
Marketing Manager: Katie Winters
Permissions Editor: Adele Hutchison

Copyright ©2012 by SAGE Publications, Inc.

Printed in the United States of America

Library of Congress Cataloging-in-Publication Data

Dhooper, Surjit Singh.

Social work in health care : its past and future/Surjit Singh Dhooper.

p. cm. — (SAGE sourcebooks for the human services series)

Revised ed. of: Social work in health care in the 21st century

Includes bibliographical references and index.

ISBN 978-1-4522-0620-2 (pbk. : acid-free paper)

1. Medical social work. I. Dhooper, Surjit Singh. Social work in health care in the 21st century. II. Title.

HV687.D48 2012
362.1'0425—dc23   2011036146

This book is printed on acid-free paper.

11 12 13 14 15 10 9 8 7 6 5 4 3 2 1

CONTENTS

PREFACE

In early 2010, Kassie Graves of SAGE Publications approached me to revise *Social Work in Health Care in the 21st Century*, which I had published in 1997. I agreed, and the result is a new product. It is based on the same premise and promise and has the same format and structure, but is much richer in content. I have chosen to call it *Social Work in Health Care: Its Past and Future*.

The health care scene is changing. The health care system is being forced to recognize the need for change and is changing in many ways on many fronts—some changes being more obvious than others. For example, the September 11 attacks, anthrax, SARS (severe acute respiratory syndrome), flu vaccine shortages, fear of avian flu, and Hurricane Katrina have highlighted the inadequacy of the public health sector's preparedness for dealing with man-made and natural disasters. These changes have forced the federal government to attend to state public health departments' need for appropriate resources. Thus, a neglected sector of health care is receiving much-needed attention for revitalization.

The Patient Protection and Affordable Care Act of 2010 is the law of the land. It will provide health care to 32 million more Americans and bring about important changes in the way health care is delivered. It affects people, employers, and health insurance companies in significant ways. Its provisions will go into effect over a period of several years. Hundreds of thousands of young adults already are taking advantage of

the provision that allows persons younger than 26 to remain on their parents' health plans. The Health and Human Services Department estimates that about 1.2 million young adults will sign up for coverage in 2011 (Galewitz, 2011). The act was passed exclusively with the votes of Democrats in the two houses of Congress; Republicans opposed it and are vowing to undo it. Attorneys general of several states have sued the federal government, citing the law as a violation of state sovereignty. Legislators in many states have introduced measures to amend their constitutions to nullify portions of the new law. Governors are afraid that adding millions of people to their states' Medicaid rolls will add billions of dollars to state health care costs.

Republican members of Congress are planning to repeal or roll back the new law, or chip away at it if they cannot dismantle it. *Repeal*, *replace*, and *revise* are the buzzwords. The probability of their plans' success is low because (1) the law is a response to a genuine need, (2) its popular and unpopular provisions are intertwined, (3) it will save $143 billion over a 10-year period, (4) opponents do not agree on what to replace it with, and (5) they are not likely to gain the two-thirds majority needed in both houses of Congress to overcome a veto (Pear, 2010). Nevertheless, there is an air of uncertainty.

Changes independent of the politics of health care are also taking place. Advances in biomedical knowledge and health care technology are the most obvious and impressive. Americans appreciate and take pride in the medical miracles being achieved in the nation's hospitals. They are also spending billions on alternative methods of treatment that are not dependent on high technology—methods such as acupuncture, yoga, tai chi, homeopathy, massage therapy, and aromatherapy. Physicians are learning to coexist with those practicing nontraditional forms of medicine.

Advances in medical science and technology have the potential to turn physicians into super-technicians. The pecking order within the medical profession is changing. Specialties such as family practice, geriatrics, rehabilitation medicine, psychiatry, and general medicine are becoming more prominent. Hospitals are diversifying activities horizontally as well as vertically. They are integrating into outpatient facilities that diagnose patients prior to admission, into subacute facilities that shelter patients after discharge, and into many other forms of health care not directly linked to acute care. Ambulatory services are grabbing center stage. The ideas of prevention and early detection of illness, health maintenance, and wellness have started appealing to patients and physicians alike. The medical establishment is encouraging medical students and residents to choose generalist careers. Cost-containment efforts, exemplified by the practices of managed-care organizations, are changing the age-old concepts of "physician-patient relationship," "professional judgment," and "autonomy."

Yes, change is taking place. From the perspective of the social work profession, we need to acknowledge that (1) social work has an impressive history of significant contributions to the field of health care, which should goad and guide us to make our future in health care even more impressive; (2) social workers operate in host settings in all sectors of health care, and our place in those settings depends on our ability to affect them positively by meeting their needs; and (3) social workers have to be creative in retaining their existing roles and taking on new ones that other professionals are ill-equipped to perform. Thus, the vital questions are (1) *Should we anticipate and prepare for the future?* and (2) *How should we prepare for an uncertain future?*

My answer to the first question is that social workers do not have a choice. If we are ever to be proactive—and social workers are often accused of being reactive—we must not passively wait for the future to unfold. The answer to the second question is that we should prepare for the future by reducing the degree of uncertainty and using the uncertainty to our advantage—by anticipating the future, preparing for it, and venturing into it with faith in ourselves, with creativity, with imagination, and with the willingness to take risks.

This book is built on a threefold belief: (a) the future is never completely divorced from the past, (b) coming events cast their shadows before them, and (c) people have power over the future—we build it both by what we do and by what we do not do. This book is based on the premise that social work has much to give the health care world—and in many ways, both traditional and innovative. The book (1) looks at the four major sectors of health care—acute care, ambulatory care, illness prevention and health promotion work, and long-term care; (2) reviews the past and present of the organizations within these sectors; (3) makes projections about their future in light of realistic assessments of their current situations; (4) identifies their major needs; and (5) discusses how social work can step in and help meet those needs.

The book is divided into eight chapters. Chapter 1 describes and discusses the already-happening and likely to continue demographic and other sociological changes; advances in biomedical knowledge and health care technology; and changes in health care financing, structure, and services. It discusses persisting health and health-related problems, the significance of all these changes for the social work profession, and the profession's assets for taking on relevant future roles. Chapters 2 and 3 orient the reader to the history of the major health care organizations in the four sectors mentioned above and identify the emerging and future needs of those organizations, as well as needs of health care providers across those sectors. Chapters 4 through 7 provide a brief history of social work in each of the four sectors, propose future social work roles, and discuss the required knowledge and skills for the performance of those roles. Chapter 8 presents a set of general strategies that will, over and above the role-specific skills discussed in earlier chapters, enable social workers to thrive in the health care world of the future.

Throughout the book, effort has been made to point out or suggest appropriate theoretical concepts, practice principles, and practical "shoulds." Overall, an approach is recommended that incorporates (a) general systems theory, which helps in grasping the complex realities and relationships of systems at all levels, from individual clients to organizations and institutions; (b) the problem-solving methodology; and (c) such powerful social work concepts as "enabling" and "empowerment." Practitioners in other professions are embracing social work perspectives and methodology to enrich their theories and models for explaining health-related phenomena and to strengthen their strategies for intervening in the lives of people at individual and community levels.

It is hoped that the current and future social work practitioners in health care will take the initiative and expand the scope of their jobs, take on roles traditionally not seen as social work, help their agencies anticipate the future, plan future-relevant programs and activities, and thereby create innovative positions for themselves and other social workers. No other profession has the breadth of scope, richness of perspective, and array of skills appropriate for different levels of intervention. Social workers should seek positions that are not likely to be advertised clearly as social work positions, because many employers are likely to have a restricted view of their expertise. If this book provides some direction, guidance, and a nudge to explore the unknown, it will have served its purpose.

I am thankful to Kassie Graves, my editor at SAGE Publications. I am ever grateful for the understanding and support of my wife, Harpal. My youngest son-in-law, Theodore Kopp, a physician, checked for accuracy the material in the "Advances in Biomedical Knowledge and Health Care Technology" section in Chapter 1. His input is deeply appreciated.

—Surjit Singh Dhooper

Dedicated to my grandchildren

Maya, Matias

Mantegh, Sachleen

Tej, Amik

and

Liv

who are a source of joy.

1

INTRODUCTION

Social work has been a part of the health care scene for more than 100 years. It has an impressive history of significant contributions to the field of health care in settings such as hospitals, clinics, rehabilitation centers, nursing homes, health departments, hospices, and home health agencies. Social workers have been involved in health care at all levels: preventive care, primary care, secondary care, tertiary care, restorative care, and continuing care. Depending on the major purposes and functions of each health care setting, their roles have varied, requiring differential professional skills. Their professional organization, the National Association of Social Workers, has not only promulgated standards of social work practice in health care but also has been in the forefront of the movement for reform of the health care system.

For a hundred years, many political leaders—including U.S. presidents—have talked and tried to bring about major changes in the nation's health care system. They either failed in their efforts or succeeded in affecting some dimensions of the system in piecemeal ways. In 1912, Theodore Roosevelt promised national health insurance in his campaign for presidency. In 1945, Harry Truman came up with a plan for health care overhaul, but that fizzled after his critics started warning

him of "socialized medicine." In 1962, John F. Kennedy promoted health benefits for the recipients of Social Security, but the powerful medical industry succeeded in stalling his plan in Congress. In 1965, Lyndon Johnson succeeded in creating the Medicare and Medicaid programs. In 1971, Richard Nixon backed a proposal requiring employers to provide a minimum level of health insurance to their employees, but Senator Edward Kennedy counter-proposed a universal, single-payer reform plan and nothing happened. In 1976, Jimmy Carter called for a "comprehensive national health insurance system with universal and mandatory coverage," but as the nation fell into a deep recession, that call was neglected. In 1986, Congress passed the COBRA (Consolidated Omnibus Budget Reconciliation Act), which allows employees to continue their group health plans up to 18 months after losing their jobs. In 1988, Ronald Reagan signed the Medicare Catastrophic Coverage Act, which was repealed the following year. In 1994, Bill Clinton led a major effort to reform the health care system but failed. In 1997, he did create the State Children's Health Insurance Program. In 2003, George W. Bush signed the Medicare Modernization Act, which expanded Medicare to include prescription-drug coverage ("History of Reform," 2010).

President Barack Obama has signed into law the Patient Protection and Affordable Care Act of 2010. It is far from an overhaul of the health care system but provides health care to 32 million more Americans, brings about some significant changes, and has the potential to give a new direction to the way health care is delivered. The act was passed exclusively with the votes of Democrats in the two houses of Congress; Republicans opposed it and are vowing to undo it. They also have been able to win large segments of the general population to their view of the health care law. Before discussing the nature of this opposition and its likely consequences, we will list the main provisions of the act.

The Patient Protection and Affordable Care Act of 2010 is divided into 10 titles. Its provisions will go into effect over a period of several years—some immediately (i.e., 90 days after enactment), others 6 months after enactment, and still others in the years 2011, 2013, 2014, 2018, and 2020. The law affects people, employers, and health insurance companies in significant ways. Following the example of Tumulty, Pickert, and Park (2010) and using some of their material, we present below a timeline of the new law's provisions as they affect different entities.

2010

Americans who are uninsured because of preexisting conditions get immediate coverage through high-risk pools. They pay premiums for a standard population, not for one with higher health risk. Young adults can remain on their parent's plan until their 26th birthday. Individuals affected by the Medicare Part D coverage gap receive a $250 rebate.

Insurers are barred from (1) dropping coverage when a person gets sick, (2) denying coverage to children with preexisting conditions, (3) imposing caps in lifetime coverage, and (4) charging copayment or deductibles for preventive care and medical screening (on all new insurance plans). They are required to reveal details about their administrative and executive expenditures.

Employers: Small businesses (those employing 25 or fewer workers) can receive tax credits to purchase health insurance for their employees.

2011

Americans on Medicare Part D receive a 50% discount on brand-name drugs while they are in the doughnut hole; 50% of the Part D coverage gap is eliminated.

Insurers are required to (1) spend at least 80% of premiums on medical services or on improving the quality of health care, or (2) return the difference to the customer as a rebate.

2012

Employers must start disclosing the value of the benefits they provided for each employee's health insurance coverage on the employee's annual W-2 Form.

2013

Americans: Self-employment and wages of individuals above $200,000 annually (or of families above $250,000 annually) become subject to an additional tax of 0.5%.

2014

Americans: Most are required to get health care coverage or pay an annual penalty of $95 or up to 1% of income, whichever is higher. Families can get subsidies to buy insurance if they earn up to four times the federal poverty level.

Individuals with income up to 133% of the poverty line become eligible for Medicaid. Individuals and small businesses can buy insurance packages from the state-run "exchanges" that will offer nonprofit health insurance plans.

Employed individuals who pay more than 9.5% of their income on health insurance premiums are permitted to purchase insurance from a state-controlled health insurance option.

Insurers *are* prohibited from (1) discriminating against or charging higher rates for individuals based on preexisting medical conditions and (2) establishing annual spending caps. They become subject to a new excise tax based on their market share.

Employers: Businesses employing 50 or more full-time workers must provide health insurance coverage or pay a $2,000-per-employee tax penalty.

Others: Pharmaceutical companies and manufacturers of medical devices start paying an excise tax.

2018

Insurers: All existing health insurance plans must cover preventive care and checkups without payment. High-cost, employer-provided policies ($27,500 for family or $10,000 for single coverage) become subject to a 40% excise tax.

2020

Americans on Medicare Part D: The prescription-drug coverage gap is eliminated.

Other important provisions of the act are aimed at transforming the features of the health industry that reward volume of services and not value. These direct the federal government to experiment with ways providers can be compensated for quality of care. The experiments will include (1) pilot projects exploring different payment reforms within the Medicare program; (2) comparative-effectiveness research; (3) cuts to the Medicare program (eliminating waste in the system); (4) an independent board to study clinical outcomes and evidence; (5) penalizing hospitals with the highest rates of avoidable infections and unnecessary readmissions; (6) bonus payments to Medicare Advantage plans with the best clinical outcomes and highest patient ratings; (7) program funding for further training, scholarships, and loan repayments for physicians, nurse practitioners, and dentists entering primary care; (8) creating health centers based in communities and schools; and (9) support for programs such as "medical homes," a team-based approach to health care that emphasizes maintenance of health rather than treatment of disease.

Although the new law does not directly change the health care system's shape and structure, its functions and priorities, and the roles and responsibilities of its functionaries, it will affect the lives of millions of Americans. It will provide health insurance coverage to young adults between the ages of 19 and 29, who represent the largest segment of the uninsured—numbered at about 13.7 million in 2008 (Collins & Nicholson, 2010). Up to 15 million women who are uninsured will gain subsidized coverage, and another 14.5 million who are insured will benefit from the provisions that improve coverage or reduce premiums. Women who are charged higher premiums than men, who cannot secure coverage for the cost of pregnancy, or who have preexisting conditions excluded from their benefits will ultimately find themselves on a level playing field with men (Collins, Rustgi, & Doty, 2010). Several short- and long-term provisions will help small businesses pay for their workers' health insurance. Over the next 10 years, small businesses could receive an estimated $40 billion in government support through the premium credit program. Up to 16.6 million workers are in business establishments eligible for tax credit (Collins, Davis, Nicholson, & Stremikis, 2010).

Despite the anticipated benefits listed above, the health care law is being challenged. Opponents, mostly Republicans, are opposing it on several grounds. Attorneys general of several states have sued the federal government, citing the law as a violation of state sovereignty. They claim that Congress has no authority to require individuals to purchase health insurance. Legislators in many states have introduced measures to amend their constitutions to nullify portions of the new law. Governors are afraid that adding millions of people to their states' Medicaid rolls will add billions of dollars to state health care costs, even after the federal government picks up the tab for the newly eligible. There are those who believe that health care reform should be left to the states. However, the reality is that a state-by-state approach would make it harder to rein in health costs with system-wide reforms. In the current economic climate, states are in no position to launch initiatives. Even in better times, states with the highest rates of uninsured have shown little interest in expanding coverage (MacGillis, 2010). Furthermore, having 50 different health care delivery programs would create a nightmare of varying coverage and bureaucracy (Seward & Todd, 1995). And as Ignagni (1995) put it,

If I am a Medicaid recipient, why should I be deprived of benefits in one state and entitled to them in another, or protected by quality assurance standards in one state and left unprotected in another, simply by accident of birth or residence? Similarly, should a health plan operating in 50 states be subjected to 50 different sets of regulatory requirements? And should different kinds of health care delivery systems be held to different levels of accountability? (pp. 223–224)

Many legal authorities are of the opinion that the legal challenges to the new law have no merit and are unlikely to succeed (Jost, 2010). Instead of beginning the work of developing systems to implement the expansion of Medicaid, state governments are allowing themselves to be distracted from the real work ahead. Many of the states opposing expansions are those whose Medicaid-eligible patient populations have the most to gain from health reform (Ku, 2010). Republican members of Congress are planning to repeal or roll back the new law, or to chip away at it if they cannot dismantle it. *Repeal, replace,* and *revise* are the buzzwords. Their strategies include (1) withholding money needed to administer and enforce the law; (2) going after specific provisions of the law, such as the requirement for most Americans to obtain health insurance and for employers to offer insurance to their employees or pay a tax penalty; and (3) scaling back the expansion of Medicaid if states continue to object to the cost of adding more people to the program. The probability of their plans' success is low because (1) the law is a response to a genuine need, (2) its popular and unpopular provisions are intertwined, (3) it will save $143 billion over a 10-year period, (4) opponents do not agree on what to replace it with, and (5) they are not likely to gain the two-thirds majority needed in both houses of Congress to overcome a veto (Pear, 2010). Nevertheless, there is an air of uncertainty.

On the other hand, trends in demography, patterns of morbidity, and advances in the technology of health care are like straws in the wind, indicating the direction of future changes despite the politics of health care. Shapes of things to come already are visible, validating the truth of the adage that coming events cast their shadows before them. It is reasonable to think that the future U.S. health care system will be different from what it is today. It will be different in the philosophy, approaches, priorities, and rewards of its organizations and in the attitudes, knowledge, and skills of its care providers. Social work must prepare for those changes and turn the prevailing uncertainty into an opportunity for meaningful contributions to the health care of tomorrow. This book is a partial response to that professional need.

This chapter (a) reviews the past and present of social work in health care; (b) forecasts the future of health care by looking at the anticipated demographic and other sociological changes, advances in biomedical knowledge and health care technology, and changes in health care financing, structure, and services; (c) identifies the health and health-related problems that are likely to persist; (d) discusses the significance of the changing health care scene for social work; and (e) identifies the assets that the social work profession can build on for its future roles.

A BRIEF LOOK AT SOCIAL WORK AND HEALTH CARE

In all health care settings, social workers have provided a holistic perspective on problems and situations, highlighting the social antecedents and consequences of illnesses and the need to deal with the larger picture along with the immediate concern. At the level of the individual's acute or chronic illness, a social worker's focus is on the patient's physical, psychosocial, and environmental health needs. In the second half of the 19th century, social workers were in the forefront of the movement for reform in labor, housing, relief, sanitation, and health care. They were acutely aware of the interdependence of all dimensions of human life. They saw how such social factors as poor housing, neighborhoods, work conditions, family situations, and diet adversely affected health and how poor health, in turn, produced a host of social problems. They viewed health as more than the mere absence of illness and considered physical health as necessary for social, psychological, and economic well-being. The following quote illustrates this interrelationship:

> It is bad enough that a man should be ignorant, for this cuts him off from the commerce of men's minds. It is perhaps worse that he should be poor, for this condemns him to a life of stint and scheming in which there is no time for dreams and no respite from weariness. But what is surely worst, is that he should be unwell, for then he can do little about either his poverty or his ignorance. (Kimble, as quoted in Haughton, 1972, p. 28)

This recognition of health care's importance for the total well-being of the individual and the ability of social workers to make unique contributions to patient care resulted in health social work becoming the largest field of social work practice. Of all the health care sectors, social work in hospitals became the most remarkable in terms of the number of social workers employed, variety of professional social work roles performed, richness of the practice models used, strategies and approaches developed, and tasks performed—tasks aimed at enhancing the quality of patient care, as well as at contributing to the institutions' efficiency and cost-containment efforts.

The emergence of social work roles and responsibilities and the development of appropriate knowledge and skills have been partly the result of an evolutionary process and partly that of the profession's reaction to the changing situation and needs of the health care system. Many factors have affected the development and practice of social work. The complexity of health care organizations along with a number of variables such as their perception of social work practice, their resources, the organizational climate, the competencies of social workers, and administrative and interdisciplinary support (Holosko, 1992) resulted in the differential use of social work skills. There is also much variation in the nature and functions of various health care organizations, even within each health care sector. Here, we look at hospitals as an example of this variance and how hospital-related variables affect the practice of social work.

Marked differences exist between, for example, a small community hospital and a large university-based teaching medical center or between a public general hospital and a for-profit private specialty hospital. Such differences have demanded variations in the nature and degree of social work involvement. The standards of the Joint Commission on Accreditation of Health Care Organizations require that every hospital make social work services readily available to patients and their families; that these services be well organized, properly directed, and staffed with a sufficient number of qualified individuals; and that social work services be appropriately integrated with other units. Hospital social work departments vary considerably, however, in terms of the number of social workers employed and the extent and nature of their work. The dominance of the health care field by physicians and their perspective of and approach to health care is also an important reality. Physicians and others often have tended to define social work roles and functions. Social workers have carried out the expected roles and performed the required functions, but while doing so, they also have sensitized other health care professionals to the psychosocial aspects of illness and treatment and the need for dealing with the total patient rather than merely his or her illness or disease.

> In reviewing social work's goal of making the health care delivery system more sensitive to the needs of its clients, one finds that social work professionals have met with infinite success in their ability to have other professions adapt to their ways of helping, such as by considering the whole person and his or her life outside the institution. (Kerson, 1985, p. 301)

This success has had an important side effect. Professionals from other disciplines have accepted part of the "what" and "how" of social work and incorporated it into their philosophies and practices. Meyer (1984) said that we should be glad "that some of our special values are now held in esteem by others; it means that clients will reap the gains" (p. 7). However, this loss of distinctiveness of social work perspective and methodology has weakened, to a large extent, social work's claim to its own "turf" within the hospital. Social work functions in hospitals have included work with patients and their families involving provision of both concrete services and intangible psychotherapy; work on behalf of patients and their families, both within the hospital and outside; work regarding the hospital's mission and overall functioning; work regarding the community's health needs and resources; and education of social work students and other health care professionals.

Most social work units in hospitals have been responsible for at least the following functions: (a) high-risk screening, (b) psychosocial assessments and intervention, (c) interdisciplinary collaboration for coordinated patient care, (d) discharge planning, and (e) postdischarge follow-up. Despite the important relevance of these functions to the quality and effectiveness of medical care, social work has not become a core health care profession. Social workers have experienced only limited success in asserting their professional autonomy and assimilating into the medical world as occupiers of their own legitimate turf. In the words of Erickson and Erickson (1992),

> Having a place to stand within the field, with a defined area of competence, a shared and recognized domain of autonomy, are all matters that are never finally settled (other than perhaps in specific sites) in the field, but rather are continuously subject to redefinition. (p. 7)

Meyer (1984) provides an explanation of this state of affairs:

> Our professional problem is not that we are lacking in experience, knowledge and skills, but rather that we have for so long concentrated our efforts on the doing of our work, we have not articulated it, we have not evaluated it, and worst of all, we have not thought about it. We are still an emerging profession because we have used our feet and not our heads. In this regard, it would be well to follow the medical model; physicians write up what they do, and often because they claim expertise, they are perceived as having it. Social workers are too modest to claim the domain they have been working in for a hundred years. (p. 9)

The unpleasant reality is that, in the turmoil of change on the health care scene that started with the introduction of a new system of financing based on diagnosis-related groups (DRGs), social work lost ground in the hospital sector. Hospitals experienced closings, downsizings, mergers, affiliations, and other forms of restructuring, and in the process of cutting costs, departments viewed as not producing enough revenue became easy prey.

Since the late 1990s, hospital census and bed-utilization-per-staff statistics have contributed to the elimination of staff positions, which resulted in the reduction or elimination of hospital social work departments. As part of downsizing and reengineering, many hospitals eliminated the social work director's position and redeployed remaining social workers to operate under the supervision of nurses or generically trained case managers and administrators (National Association of Social Workers, 2006, p. 189).

Not only were social work positions eliminated, many social workers were replaced by nonprofessional staff and other disciplines appropriated key social work functions. In answer to the question, "Is hospital-based social work in jeopardy?" Ross (1993) said that a widespread, progressive, and serious malady was threatening this professional domain and that the prognosis was uncertain. That statement is still true. Although the status of social work in other sectors of health care has not been uncertain, social workers are not making up for the losses experienced in the hospital sector. This is where forecasting the future, and thereby hoping to influence it, becomes a desirable professional activity.

FORECASTING THE FUTURE OF HEALTH CARE

Erdmann and Stover (1993) told a story of two frogs in the meadow who fell into a pail of milk. After an hour of struggling to jump out and failing, one of the frogs gave up and drowned. The other struggled all night and churned the cream of the milk into butter and found himself sitting on a solid clump. He jumped out and went on his way. Drawing and building on the lessons from this story, the authors emphasized the importance of an optimistic outlook, hard work, perseverance, facility for assessing a situation realistically, the ability to convert facts—even inconvenient and painful facts—into a solid basis for action, and being prepared for the unexpected. We, as social workers, can add to this list the need to recognize our power over the future. "We ourselves build the future both through what we do and what we do not do" (Cornish, 1994, p. 60).

Forecasting can be done through several methods. To anticipate and prepare for the future of social work in health care, we have mixed and matched those methods and used data from the past and present, as well as projections about people and the conditions of their lives in the future. This mixing and matching has been done with the realization that forecasting the future is a risky affair. The risk of being wrong is high, and the rapid pace of changes in society is increasing possibilities of error.

The view of the health care field's future presented in this book is based on many streams of information and conjectures. These include (a) anticipated demographic and other sociological changes that will significantly affect the health care field; (b) anticipated advances in biomedical knowledge and health care technology; (c) likely changes in health care financing, structure, and services; and (d) health and health-related problems that are likely to persist. In the following section, we discuss the likely ways the health care system will respond to these changes and social work contributions to those responses. Table 1-A provides a glimpse of those forecasts.

Table 1-A Factors Likely to Affect the Future of Health Care

Demographic Changes	Decrease in the population of younger people
	Increase in the elderly population
	Nonwhites composing majority of the population
Sociological Changes	Minorities gaining political power
	More women in the workforce
	Changes in the institutions of marriage and family
Biomedical and Health-Related Technological Advancements	New drugs and diets for disease prevention and treatment
	New technologies for diagnosis and treatment
	Enhancement in the understanding of the human organism
	Changes in the approaches to health care

(Continued)

Table 1-A (Continued)

Changes in Health Care Financing, Structure, and Services	Many more people on Medicaid
	High-deductible health plans combined with health savings accounts becoming widely available
	More emphasis on outpatient care
	Illness prevention and health promotion becoming prominent
Likely-to-Persist Health-Related Problems	Medical problems
	Medicalized social problems
	Social problems

Anticipated Demographic and Sociological Changes

In order to appreciate the projected demographic changes in the country, we provide some of its current demographics below.

In 2010, the United States had a population of a little more than 310 million (310,519,000 to be exact). In 2007, people under the age of 20 made up more than a quarter (27.6%) of the population and people aged 65 and over made up about one-eighth (12.6%). Of the total population, about 156 million are female and about 152 million are male. The total fertility rate (estimated in 2009) is 2.05 children per woman, which is slightly lower than the replacement rate of 2.1. Racially, the country has a white American majority. Minorities compose about one third (102.5 million) of the population. Population growth is fastest among minorities as a whole. In 2005, 45% of American children below the age of 5 belonged to minority groups ("Demographics of the United States," 2010).

From 80 million in 1900, the population of the United States has grown to more than 300 million in 2010 and is projected to reach 438 million by the middle of the century. The nation's elderly population will more than double by

then. The non-Hispanic white population will increase more slowly than other racial ethnic groups. That will result in white Americans becoming a minority (47%) by 2050. The Latino population, already the largest minority group, will triple in size and account for most of the country's population growth (Passel & Cohn, 2008). In 2050, the nation's population of children is expected to be 62% minority, up from 44% today. The percentage of the "working-age" population (those aged 18–64) is projected to decline from 63% in 2008 to 57% in 2050. The working-age population is projected to become more than 50% minority in 2050 (up from 34% in 2008). Immigrants and their U.S.-born descendants are expected to provide most of the population gain in the decades ahead (U.S. Census Bureau, 2010).

These projections are based on two assumptions: (1) the rate of immigration will hold steady, and (2) the different birth rates of first-, second-, and third-generation immigrants will continue. Regarding the validity of the first assumption, we agree with Haub (2008) that (1) there are no laws on the horizon that would seriously curb immigration, (2) some people view immigration as necessary for filling gaps in the aging workforce and providing support for retirees,

(3) the United States will continue to symbolize a better life for millions in developing countries, (4) populations in many sending countries and regions will continue to grow and thereby maintain a pool of potential immigrants, and (5) immigrants maintain ties with their extended families in their native lands, and family reunification provisions of the immigration law also lead to the continued inflow of new immigrants. Regarding the second assumption, there is no reason to believe that the pattern of birth rates for first-, second-, and third-generation Americans will be different in the future.

In view of the current and projected demographic changes, Irvin (2007) says that the United States is headed for a "demographic singularity," which he defines as a pace of change so fast that the American identity as we know it will be irreversibly altered. These changes are also likely to lead to many others that will significantly affect the nature, quality, and structure of health care in the future. The gradual increase in life expectancy will continue. For example, in 2007, American men could expect to live 3.5 years longer and women 1.6 years longer than they did in 1990 (National Center for Health Statistics, 2010a). More and more people will live longer and be healthier. They will be culturally more diverse, better informed, and politically more active. Social institutions will constantly make efforts to accommodate the special needs of various groups such as the elderly, minorities, and women.

As hinted above, a sizeable proportion of the population will be made up of those aged 65 and older. The U.S. Census Bureau projects that the 65+ population will double between 2000 and 2050. One in nine current baby boomers will live to at least age 90. The number of those 85 years old and over will quadruple by 2050. Based on the findings of several studies and surveys, Ervin (2000) has offered the following forecasts regarding this population.

1. *The retired will work again.* More elders will reenter the labor force because of their proficiency with computers and the new legislation that allows those 65 to 69 to earn without penalizing Social Security benefits.

2. *Tech-savvy seniors will maintain their independence.* Elder-friendly technology will help in several ways by improving the ability of frail and vulnerable seniors to access information and resources and by reducing isolation of those living in rural and hard-to-reach areas. Products such as the multifunctional pager, which alerts seniors when it is time to take a particular medication, will become readily available.

3. *The hottest fitness buffs? Seniors!* Health plans will begin offering health club memberships and personal trainers as part of their coverage for seniors.

4. *Senior-friendly cars will offer independence.* Automakers will market cars that are easier and safer for seniors to drive. The "senior-mobiles" may feature higher seats, larger numbers on the speedometer, and slower acceleration. They will help seniors retain their independence—as losing the ability to drive is, for many, synonymous with losing their independence.

5. *Seniors will be important voters.* Seniors are already the top voters; they will be the most informed voters in the future. One survey showed that four of the five TV programs most frequently watched by seniors are some type of news program. Seniors also are avid readers, with 87% ranking reading the newspaper among their most favored regular activities.

6. *More alternatives to nursing homes will emerge.* These will include assisted living, independent living, life-care communities, and adult day-care facilities. Most people do not know of the alternatives currently available. One of the government's biggest tasks in the future will be to increase people's awareness in this regard.

7. *Boomers could end up impoverished.* Many aging baby boomers may find themselves impoverished because they did not plan for the costs of long-term care.

8. *Elder care shortage is coming.* As the population of those 85 and older doubles to 8.4 million by 2030, the demand for professional home-care aids will skyrocket.

9. *Aging boomers will force health care policy changes.* There is power in numbers. About 76 million boomers born between 1946 and 1964 soon will join the ranks of older Americans. Many of them are providing care for their aging parents. They also have a vested interest in ensuring that quality health care will be available for them as they grow older.

10. *Elder care will hurt women's careers.* Despite their advancement up the corporate ladder, women are disproportionately affected by elder care. A study by the National Alliance of Caregiving and the AARP found that 31% of caregivers significantly alter their career paths, and some leave the workforce altogether.

11. *Telecommuting will assist family caregivers.* Increased telecommuting will ease the burden of long-distance caregiving by allowing working adults to move closer to their aging parents. As more and more companies offer telecommuting, their employees will be able to work from anywhere in the country and, thereby, also meet eldercare responsibilities.

12. *More employers will offer eldercare.* Eldercare benefits will become a major issue as increased eldercare-related absences and falling productivity begin to take a toll in the workplace. Employers will offer more eldercare benefits to combat employee turnover.

13. *Caregivers will need interviewing skills.* As the senior population grows, there will be a constant stream of new products and services for them. Caregivers will be forced to make decisions on whom to hire and which organization to use. Employers will provide training to their employees on how to make good decisions about hiring home aides and choosing eldercare service providers.

14. *Working families will gain state allies.* California, Minnesota, Oregon, and Washington already have passed laws that allow workers not covered by union contracts to use up to one half of their paid sick leave to care for an ill child, spouse, or parent. Other states will take similar steps to ensure that companies accommodate the caregiving responsibilities of their employees.

An increasingly large number of the elderly will lead generally healthy and independent lives.

More and more of them will respond to society's call to continue using their knowledge and skills by staying in the workforce longer or reentering it. As a group, however, the elderly will continue to be heavy users of health and social services as they survive such illnesses as heart attacks and strokes. At present, about 6.5 million older people need assistance with activities of daily living (e.g., bathing, cooking, cleaning, dressing). That number is expected to double by 2020. How best to meet the needs of the elderly and where—particularly the issue of community-based versus institutional long-term care—will continue to be important societal concerns.

The increased diversity *in* aging as well as *of* the aged population will be an important element adding complexity to that social reality. Even today, 40 years and three generations may separate the younger from the older "elderly." Different subgroups of the elderly have differing needs. The number of elderly from different racial, ethnic, and otherwise culturally diverse groups will grow, making it impossible to ignore their needs. Meeting these differential needs will be a significant challenge to policymakers and program planners. The attention given to the needs of the elderly and the resources devoted to meeting those needs possibly will generate animosity toward them on the part of younger generations. Feelings of neglect and social starvation may become part of the experience of more and more elderly. The suicide rate of the elderly is higher than that of the general population. People over age 65 make up only 12% of the population but are responsible for 16% of all suicides. While the suicide rate in the general population is 11 per 100,000 persons, it climbs to 14 per 100,000 in the elderly age group ("Suicide in the Elderly," 2009). This is despite the availability of powerful antidepressant medications and various psychosocial therapies for dealing with depression, which is considered to be the major cause of suicides in the elderly. The causes of depression in the elderly will not likely be reduced in the future.

As forecast above, the United States is moving rapidly from a white society of European origin to a multiracial and multicultural one. Many major cities already have nonwhite majorities, and this trend is rippling out from urban centers to suburban and rural areas. With today's minorities making up almost half the U.S. population by 2050, not only will the country's complexion have changed but its cultural norms and power structure will have as well. Spanish language will vie with English for prominence as the medium of communication. Los Angeles is now the second-largest Spanish-speaking city in the world, after Mexico City. One can prosper in southern Florida even if one speaks only Spanish. Some 1,000 publications already cater specifically to Latino audiences ("Latinos on the Rise," 1993). Similarly, Asian Americans will become much more visible and active. In the future, the various minority groups—ethnically different, culturally varied, and religiously diverse—will assert their claim to their share of political and economic power more successfully than they are now.

The same will be true of women. Their participation in the labor force will continue to increase. In 2008, 59.5% of women aged 16 and over were employed, compared with 73% of men (U.S. Bureau of Labor Statistics, 2008). In the future, women will reach a critical mass in virtually all white-collar professions. They will exercise more political power and ensure the elimination of gender-based disadvantages for themselves in the educational, occupational, and political arenas. They will not only have greater employment opportunities with equal pay for equal work under conditions favorable to them but will also occupy positions of leadership at all levels of management. Traditionally "feminine" attributes, such as the willingness to share power and information, will be seen as necessary to lead in a time of rapid change (Rosener, as quoted in Field, 1993). Their influence on the health care field will be manifold. This statement is truer today than it was 20 years ago: "Women who have been the backbone of medical institutions in menial and powerless roles are now claiming more influential positions as well as seeking different attitudes and behaviors from male physicians who have dominated the health care field" (Rehr, 1991, p. 11). In the future, they will have secured not only an easy entry into the fields of medicine and health care management but also positions of leadership. They will also be important for the application and success of many new health care technologies, such as gene therapy and chromosome manipulation, that will involve women more than men as patients.

Changes in marriage and family will continue at a mind-boggling pace. Fisher (2010) says that marriage has changed more in the past 100 years than it did in the 10,000 years before that and it could change more in the next 20 years than in the past 100. She has described the already occurring changes in this way:

> Let's look at virginity at marriage, arranged marriages, the concept that men should be the sole family bread winners, the credo that a woman's place is in the home, the double standard for adultery, and the concepts of "honor thy husband" and "til death do us part." These beliefs are vanishing. Instead, children are expressing their sexuality. "Hooking up" (a new term for a one-night stand) is becoming commonplace, along with living together, bearing children out of wedlock, women-headed households, interracial marriages, homosexual weddings, commuter marriages between individuals who live apart, childless marriages, betrothals between older women and younger men, and small families.
>
> Our concept of infidelity is changing. Some married couples agree to have brief sexual encounters when they travel separately; others sustain long-term adulterous relationships with the approval of a spouse. Even our concept of divorce is shifting. Divorce used to be considered a sign of failure; today it is often deemed the first step toward true happiness. (p. 27)

Before the 1960s, divorce was uncommon, laws made it difficult to divorce, and the general public disapproved of divorce. During the 1960s, 1970s, and 1980s, divorce rates increased, the legal system made it easier to get a divorce, and the general public became more accepting of divorce. In the 1990s, the divorce rate declined, state governments enacted programs to strengthen marriage, and the general public started supporting the norm of lifelong marriage. The present stage is likely to continue for some time (Amato, 2004).

Are the divorced better off than their married counterparts? Using data from the General Social

Survey, Forste and Heaton (2004) examined mean differences in measures of well-being, family attitudes, and socioeconomic status of individuals divorced, remarried, or in first marriages. Those first married between 1965 and 1975 were sampled, and 48% reported being divorced or separated. The divorced/separated reported the lowest level of well-being relative to those in their first marriage, and those who had remarried reported higher levels of well-being than those who were still divorced or separated. Lichter, Graefe, and Brown (2003) used data from the 1995 National Survey of Family Growth to examine marital histories of at-risk women. They found that poverty and welfare receipt are substantially lower for those who married and stayed married than for those who never married or were divorced.

Children who experience family disruption in the form of divorce and conflict are adversely affected. A number of studies have shown that divorce affects children through several mechanisms: (1) the stress of divorce tends to disrupt the quality of parenting from custodial parents; (2) living in a single-parent household undermines the quality of relations with noncustodial parents; (3) divorce typically is followed by a decline in household income; (4) divorce tends to exacerbate conflict between parents, causing many children to feel that they are "caught in the middle"; and (5) divorce is frequently followed by other stressful events, such as moving, parental remarriage, and additional parental divorce (Amato, 2004). A study by Kirk (2002) compared young adults who had experienced family divorce with those who had not. Parental divorce did not affect relationship competence, but the level of perceived family conflict did influence self-esteem, fear of intimacy, and romantic relationship satisfaction. Those who reported more conflict in their childhood families reported more fear of intimacy, less self-esteem, and lower romantic relationship satisfaction. Parental divorce did affect fear and expectations of divorce for those who had experienced it more than for their intact counterparts.

American families will become even more diverse in the future. With the decline of the traditional family of husband, wife, and children, it will become impossible to determine what a "typical" family is. The current picture of the American family includes nuclear families, single-parent families, remarried and stepfamilies, nonmarital heterosexual and homosexual cohabitation families, foster and adoptive families, and multiple-adult households. In 2008, 41% of babies were born to unmarried mothers, which is an eightfold increase from 50 years ago, and 25% of children lived in single-parent homes, almost three times the number from 1960 (Luscombe, 2010). Medical advances in the form of newer reproductive technologies are adding complexity to the familial picture. Genetic, gestational, and nurturing parents can now be separated or combined in numerous ways by various combinations of artificial insemination, in vitro fertilization, embryo transfer, and freezing (Chell, 1988).

This picture of the family will become even more complex in the future. "More individuals will experience a greater variety of family situations over their lifetime. For many this will include growing up in single- and multiple-parent situations, living singly, cohabiting, remarrying, and widowing" (Rubin, as quoted in Olson & Hanson, 1990). Child custody issues and disputes will become more tangled and difficult to deal with. Already, we are seeing biological parents fighting against stepparents for custody of children, grandparents suing for visitation rights even when a child has been adopted, and an estimated 1.5 million lesbian mothers living with their children (Herman, 1990). For the first time in its history, the U.S. Census Bureau counted gay marriages in its 2010 surveys. According to a 2007 study of adoption trends, more than 50% of gay men said they desired to be parents, compared with 41% of lesbians surveyed. Same-sex couples and homosexual singles applying for adoption tend to be older, better educated, and economically more resourceful than their heterosexual counterparts (Wagner, 2010). However, family policy, particularly adoption policy, has been slow in catching up to the reality of the new forms of family. As a result, same-sex couples are forced to manipulate the words of the law and "go in the back door" to adopt children (Crawford, 1999). This situation will change in the future.

Rates of marriage and divorce may become meaningless in the future. In view of the multiple forms of the family, such information will have little explanatory and predictive value. A recent survey by the Pew Research Center revealed that nearly 40% of Americans think marriage is obsolete (Luscombe, 2010). If the number of single-parent households continues to increase, the associated problem of disproportionately higher rates of poverty among single mothers and their children will continue.

The average number of children per family will continue to shrink, and childless families will become more common. Overall, fewer children in the country does not mean that those children are more adequately cared for. Since 1974, children have been more likely than adults to be living in poverty. In 2007, children represented 35.7% of all Americans living in poverty. As many as 13.3 million (18%) children lived in poverty, and another 15.7 million (21.2%) were classified as near poor with a family income between 100% and 200% of the poverty level. The proportions of Hispanic and black children in poverty are much higher than the above overall percentage. In 2007, 29% to 35% of Hispanic and black children were poor, compared with 10% to 13% of white and Asian children (National Center for Health Statistics, 2010a). Hence, this problem is not only persisting but getting worse. Poverty will continue to breed numerous other problems.

The complexity of life in the future will be reflected not only in the diversity of family forms but also in economic and work situations. America's large companies already have gone global.

> The companies on the S&P 500 generate 46% of their profits outside the U.S., and for many of the biggest American names, the proportion is much higher. . . . Nearly 80% of Coca-Cola's revenue comes from outside the U.S., and an even greater percentage of its employees are in foreign countries. (Zakaria, 2010, p. 32)

This phenomenon will affect not only the overall availability of jobs but also the nature and quality of jobs in the country. The U.S. industry will face tougher competition from abroad and will have to satisfy much more informed and sophisticated consumers while accommodating the needs and demands of its workers. Worker benefits will include insurance for or provision of health care, mental health care, child-care, and eldercare services. Case management and comprehensive counseling will be included in benefits packages.

In the future, the importance of groups and group work in the lives of people will grow. Kessler, Mickelson, and Zhao (1997) conservatively estimated that more than 25 million Americans have participated in a self-help group at some time in their lives—more than 10 million of those in the past 12 months. They excluded groups organized or facilitated by professionals. Not only are people part of self-help or mutual-aid groups that meet face to face, they also are participating in online support networks. The latter operate on message boards, newsgroups, and bulletin boards, and through chat groups, discussion mailing lists, and interactive websites (Madara, 1997). Nearly half of all Americans have a Facebook account (Grossman, 2010). People who belong to these groups feel better emotionally and physically than those who face their problems alone. This trend will persist in the future as people continue to appreciate the benefits of acting together in groups, as well as the benefits of forming coalitions for mutual support and empowerment. Further improvements in communication technology will make it even easier for people to realize those benefits.

Advances in Biomedical Knowledge and Health Care Technology

Advances in social workers' understanding of human health and illness and their ability to affect those phenomena positively will continue at an astonishing pace. Already, advances in neonatal care are resulting in the survival of live-born infants weighing less than 1,000 gm. (2.2 lb.), who would more often die than live even 40 years ago. Techniques such as cardiopulmonary resuscitation, mechanical ventilation, renal dialysis, artificial feeding, and antibiotics are prolonging the lives of adults. Experiments being conducted in laboratories and clinics all over the world provide examples of future advances. In his book *Rx 2000: Breakthroughs in Health, Medicine, and Longevity in the Next Five to Forty Years,* Fisher (1992), a physician, predicted not only specific improvements, inventions, and developments but also the time frames during which they were likely to take place. Some of these have happened already; others are happening or are expected to happen in the near future; and still others will involve some waiting for. We have divided the recent and anticipated changes into four groups: (a) development and discovery of drugs and diets for the prevention and treatment of diseases; (b) improvements in the technology of diagnosis and treatment, both medical and surgical; (c) enhancement in the basic understanding of the human organism; and (d) changes in the approaches to health care.

New Drugs and Diets for Disease Prevention and Treatment

In the future, (a) a drug for the prevention of breast cancer will be released, (b) an AIDS vaccine will be developed, (c) drugs will be able to prevent or correct osteoporosis by regulating calcium metabolism and bone formation, (d) drugs will be able to inhibit the growth of the prostate gland, (e) a vaccine against bacteria that cause cavities and periodontal disease will become available, and (f) drugs that slow cell metabolism (and thereby keep the cells alive longer) and, thus, slow the aging process will become available (Fisher, 1992).

Of all American deaths, 60% are attributable to behavioral factors, social circumstances, and physical environmental exposures (Kindig, Asada, & Booske, 2008). People will become more conscious of this reality and realize that they do have some control over these aspects of their lives. For instance, there will be a greater appreciation of the relationship between improved diet and good health. "Nutraceuticals"—nutritional products with disease-related benefits—will come into the mainstream of medical practice and thereby become an important part of health care in the future. Examples of these nutraceuticals are calcium for possible prevention of colon cancer, nicotinic acid for reduction of serum cholesterol, beta carotene for possible prevention of lung cancer, and magnesium for the treatment and prevention of certain types of hypertension ("Foods That Bring Better Health," 1991). Gottlieb (1995) recommended food therapies for maladies as diverse as colds and prostate problems.

Not only will newer and more effective drugs prevent and cure diseases, but they also will be administered in easier ways. The following are some examples of future approaches to drug delivery.

A new form of oral drug delivery using hydrogel has been developed at Purdue University. Hydrogel is capable of remaining in the stomach and releasing drugs into the bloodstream for up to 60 hours, which is five times longer than the capability of current drugs ("A Spoonful of Hydrogel?" 1991).

The use of tiny pumps implanted in a patient's body to send a drug to the target site will become common. The pump can be reprogrammed by a computer and radio signals to alter the dosage of the drug released and can be refilled by hypodermic syringe when its reservoir is empty. It will help treat diabetes and heart disease as well as Lou Gehrig's, Alzheimer's, and Parkinson's diseases ("Tiny Pumps for Drugs," 1988).

Medicines will be delivered through a tiny array of hundreds of microscopic needles rather than through a single hypodermic needle. Researchers at the Georgia Institute of Technology are developing such a device. The microneedles penetrate only the outermost layer of skin, which contains no nerve endings, delivering drugs that cannot be administered orally ("Tiny Needles," 1998).

Smart drug delivery systems that deliver medicines to the body at a precise location could arrive before the end of the decade ("Tomorrow in Brief: Nanotubes," 2005).

New Technologies for Diagnosis and Treatment

Technology is reshaping health care by providing more sophisticated diagnostic tools and treatment options. Already available diagnostic technologies include the following:

- *Three-dimensional and cine-computed tomography (CT),* which is a vast improvement on the conventional CT. Three-dimensional CT has increased the utility of CT imaging, and cine-CT provides images at four times the speed of conventional CT.
- *Two-dimensional Doppler echocardiography,* which combines two-dimensional imaging with Doppler display of blood flow. This technique allows for a safe and definitive diagnosis of a number of cardiac problems.
- *Low-osmolality radiographic contrast agents,* which are safer than the standard media used in such procedures as angiography and myelography.
- *Magnetic resonance imaging*, which is the top-rated modality for imaging the central nervous system. Newer, low-strength magnetic resonance imaging units can even be installed in mobile labs.
- *Mammography*, which is considered a "must" technology for the diagnosis of breast cancer.
- *Single photon emission computed tomography*, which merges nuclear medicine and CT technology and is an improvement on conventional imaging in the fields of cardiology and oncology.
- *Tumor markers*, on the basis of advances in monoclonal antibody production, are likely to improve cancer diagnosis.
- *Chorionic villus sampling*, a promising replacement for amniocentesis for prenatal diagnosis.
- *Ultrasound,* which is being used in combination with other diagnostic approaches such as endoscanning, which combines ultrasound and endoscopy (Coile, 1990).

Even more powerful diagnostic techniques and tests will become available in the future. At Battelle's Medical Technology Assessment and Policy Research Center, researchers have developed a machine that can measure gases in parts per trillion. Even at the very early stage of many diseases, the patient's breath contains small amounts of certain chemicals. If physicians can detect these chemicals by analyzing the patient's breath, they may be able to detect a disease (Olesen, 1995).

A simple blood test will predict heart attack in the future. Measuring plaque buildup within the blood vessels of the heart is the best way to identify those at greatest risk of having a heart attack. At present, this is done through an invasive angiogram. A study has found that a blood test can forecast with 83% accuracy how much plaque is present. More research will determine the validity of the test (Park, 2010a).

Sudden cardiac death claims more than 400,000 American lives each year. It will become possible to prevent sudden cardiac death through the use of a portable heartbeat monitor. Researchers at Northwestern University are working on such a noninvasive monitor. It will record heart rate variability 24 hours a day and enable physicians to identify and treat patients at high risk of sudden cardiac death early enough to prevent death ("Preventing Sudden Cardiac Death," 1990). While describing telemedicine already in practice, Blanton and Balch (1995) said that patients recovering at home from heart attacks can put on a headset, connect the electrocardiogram wires to their chests, and ride their stationary bikes. The electrocardiogram information is carried to a medical technician in a hospital through telephone wires. Physicians at East Carolina University have set aside a cable channel to enable cardiac rehab patients to make visual contact with the hospital staff.

Physicians and other medical care providers will be able to monitor their patients' conditions more easily and reliably in the future. Devices that will enable them to do so include the following:

- A wireless digital "bandage" that continuously monitors a patient's vital signs and transmits data in real time to health care professionals. Such a device is being tested in the United Kingdom (Cohen, 2010).
- The iStethoscope, developed by English computer scientist Peter Bentley, is an iPhone application that uses an audio amplifier to filter sounds from the phone's built-in microphone to transmit clear signals of a patient's heartbeat to his or her cardiologist ("Heartbeat Monitor by Phone," 2010).
- The outpatient health monitoring system uses wireless sensors to constantly monitor asthma patients and check environmental factors in patients' homes, such as the presence of allergens,

pollution, and humidity. This is like a physician giving his/her patient constant online checkups ("World Trends & Forecasts: Your Doctor," 2009).

- Wireless technologies such as wearable computers and hospital mattresses embedded with sensors will allow for more constant and reliable monitoring of patients' vital signs by physicians and other health care workers ("World Trends & Forecasts," 2004).

- A monitoring device developed at the University of Florida detects sanitizer or soap fumes from people's hands, offering real-time monitoring of hygiene compliance ("Soap Sniffer," 2009).

Similar devices will help patients monitor their bodies' workings and will help in other ways.

- A small device called the Fitbit tracks how fast you are walking, your heart rate, and even how well you are sleeping, and then uploads that information directly to a publicly viewable database. The Fitbit Tracker became available for purchase in January 2009 ("Be Your Own Big Brother," 2009).

- Laptop "doctors" will monitor your vital signs on the go ("Futurist Update," 2005).

- Radio-frequency identification technology is being embedded in the traditional white cane used by people with little or no vision. The SmartCane incorporates an ultrasonic sensor, and the user carries a miniature navigational system in a bag. The device detects obstacles in the user's path and provides navigational cues with voice as well as vibration-based alerts. The SmartCane is under development at Central Michigan University ("Smart Cane Will Help," 2009).

- Lyme disease can cause neurological problems, cardiac distress, facial paralysis, and arthritis. Cases of this disease have increased over the past few years. It has symptoms similar to those of other diseases and is, therefore, often misdiagnosed. A specific test for this disease, which Fisher (1992) forecast, has become available.

Among the therapeutic technologies already being used are (a) balloon angioplasty, which is replacing cardiac bypass surgery for the treatment of blockages of cardiac vessels; (b) continuous arteriovenous hemofiltration, which is used as an alternative to conventional hemodialysis for the treatment of acute renal failure; (c) cochlear implants, which are a multichannel, significant improvement over single-channel devises for those with profound hearing loss; (d) gallstone pumps, which are used for flushing chemically dissolved gallstones, a nonsurgical approach to that problem; (e) lithotripsy, which uses sound waves to shatter kidney and urethral stones and is fast replacing conventional surgery as a treatment choice; and (f) lasers, which are used for a number of therapeutic purposes such as closing surgical wounds and unblocking coronary arteries (Coile, 1990).

Radiation treatments will use newer devices and techniques such as the gamma knife, a noninvasive devise that delivers a single high dose of ionizing radiation from 201 cobalt-60 sources to previously inoperable brain tumors. At the point where all 201 beams intersect simultaneously, gamma radiation is dispensed to the tumor without affecting the surrounding tissue ("Invisible Scalpel," 1989).

Physicians at Clatterbridge Hospital in northwest England are testing the use of proton therapy for treating eye cancer. It is believed that beams of subatomic particles other than X-rays can be used effectively against cancer. The more precise targeting of doses allows physicians to treat a tumor without affecting the surrounding tissues ("Proton Therapy," 1989).

Newer, more effective, and safer treatments for cancer will be developed. In their search for new strategies, scientists are focusing on genomic research.

Cancer occurs when changes in a cell's genome, or DNA instruction manual, trigger uncontrolled growth. New drugs target such molecular changes—blocking the effects of a factor that promotes cancer cell growth, for example, or inhibiting the formation of blood vessels that feed the tumor. Different cancers have different patterns of genome changes, and patterns differ even among those with the same type of cancer. So researchers are devising ways to tailor chemotherapy to each patient's tumor—which should be more effective and less toxic than the current one-size-fits-all approach. (Collins, 2010, p. 8)

It will become possible to cure allergies, reverse baldness, and even manipulate biological rhythms (to combat such problems as jet lag).

Researchers at the University of Cincinnati have developed an implantable hearing aid no bigger than an eyeglass screw. This micromachine holds more than 10,000 transistors and requires only 20 microamps of power from its battery to operate. Replacement of the battery once every 5 years can be done through a simple surgical procedure ("Tiny Hearing Aid Developed," 1995).

Couples suffering from infertility will benefit from newer and more sophisticated noncoital reproductive technologies. Two new approaches to treating infertility—in vitro fertilization and gamete intrafallopian transfer—already are being used. The practice of embryo freezing as an adjunct to in vitro fertilization has become commonplace.

Researchers at Stanford University have found a way to film the development of embryos in the first 48 to 72 hours after fertilization in a lab dish. This early peek may be crucial in embryo selection (Park, 2010b).

A new field of fertility medicine that helps cancer survivors have babies after treatment already has emerged. It is called oncofertility, as it is at the intersection of oncology and reproductive medicine. In the case of women, it uses a cutting-edge technique called ovarian tissue cryopreservation. An ovary or a piece of an ovary is laparoscopically removed and frozen before cancer therapy and later transplanted when the woman decides to get pregnant. More than a dozen live births have been reported from transplanted frozen ovarian tissue (Rochman, 2010).

New technologies also will save many more premature babies. A new ventilator developed in England monitors a baby's breathing pattern and works in harmony with it, rather than forcing air into the lungs haphazardly. By permitting these infants to breathe normally, the ventilator promotes full development of the babies' brains and bodies.

Advances in surgical approaches to treatment will be equally impressive. These will be in the areas of improved surgical techniques with fewer surgery-related risks, use of more sophisticated artificial devices, and transplantation of human organs and tissues. The following examples provide an idea of future possibilities.

Under microscopic surgery, surgeons are able to suture veins and nerves as small as the period at the end of this sentence (Ross & Williams, 1991).

The linking of new imaging technologies with robotic surgery will become common (Coile, 1990).

Robot-assisted surgeries already are happening. The first robot-assisted closed-chest coronary bypass graft procedure was performed in 1998 in Germany, and the first all-robotic-assisted kidney transplant was done at St. Barnabas Medical Center in Livingston, New Jersey, in 2009 (Mironov, 2011). Kolata (2010) reports that robot-assisted prostate surgery has grown at an unprecedented rate. Last year, 73,000 American men—86% of those who had prostate cancer surgery—had robot-assisted operations. In the future, not only will the surgical robotic systems perform operations with great precision without requiring surgeons to be present in the operation room, but they also will create new tissue that helps in rapid and complete healing (Mironov, 2011).

Doctors will use sonar to detect bone fractures ("Health & Medicine: Doctors Use Sonar," 2007).

A bone-substitute material that stimulates natural bone growth has been developed. It promises to revolutionize surgery for hip and knee replacement, bone cancer, and damage caused by accidents ("Bone Substitute," 1994).

The use of artificial skin, hips, knees, finger and toe joints, Teflon ligaments, and heart valves already is taking place. These artificial body parts will be further improved, and others will join this list in the future. Research at Germany's Frauhofer Institute for Interfacial Engineering and Biology and its use of factory-like techniques may lead to the production of skin, cartilage, and other body parts quickly and in large quantities ("Tomorrow in Brief," 2009).

Another example of future improvements in artificial body parts is found in the work done at the Oxford Orthopaedic Engineering Centre in England. Researchers there have developed a new standard for artificial-hip design and manufacture that can predict how such a hip will settle in the body over the next 10 years. Artificial-hip replacement markedly improves the quality of life for patients, but in up to 30% of cases, the surgery must be redone. The design of artificial hips in the future will be based on specific factors such as body weight, inertia, forces from the muscle, and the way the patient walks so that those hips can last the patient's lifetime ("Longer-Lived Artificial Hips," 1994).

People undergoing amputations will be able to wear more comfortable, natural-looking prostheses. For instance, the Endolite lightweight prosthesis enables its wearer to take part in strenuous activities such as squash, rock climbing, and cycling. Even those who have lost both legs can run again ("Amputees Get Back on Their Feet," 1990). Such prostheses may be crude examples of what will be available in the future.

Repairing of injuries to the nervous system will make significant progress in the next 10 years ("Health & Medicine: Repairing Injuries," 2007).

Use of nanotechnology in medicine will increase. Nanotechnology is a branch of engineering that deals with the manipulation of individual items and molecules. Current imaging methods detect cancers only after they are large enough to be visible. Nanotechnology will enable physicians to spot a single cancerous or even precancerous cell. The Center for Cancer Nanotechnology Excellence at Stanford University has developed a technique that attaches gold nanoparticles to molecules that have a special affinity for cancer cells (Collins, 2010).

"Artificial blood" will become the answer to the ever-present scarcity of donated human blood and the danger of contamination. Researchers at the University of Sheffield, England have developed a sterile synthetic blood made up of millions of plastic molecules that resemble hemoglobin. It contains iron atoms that help transport oxygen through the body. This plastic blood can be used with any blood type, and unlike donated blood, it can be stored for months at room temperature. This may one day be used as a blood substitute in emergency situations ("Tomorrow in Brief," 2007).

In the field of transplantation, some things that existed only in human fantasy not long ago have become a part of regular medical practice. Surgeons are able to transplant some 25 tissues and organs. Tissues used in transplantation include bone, bone marrow, corneas and other eye parts, ligaments, tendons and other connective tissues, blood, blood vessels, and heart valves. Organs include kidneys, livers, hearts, lungs, pancreases, testis, stomachs, and intestines, and their transplantation already is giving thousands of sick people a new lease on life [1]. In the words of Humar, Matas, and Payne (2006),

> The field of organ transplantation has undergone remarkable changes in the last decade. The growing number of agents available for immunosuppression have played a significant role in the advancement of this field. However, just as important has been the development of surgical innovations in the field. This includes not only the development of new surgical procedures, but also modification of the existing ones. This has involved all areas of organ transplantation including deceased-donor procurement techniques, living-donor transplantation, and transplantation of individual organs including kidney, liver, pancreas, and intestine. Examples include procurement from non-heart-beating donors; living donor transplants involving the liver, pancreas, or intestines; laparoscopic donor nephrectomy; split-liver transplants; and multivisceral transplants. All of these represent new, innovative procedures that are being performed on a regular basis in the last few years. (p. v)

Not long ago, a face transplant was performed at the Cleveland Clinic (McCarty, 2010), and a Belgian team used a novel method to make an organ acceptable to a recipient's body. The surgeons implanted the windpipe from a dead man into the arm of a young lady whose own windpipe had been smashed in an accident. After about 10 months, when enough tissue had grown around the implanted organ, they let her stop taking antirejection drugs and transferred the windpipe to its proper place (Cheng, 2010). Spain has opened the world's first organ-growing laboratory for human transplants. The laboratory will "empty" human hearts or other organs unsuitable for transplantation and recolonize their cell content with the transplant patient's stem cells, allowing the organs to grow anew and readying them for transplant into the patient's body ("Spain Opens," 2010).

In the future, researchers will have added to the types of transplants being performed, including brain "implants." The ability to maximize the success of transplants will be further improved by such developments as the following:

- New approaches to keeping people alive while they wait for organs will be found.
- A suitable mechanical heart will be used in the interim to prevent death from heart disease during the wait for a transplantable heart.
- Transplanting organs from animals into humans will become possible.
- It will become possible to treat kidney failure by transplanting half a kidney instead of a whole organ, thereby maximizing the use of available organs.
- Maintaining the viability of recovered organs for transplantation for long periods of time will improve.
- Inducing transplantation tolerance in organ recipients will become possible.
- Transplantation of organs also will be used as a preventive measure.

Enhancement in the Understanding of the Human Organism

In the future, medical scientists will have added to human knowledge an understanding of life at the cellular level. Physicians of the future actually will be able to look inside every one of the trillions of cells of the human body and detect abnormalities at the most basic molecular level long before symptoms of disease appear (Fisher, 1992). That ability will empower them to attack disease at that most basic level and thereby make the prevention of disease the most important aspect of medical practice.

Genetics will be another area in which tremendous progress will be made. It will become possible to genetically engineer and artificially construct human organs. Similarly, the genetically engineered replacement for damaged brain cells in patients such as those with Alzheimer's disease will become a viable approach to treating those patients (Fisher, 1992). All human diseases and disorders will have their linkages, if any, to the human genome identified. The intermediate biochemical processes that lead to the expression of the disease and its interaction with a person's environment and personal history also will be explicated (Coates, 1994). A team of European researchers with EUREKA consortium has developed a novel chemical compound—a new type of synthetic DNA-carrying agent that brings the treatment of illness on the genetic level closer to reality. Gene therapy involves transferring new genetic information into the nucleus of damaged or deceased cells to reprogram those cells and thereby repair them (Tucker, 2010). In the future, research will help in the understanding, more effective treatment, and even prevention of such complex diseases as schizophrenia, heart disease, and inherited cancers. It also may lead to programs to enhance people's overall physical and mental abilities.

On the other hand, promises of genetic therapies will tempt people into tampering with their DNA. The Genetic Age will create a host of ethical issues that will defy our existing approaches to dealing with ethically challenging situations. Authors of *Chance to Choice: Genetics and Justice* (Buchanan, Brock, Daniels, & Wikler, 2000) have provided the following scenarios of the Genetic Age: (1) *Parents demand perfect babies,* babies who have no future risk of such diseases as breast cancer and Alzheimer's and who will fall in the highest quintile of intelligence. (2) *Jobseekers gain a genetic edge* by adding genetic credentials to their résumés. (3) *Genetic gridlock occurs* when an inexpensive blood test can detect for prospective parents all serious genetic disorders and susceptibilities for illnesses. Advocates and opponents of mass genetic screening have equally convincing arguments for their stances. (4) *Cult leaders clone multitudes of followers.* (5) *Genetic technology transforms the insurance industry.*

A field known as *fetal origins* will grow in importance and influence.

> Pioneers [of this field] assert that the 9 months of gestation constitute the most consequential period in our lives, permanently influencing the wiring of the brain and the functioning of organs such as the heart, liver, and pancreas. The conditions we encounter in utero, they claim, shape our suscepti-bility to disease, our appetite and metabolism, our intelligence and temperament. (Paul, 2010, p. 51)

Everything in the daily life experience of a preg-nant woman, including the air she breathes, food she eats and drinks, conditions she deals with, and emotions she feels, is shared with the fetus and becomes a part of its body. Several research studies are being conducted to test the hypothe-ses generated by this field and the validity of the interventions based on those hypotheses. Parti-cularly notable is a massive federally funded study, the National Children's Study, which will involve 100,000 pregnant women and follow their offspring until the age of 21 (nationalchild-rensstudy.gov). This will lead to better services for the physical and mental health needs of preg-nant women.

Changes in Approaches to Health Care

Approaches to health care will not be restricted to the traditional medical model of treatment. Already, Americans are spending billions per year on alternative medical methods, and agencies that offer nontraditional health care services have cropped up. The complementary and alternative medical treatment practices, as they are called, include "approaches such as aromatherapy, special diets, homeopathic and naturopathic medicine, traditional Chinese medicine, ayurveda, Qi gong, Reiki, therapeutic touch, light and sound therapy, energy healing, distant healing, and other modali-ties" (Huff & Yasharpour, 2007, p. 35). More than one third of American adults and 12% of children

are using some form of complementary or alterna-tive medicine. Therapies showing significant increase in popularity in the past 5 years are deep-breathing exercises, meditation, massage therapy, and yoga. Hospitals are responding to increased patient demand for these services ("Hospitals and Patients Seek Alternatives," 2009).

The federal government has established the National Center for Complementary and Alter-native Medicine within the Institute of Health to explore these practices, train complementary and alternative medicine researchers, and share research findings with public and health profes-sionals. In 1994, 30 researchers and institutions were selected from among 452 grant applications for such projects as testing acupuncture and hyp-nosis to relieve pain and heal bones, massage therapy for surgical patients, dance movement for cystic fibrosis, macrobiotic treatments for cancer, biofeedback for diabetes, yoga for heroin addic-tion, tai chi for balance disorders, and massage therapy for AIDS babies ("Mainstream Takes New Look," 1994). Another example of newer therapies is aromatherapy. Research on the sense of smell by Shizuo Torii at Toho University in Japan has revealed that different fragrances produce different effects; some are calming and relaxing, others stimulating, and still others improve concentration ("Aromacology," 1990). "As life expectancy increases, people will not only be greatly con-cerned about their outer aging signs but about learning the techniques for keeping all of their senses at peak performance" (Green, 1993, p. 17). The growing acceptance of nontraditional thera-pies by even the medical establishment is reflected in the appearance of the journal *Alternative Therapies in Health and Medicine.*

In the future, health care personnel will not be dominated by those trained in allopathic medi-cine. These physicians will coexist with those practicing nontraditional forms of medicine such as acupuncture, homeopathy, and other approaches to treatment and care.

In the future, the current health care profes-sionals will have redefined their roles in several ways. Landers (2010) has talked about physicians in San Diego, California, going to patients' homes with a new version of the black bag that includes a mobile X-ray machine and a device that can perform 20 laboratory tests, and Massachusetts General Hospital in Boston is experimenting with Internet videoconferencing to permit virtual visits from patients' homes. Medical establishments will strive to provide accessible, patient-centered, coordinated care. The concept of patient-centered medical homes is being accepted as a viable approach to primary care. In 2007, four primary care specialty societies, representing more than 300,000 internists, family physicians, pediatricians, and osteopaths, agreed on the joint principles of the patient-centered medical home: (1) personal physician, (2) whole-person orientation, (3) safe and high-quality care, (4) enhanced access to care, and (5) payment that recognizes the added value provided to patients (Abrams, Davis, & Haran, 2009).

Gender change in the health care workforce, with more women in positions of authority, will be a significant feature of the future health care scene. Within the existing medical profession, pecking order will change among specialists. Specialties such as family practice, geriatrics, rehabilitation medicine, and psychiatry will become more prestigious. Newer specialties such as environmental medicine and addiction medicine, and subspecialties such as child abuse pediatrics (Lane & Dubowitz, 2009) will emerge. The resultant knowledge gaps and communication difficulties between specialties and subspecialties will become larger and bigger (Tow & Gilliam, 2009). On the other hand, general practitioners will regain a place of honor among their colleagues. Overall, focus of health establishments will be on primary care with a commitment to prevention and wellness. The need for generalist physicians will become even greater under the new law.

Schools of medicine and teaching hospitals already are being challenged to encourage students and residents to choose generalist careers. In 1992, the Association of American Medical Colleges created a task force to develop a policy statement for that purpose. That policy statement says:

The Association of American Medical Colleges (AAMC) advocates as an overall national goal that a majority of graduating medical students be committed to generalist careers (family medicine, general internal medicine, or general pediatrics) and that appropriate efforts be made by all schools so that this goal can be reached within the shortest possible time. ("AAMC Policy," 1993, p. 2)

The task force also recommended several strategies for accomplishing this goal. Others since have added suggestions to these recommendations. However, there has been next to no success in this regard. The number of medical school graduates choosing careers in family medicine dropped by 50% between 1995 and 2005 (Bodenheimer, 2006). Among third-year internal medicine residents in 2003, only 27% planned to practice general medicine—a rate just half that in 1998 (Garibaldi, Popkave, & Bylsma, 2005). Government incentives will reverse this trend.

Health care retail outlets, which are more patient centered than physician centered, will become a part of the mainstream. These are located in drug stores, food stores, and department stores such as Target and Walmart and provide medical care for minor ailments 24 hours a day, 7 days a week. Certified nurse practitioners and physician assistants staff these mini-clinics and see walk-in patients quickly (in about 15 minutes) and affordably (for $39 to $110, covered by most insurers). The first of such clinics, called MinuteClinic, was opened in Minneapolis in 2000. Others are cropping up all over the country. Medical associations do not disapprove of them (Reece, 2007).

Within the diversity of professionals and approaches, unity will gradually grow. Considering and treating the patient as a partner will be the common theme reflected in the behaviors of all health care workers and their approaches. The informed consumers of future health care will not tolerate any other type of relationship. "Today's health care consumer is a sleeping giant—one who is awakening to his power. Fully awakened, he will be the master and health care providers will be the servants" (Leland R. Kaiser, as quoted in Coile, 1990). According to Veatch (2009), a new medicine is on the horizon in which patients will capture responsibility for their health choices. They will need to know the current medical facts—facts about diagnosis, prognosis, and expected treatment outcomes—but will become the experts in deciding which among the expected outcomes is best for them. Changes in the world of this new medicine will include the following:

1. The language of medicine will change. Veatch (2009) provides the following examples:

   a. Doctors don't give orders. (They provide assessment of the medical facts.)

   b. Patients are not discharged from hospitals. (Hospitals are not prisons.)

   c. There is no such thing as "medically indicated treatment."

   d. There is no such thing as "treatment of choice."

   e. No treatment is ever "medically necessary."

2. Informed consent will be abandoned. (Patients need choice, not consent to the physician's recommendation.)

3. There will be no justification for physicians to prescribe medications (if they cannot know what is best for the patient).

4. Patients will no longer be stigmatized by labels created by health professionals.

5. Every person will be entitled to a decent amount of health care.

6. Hospice care will be a right of every person at the end stage of life. (It is not medical care and should not be part of health insurance.)

Ferguson (1992) presented a physician's forecast about how a health-active and health-responsible patient of the future will behave under what he called the "information age model of care." It is a six-step model. At Step 1—using individual self-care—the person tries to deal with his or her health problem or concern on his or her own. At Step 2—tapping into one's network of family and friends—he or she asks loved ones for help and advice if self-care does not work. At Step 3—using formal self-help networks—if advice from loved ones does not solve the problem, then he or she may seek help from community self-help programs such as a self-help hotline or self-help support group. At Step 4—using a professional as an adviser—the person seeks appropriate information, tools, skills, and support. This does not result in the health professional stepping in and taking over. At Step 5—using a professional as a partner—the health professional does the things the person cannot do for him- or herself, such as ordering tests, prescribing drugs, and performing surgery. At Step 6—using a professional as an authority—the patient is unconscious or incapacitated and would want the professional to step in and manage the situation.

This health activity and health responsibility on the part of the patient will result from an easy access to information. Online technology already is making it possible for people to research information about their diseases and access disease support groups. Furthermore, patients are taking advantage of the growing self-help literature. For example, in one self-help book, Louria (1989), a physician, proposed a 17-point lifestyle regimen for what he called "taking control of your medical destiny." Included in the 17 points are specific medical tests (e.g., blood pressure, cholesterol level, mammogram) and the recommended frequency for running these tests. To these tests, he added a number of actions that people should take themselves, such as testicular or breast self-examination, daily back exercises, and seat belt use. For those over 65, his program includes yearly tests for taste, smell, hearing, and vision, as well as an evaluation of social support systems and disabilities.

Many more devices than blood pressure kits (commonplace today) will help in such self-performed or self-directed programs. A meter that determines a person's percentage of body fat is available. This handheld device uses infrared light to analyze the muscle-to-fat ratio in five places on the body. It compares the user's weight, height, age, and gender with medically established values and produces a customized health and fitness plan. Those who are ill but not in need of acute care will have personal emergency response systems based on implantable biosensors. They also will use a number of techniques and devices at home as part of their treatment. This home care already is happening to an extent. "Cancers and pneumonias are now routinely treated with home chemotherapy and portable infusion therapy. Indwelling catheters allow home administration of hyperalimentation formulas and antibiotics" (Coile, 1990, p. 115). When they need the services of health care practitioners and facilities, patients in the future will have researched their background, experience, resources, quality of care, and cost beforehand. In the words of Reece (2007),

> Given the size of the self-care movement, the electronic data entry self-services already common in U.S. retail establishments and widespread use of Internet search engines, innovations in self-care, self-service, and self-empowerment are powerful and inevitable. (p. 323)

For those needing hospital-based acute services, the *cure* will be accomplished through the use of sophisticated medical and surgical techniques and equipment, and *care* will be marked by patient-centered approaches and environment. To satisfy the patients of tomorrow, hospitals will have an atmosphere of openness and informality. Ferguson (1992) described some pilot programs [2] in patient-centered health care that are turning out to be the forerunners of hospitals of the future. Reece (2007) listed the following characteristics of hospitals being built for aging boomers and their children.

- *Hospitals designed for safety.* Designs include one-bed rooms, better lighting, rounded corners on all objects in the room, no-slip floors, soundproof walls, and hand-washing basins in every room.
- *Hospitals designed for rapid information transfer.* Designs include information kiosks in every room for both patient and hospital staff use. Hospitals are linked with community-wide information systems.
- *Hospitals designed to create a culture of caring and healing.* Designs include "spacious receptive atriums, colorful decorating schemes, pastoral paintings on walls, entertainment and information centers, roof-top gardens, plants in the room, gourmet menus, and beds for relatives—even quarters for favorite pets" (p. 135).

- *Hospitals designed for convenience.* Designs include "ample parking; electronic check-in sites; websites showing medical staff backgrounds, nurse/patient ratios, and outcomes for major procedures; and one-stop shopping for doctors, lab tests, X-rays, imaging studies, and retail sites for 24/7 care manned by hospital-employed nurse practitioners" (pp. 135–136).

The recognition of special needs of older patients also is generating "senior emergency rooms" in hospitals across the country. Senior emergency rooms feature a quiet environment, dimmable light, extra-padded mattresses, nonglare floors, and blanket warmers. Doctors and nurses in these emergency rooms are trained in geriatrics. Every visit is followed by a call from a geriatric social worker or nurse ("An ER Just for Older Patients," 2011).

On the long-term care front, some nursing homes are changing in ways that will enhance their residents' quality of life. Labeled as "culture change in nursing homes," a group of providers—the Pioneer Network in Long-Term Care—is dedicated to making nursing homes exemplify the following values: (1) responding to spiritual as well as mind and body needs; (2) putting persons before tasks; (3) seeking to enjoy residents and staff as unique individuals; (4) acting on the belief that as staff are treated, so will residents be treated; (5) beginning decision making with residents; and (6) accepting risk taking as a normal part of adult life (Fagan, Williams, & Burger, 1997). While discussing the physical environments of long-term care facilities, Kane (2001) says,

> But on the positive side, currently there is unprecedented interest in physical design of living quarters for care, as well as specialized furnishings, fixtures, and equipment to enhance functioning. Long-overdue attention is being paid to chairs, switches, knobs, fabrics, colors, and materials. (p. 301)

The provision of *patient-as-a-partner–focused* comprehensive and well-coordinated services aimed at enhancing the patient's quality of life will become the overall goal of the system at all levels of care and in all settings. Mental health and social services will have to be viewed as integral parts of this broadly conceived health care system. The futility of artificial boundaries between health and mental health and health and social welfare will become obvious. Comprehensiveness of services will be the feature distinguishing that system from what we have today. Social and psychological disorders and social diseases resulting from lifestyle, environment, substance abuse, and stress will be as much the focus of that system as the treatment of physical diseases.

Understanding of mental illness will improve, and perspectives on and approaches to dealing with mental health problems will change. The belief in the biological bases of psychiatric disorders will continue to propel the search for more effective medicines for these disorders. Already, drugs capable of targeting specific mechanisms in the brain have been developed (White, 1993). Important changes in the theoretical perspectives on mental health problems are happening already. Friesen (1993, p. 12) listed the following among the advances in child mental health:

- *From* psychological models focusing mostly on intra- and interpersonal phenomena *to* more complex biopsychosocial and ecological models
- *From* a focus on pathology and deficits *to* a focus on strengths and empowerment
- *From* a focus on "child saving" *to* a focus on preserving and supporting families
- *From* a primary view of families as objects of intervention (client, patients) *to* families as partners in the design, delivery, and evaluation of services

Similarly, the concepts of "service delivery" and "practice roles" are changing (a) from a paradigm of program-centered services to person- and family-centered services; (b) from a solely therapeutic focus on the sick person's behavior, emotional life, and family dynamics to comprehensive services that address the full range of the person's needs; (c) from an exclusive focus on formal services to a larger view inclusive of formal and informal sources of help; (d) from limited service options to a wide array of services; (e) from agency-based "expert" roles to professionals working collaboratively with families; and (f) from a specialized, fragmented set of services to the ones that are truly coordinated at the interprofessional and interagency levels, with the sick and their families as full and active members of the therapeutic team (Friesen, 1993). Such approaches will be built into the system, encouraged, and rewarded.

Changes in Health Care Financing, Structure, and Services

The Patient Protection and Affordable Care Act of 2010 will bring health care within the reach of many more Americans, but a comprehensive reform of the health care system is not likely within the foreseeable future. The historical and economic factors responsible for the current system will continue to exert their influence.

Historically, how Americans financed health care was based on the goal of protecting health care providers and not on serving the consumers. Economically, the health care system is a pervasive force in society (Merrill, 1994). Health insurance in the United States is a child of the Depression and the American Hospital Association, or AHA (Law, 1976). Because of the ravages of the Depression, when people could no longer pay for their hospital care, hospitals developed what later became Blue Cross plans. As Merrill (1994) put it, "It is interesting to note that, until 1971, the logo for Blue Cross was owned by the AHA and, historically, hospital representatives tended to dominate the boards of these plans" (p. 17). Although other motivations and concerns led to the creation of Blue Shield, the major motivation was physicians' need for "a mechanism by which they could also get reimbursed by patients who were financially strapped as a result of the Depression" (p. 18).

The health care industry is a vital economic force. In 2007, it represented 16.2% of the gross domestic product, or about $2.2 trillion (AHA, 2009a). It directly employs millions of people and indirectly creates jobs for millions more—the people who manufacture products or provide services that are health related. Any prospect of major changes in the financing and structure of the health care system threatens the profits and positions of powerful groups and the bread-and-butter sources of millions of people. However, health care in the United States at the beginning of the 21st century is becoming characterized by a single-minded quest for profitability (Bodenheimer & Grumbach, 2002). This is reflected in the consolidation of the health care market—large insurance companies buying smaller ones, hospitals merging into hospital systems, and physicians forming specialty groups (and opening their own ambulatory surgery, diagnostic, and imaging centers). "Consolidation went hand in hand with organizations converting from nonprofit to investor-owned 'for-profit' status as they sought to raise capital for buy-outs, market expansion, and organizational infrastructure" (p. 190). These phenomena are a threat to the notions of professionalism and community service; however, they are leading to innovations in various sectors of health care.

In the future, the recipients of health care will continue to fall into the following four groups:

1. Insured through Medicare providing universal access to those 65 and older

2. Insured privately through employment or individual purchase

3. Insured publicly through Medicaid

4. Uninsured (the number in this group will be much smaller than before the passage of the new law)

States will continue to be heavily involved in the needs of those in Groups 3 and 4, with varying degrees of success. Society will gradually accept health care as a societal obligation and not as an individual responsibility.

The increased access to health care will result in (a) the demand for medical services exceeding the available resources, (b) growth in cost-containment measures, and (c) rationing of expensive medical technology (Barzansky et al., 1993). A cultural paradigm shift from "don't worry about it, the insurance will pay for it" to "we're only going to do this if you really need it and we're fairly convinced it will help" (Lundberg, 1994) already is taking place. However, it will become more difficult to decide what the minimal but adequate care is. Gradually, a consensus will emerge that "an adequate level of care should be thought of as a floor below which no one ought to fall, not a ceiling above which no one may rise" (Abramson, 1990, p. 10).

The problem of high cost of care will continue. So far, cost-containment efforts have essentially been cost-shifting strategies, each entity trying to contain its costs by shifting them to someone else. Society has not had the political will to reduce health care costs. As Merrill (1994) put it,

> It may not be in anyone's best interest to see overall costs contained and, thus, there never was the consensus needed to ensure that any of these efforts would prove successful, whether they involved regulatory approaches or more competitive strategies. (pp. 51–52)

Managed care and managed competition will continue being used as approaches to controlling costs and regulating access to health care but will be supplemented by consumer-driven approaches. Managed care is a generic term for organized systems of care that feature precertification requirements, a limited network of providers, and risk-based payment. Managed care is not new. In 1932, the Committee on the Cost of Medical Care called for the reorganization of medical practice from fee-for-service provided by solo practitioners to prepaid group practice. Kaiser Permanente started the first prepaid group practice more than 70 years ago, and health maintenance organizations (HMOs), the traditional form of managed care, grew after the passage of the HMO Act of 1973.

HMOs and preferred provider organizations (PPOs) are popular examples of managed health care. There are various models of HMOs and PPOs. All forms of HMOs use a gatekeeper, a primary care physician who is the first point of contact for care and must authorize referrals for specialty care. PPOs do not require a gatekeeper and allow for self-referral to specialists. PPOs generally are formed by insurers or employers who contract with health care providers to create a network of preferred providers. These providers agree to follow certain utilization management guidelines and accept discounted fee-for-service payments in order to belong to the network. There are also point-of-service (POS) plans that offer limited coverage for self-referral outside the network of care providers. Members in plans that use a gatekeeper (HMOs) have the lowest copayments, those in plans that allow for self-referral to network providers (PPOs) have higher copayments, and those seeking care outside the network (POS plans) have the highest copayment (Kominski & Melnick, 2007). Managed competition is a system that allows health plans to compete for the enrollment of beneficiaries who can choose among those plans. "Thus, a sponsor—an employer, a government unit, a purchasing cooperative—acting for a large group of subscribers, structures and adjusts the market to overcome efforts of insurers to avoid competition" (Leukefeld & Welsh, 1995, p. 1210).

Over the years, enrollment in managed care organizations has varied. By the end of the 1990s, HMO enrollment (including enrollment in POS plans) had grown to an estimated 81 million people or about 25% of the U.S. population. Since then, the growth of HMOs has declined and PPOs have made gains. The primary driving force behind the growth of managed care has been employers seeking lower-cost alternatives to fee-for-service indemnity insurance for their employee health benefit plans. Of all individuals who obtained health insurance through their place of employment, 97% were enrolled in some form of managed care as of 2005 (Kominski & Melnick, 2007).

As a cost-containment strategy, managed care has met with limited success. Miller and Luft's (1994) extensive review of the literature on the performance of managed care plans led them to conclude that no bottom-line estimates of expenditure differences per enrollee existed between managed care plans and indemnity (traditional insurance) plans. In the fee-for-service world, providers make more by doing more; financial incentives encourage over-treatment. In the managed

care world, providers make more by doing less; the system encourages under-treatment. The primary mechanisms used by managed care organizations are strict utilization review and financial risk shifting. "These mechanisms may operate in direct conflict with the goals of improving the health status of the underserved" (Randall, 1994, p. 225). The later literature reviews by Miller and Luft (2002) supported their earlier findings that HMOs use fewer resources but that most of the effect is now attributed to shorter lengths of hospital stays rather than to lower admission rates. Thus, these managed care and managed competition approaches do not seem "capable of providing universal, comprehensive, affordable, equitable coverage" (Mizrahi, 1993, p. 89). Others see managed care as an effort on the part of many important entities to attain dominance of the health care world.

> Providers wish to protect their sources of income; industry and government are under pressure to contain health care expenditures; and the medical industry wishes to protect and increase its profitability. It is important to note that the health care consumer is conspicuously absent from this array. (Cornelius, 1994, p. 49)

Nevertheless,

> managed care has become entrenched in the health care market, and the predominant form of health care delivery, albeit in continuously evolving organizational forms. Along with its rapid growth during the 1990s, managed care has also experienced an increasing level of popular dissatisfaction and bad publicity since the late 1990s and throughout the early 2000s, as newspapers and other media constitute regular outlets for some of the most common complaints against managed care. (Kominski & Melnick, 2007, p. 564)

A new model of health care has emerged that puts the patient center stage. Employers are offering their employees high-deductible health plans (HDHPs) combined with health savings accounts (HSAs). These consumer-directed health plans are "designed to make patients and families more conscious of each dollar spent on health care by making them more responsible for the financial consequences of their health care utilization" (Brown & Lavarreda, 2007, p. 104). An HSA consists of contributions made by an employer to an employee's tax-free savings account to help pay predeductible expenses under a health insurance policy that has a high deductible. This shifts the responsibility for health care services from the employer to employees (or patients). Any money not spent from the account is allowed to accumulate tax free, and employees can take the account with them if they change jobs. This not only makes the health care plan portable but also provides incentive for people to stay healthy and shop around for the best care at the most reasonable price, because they pay upfront for health services themselves. West (quoted in Reece, 2007) gives an example of how an HDHP policy with an HSA account would work for someone whose health care is not paid for by an employer. The premium for a healthy family in his area is $1,600. His family of seven is covered by a policy with a $5,000 deductible and costs them $300 a month. They put $420 in their HSA. Thus, it costs them $720 a month instead of $1,600.

The insurance industry, health care providers, financial institutions, and employers also are helping in the success of this model. Regulations under the Medicare Modernization Act of 2004 (which had a provision making HSAs widely available) provide a list of safe-harbor benefits that an HDHP can provide. Preventive safe-harbor services covered by HSAs include periodic health evaluation, routine prenatal care, well-child care, immunizations, tobacco cessation programs, obesity weight-loss programs, and screening services (e.g., Pap smears, mammograms, and bone-density measurements; Reece, 2007). The HDHP policies provide these services for free, and insurance companies are outdoing one another by offering richer preventive services. Managed care companies are providing websites for clients to track medical records, look up information on diseases, and compare costs and ratings of hospitals, physicians, and other care providers. In 2005, Aetna started a pilot project comparing hundreds

of negotiated rates with area physicians and making those negotiated prices available online. By the end of 2006, that program had been extended to many different parts of the country (Reece, 2007). St. Luke's Health System, a 10-hospital system in Kansas City, Missouri, is making shopping easier for HSA holders by repricing its inpatient care and outpatient procedures and services. Physicians seem willing to provide services at discounted prices because they get paid at the time of service and do not have to wait months for payment by insurance companies. "Banks, credit unions, and money management firms are now quietly positioning themselves to become central players in the business of health care, offering 401(k)-type accounts to cover future medical expenses" (Dash, as quoted in Reece, 2007). Soon, these institutions will be offering debit cards to HSA account holders. Large employers are providing their employees education, encouragement, technical assistance, and technological wherewithal to take advantage of the preventive and wellness services and manage their HSA accounts (Hogan, as cited in Reece, 2007). About 3 million Americans are currently signed up for HSAs (Baum, as cited in Reece, 2007). It seems likely that the future will see further growth in HDHPs, with HSAs and even HMOs trying to regain some of their lost market by focusing on health maintenance.

The health care system of the future will continue to be marked by pluralism and diversity, but with more logic to its organization and greater integration of its services, both within the system and in the larger human services community. In health care settings, on the one extreme, hospitals will provide short-term, intensive, specialized treatment, and on the other extreme, residential facilities will provide long-term care through different service models. Between the two extremes, all kinds of ambulatory centers will provide both specialized and generic disease prevention, illness management, health maintenance, and wellness enhancement services. These centers will see more patients with more diverse problems than presently are being seen in ambulatory care settings.

Hospitals of the future will be cores of high-intensity and high-technology medical care. Most diagnostic and therapeutic technology, as well as powerful computer programs, will be within the reach of most hospitals and will turn even small hospitals into medical centers. Hospitals, however, will be for only those patients who have acute problems requiring highly specialized treatment. Hence, there will be fewer hospitals with fewer beds. The volume of acute inpatient services has begun to shrink already. Inpatient days fell from 263 million in 1982 to 206 million in 1990. In the overall scheme of things, hospitals will lose much of their preeminence in the future.

> Long the central institution of the health care delivery system, the hospital is being challenged by important developments in epidemiology, technology, and economics. Individually and collectively, these changes threaten to push the hospital to the margins of the system, leaving most medical services and dollars controlled by "accountable health partnerships" that emphasize outpatient, home health, and subacute care. Alternatively, these environmental changes could provide a window of opportunity for the hospital to embark on a new mission as a health care center without walls. (Robinson, 1994, p. 259)

Although the shrinkage in inpatient services alluded to above has not caused an appreciable reduction in the number of hospitals yet, it has led to diversification of the care provided by hospitals. "Hospitals have integrated rapidly into outpatient facilities that diagnose patients prior to admission, into subacute facilities that shelter patients after discharge, and into many forms of health care that are not directly linked to acute inpatient care at all" (Robinson, 1994, p. 262). "Ambulatory hospitals" are testing the feasibility of clustering ambulatory care services away from hospital campuses.

Hospitals of the future will embark on new ventures such as the ones mentioned above, as well as others such as alcohol and drug units, rehabilitation centers, occupational health centers, day hospitals for the elderly, and rape crisis centers. They will also be more effectively connected with other health and social services in the community. The connection with other health care organizations will take the form of integration, both horizontal and vertical. The idea of regionalization of medical care also will become a reality, whereby, for example, a CT scanner or a cataract surgery center will be located in the institution where more patients are in need of it, and others will be referred from affiliated hospitals (Rehr & Rosenberg, 1991).

Most health care will be provided through neighborhood-based outpatient programs. Ambulatory care centers—variously called emergicenters, surgicenters, and walk-in clinics—already are appearing all over the United States at a rapid rate. Over the next 5 years, under the Patient Protection and Affordable Care Act, $11 billion in funding will be provided for the construction, operation, and expansion of community health centers across the country. In the future, the various kinds of nonhospital health care settings will be better equipped to perform sophisticated diagnostic and treatment work and many of the functions of today's hospitals. These settings also will be the centers of wellness-focused prevention and early detection work.

The health care system of the future also will be guided and goaded by the need for efficiency. The use of computers will increase and significantly contribute to improving efficiency (by minimizing the time taken doing paperwork today), cutting costs, and saving lives (because of easy access to patient data). For example, computer technology will create integrated information systems for hospitals; these systems will allow hospital personnel in any department to look at and update patient records. (Possibilities of the abuse of medical information have been reduced by HIPPA [Public Law 104-191].) [3] In emergency medicine of the future, physicians will not start from the very beginning with every patient—as happens today because emergency personnel often know nothing about the patients they treat. A typical future situation might be as follows: A patient, John, with a bleeding leg, appears in a hospital emergency room and hands his "smart card" to the nurse. By inserting that card into the computer, the emergency room staff are instantly able to see onscreen all the needed information—his medical history as well as other pertinent data—and proceed with attending to his injury.

> In radiology, imaging technology allows X-rays of John's leg to be scanned and stored in digital form so that physicians in any other department can view the image. Before John is sent to surgery, physicians schedule an operating room and order the necessary materials through an online scheduling system. ("Hospital of the Future," 1990, p. 46)

Such use of computer technology already is taking place and proving its utility. Several telemedicine projects are in place in the United States, mostly serving rural areas. These projects make it possible for medical specialists from medical schools to provide consultation to practitioners in distant and remote areas. Benjamin Berg, a Hawaiian heart surgeon, dictated a complicated heart surgery over an Internet feed for a man 3,500 miles away in Guam. Berg monitored every move and heartbeat of the patient via sensors embedded in the catheter inserted into the patient's heart ("World Trends & Forecasts: The Internet," 2009). The future possibilities of use of the Internet and other technologies are enormous, and these will affect all facets of health care.

LIKELY-TO-PERSIST HEALTH AND HEALTH-RELATED PROBLEMS

In the future, as pointed out earlier, health care agencies will be more than the illness care facilities that they are today; they will be responsible for the prevention, early detection, and treatment of illness, as well as the promotion of wellness. Health care professionals will take seriously the fact that medical care accounts for only about 15% of the health status of any population, while lifestyle accounts for 20% to 30%, and other factors—such as poverty, inferior education, income differences, and lack of social cohesion—account for the other 55% (Satcher & Pamies, 2006). Professionals will realize that social and

health problems are inseparable. Our discussion of the health and health-related problems likely to persist in the future include (a) medical problems, (b) medicalized social problems such as alcoholism, and (c) social problems such as poverty, homelessness, and violence and person abuse (e.g., child, spouse, and elder abuse). These will have tremendous impact on the scope, structure, and approaches of health care in the future.

Medical Problems

Swartz (1999) forecast that most types of diseases will be virtually eliminated by 2050, thanks to a combination of improved diet, lifestyle, and environmental factors and advances in gene therapy and drugs. However, in the foreseeable future, the likely-to-emerge scene shows that some diseases have been eliminated while others are persisting and have been joined by new ones. One unintended consequence of growing immigration may be new imported epidemics. Tuberculosis already is making a comeback. Most of the diseases likely to persist and continue to tax the skills of the health care community and U.S. resources are chronic diseases, such as Alzheimer's disease, arthritis, genetic defects, heart disease, stroke, and cancer.

Alzheimer's Disease

Alzheimer's disease will not only persist but possibly will worsen in incidence as the elderly population rises. Alzheimer's disease is a family disease, and it is a slow killer. Most of its victims live from 9 to 15 years after onset of the illness, and their families must live through the painful experience of watching their self-care abilities progressively worsen. Patients pass through the phases of forgetfulness, confusion, and dementia and put increasingly greater demands on their family's emotional, physical, financial, and social resources (Dhooper, 1991). The intensity of stress on the family during the dementia phase of the disease can be appropriately described as the "funeral that never ends" (Kapust, 1982). The needs of the families and caretakers of Alzheimer's patients will continue to be a challenge to the health care community.

Arthritis

Arthritis is a common problem and a significant cause of much suffering, a fair amount of disability, and billions in cost every year. The National Health Interview Survey, 2007–2009, revealed that 22.2% of adults (49.9 million) suffer from doctor-diagnosed arthritis. Its age-adjusted prevalence is significantly higher in women than in men (24.3% vs. 18.3%). It causes functional limitations in common daily activities. Of those with arthritis, 40% report that it is "very difficult" for them to do at least one of the following nine activities: grasping small objects; reaching above one's head; sitting more than 2 hours; lifting or carrying 10 pounds; climbing a flight of stairs; pushing a heavy object; walking 1/4 mile; standing more than 2 hours; and stooping, bending, or kneeling. Arthritis and rheumatism continue to be the most common causes of disability in U.S. adults. With the aging of the U.S. population, by 2030, an estimated 67 million adults (25% of the projected total adult population) will have doctor-diagnosed arthritis. Two thirds of those will be women. It is further estimated that 25 million sufferers will report arthritis-attributable activity limitation (Centers for Disease Control and Prevention [CDC], 2010b). Despite the ability to apply sophisticated technology (e.g., use of artificial joints) to its treatment, arthritis will remain on the health care scene, claiming its share of the national resources. About 10 million Americans have osteoporosis, and 34 million have osteopenia, a precursor to osteoporosis. These numbers are projected to increase to 14 million and 47 million, respectively, by 2020 (Herson, 2007).

Cardiovascular Disease

Heart disease and stroke are continuing to extract a greater toll than any other conditions—a toll in the form of early deaths, disability, personal and family disruptions, loss of income, and medical care expenditures. Although the overall age-adjusted death rates for heart disease and stroke have been declining since 1950, the actual number of deaths from these diseases has changed little in 30 years and has increased within the past decade. In 2006, heart disease and stroke were the first and third leading causes of death (National Center for Health Statistics, 2010a). *Cardiovascular disease* (CVD) is a term often used to refer to coronary heart disease, heart failure, and stroke. The burden that CVD imposes on the country is reflected in the following year 2000 figures.

Number of deaths:

2,600 deaths occur every day (i.e., one death every 33 seconds).

150,000 deaths occur each year among people younger than age 65.

250,000 coronary heart disease (CHD) deaths occur each year without hospitalization.

50% of men and 63% of women who suffered a sudden CHD death lacked any previous CHD history.

Survivors:

450,000 people had survived a first heart attack for more than 1 year.

450,000 people had survived with heart failure for more than 1 year.

375,000 people had survived a first stroke for more than 1 year.

Prevalence:

12.9 million people were living with coronary heart disease.

4.9 million people were living with heart failure.

4.7 million people were living with stroke.

Risk factors:

105 million people had high cholesterol.

50 million people had high blood pressure or were taking anti-hypertension medication.

Nearly 48.7 million people aged 18 and older were current smokers.

More than 44 million people were obese.

10.9 million people had physician-diagnosed diabetes.

Projected costs for 2003 were $351.8 billion. This included direct costs (medical expenses) of $209.3 billion and indirect costs (loss of income) of $142.5 billion.

The aging of the U.S. population will make CVD an even greater burden in the future. Heart disease deaths are projected to increase sharply between 2010 and 2030, and the population of heart disease survivors will grow at a much faster rate than the U.S. population as a whole. A marked increase in the number of stroke deaths is also predicted. The disparities based on factors such as sex, race and ethnicity, education, and income will continue (CDC, 2010a).

The future will see noticeable improvements in the heart disease and stroke picture as a result of advances in medical care and changes in lifestyle. Battelle's Medical Technology Assessment and Policy Research Center forecasts that by 2015, these changes *could* prevent as many as 23 million cases of and 13 million deaths from these two illnesses. It is estimated that about half this improvement will be a result of behavioral changes, 40% a result of pharmaceuticals, and 10% a result of other biomedical advances. Despite the decline in heart disease and stroke cases, these illnesses will continue to occupy important positions among major health care concerns of the future because more than 600,000 U.S. children now have some form of heart disease.

The same will be true of a number of cancers. Some cancers will decline, but others will persist. Even with newly developed preventive vaccines and simple tests for mass screening, the United States will lag behind in its ability to bring about the drastic lifestyle changes necessary to reduce these illnesses to insignificance.

Diabetes and Obesity

Conditions associated with CVD, such as diabetes and obesity, will continue posing challenges to the health care community. Diabetes was the nation's seventh leading cause of death in 2007. It affects the body's ability to metabolize blood glucose (sugar). A healthy person's pancreas produces enough insulin for cells to absorb and convert food into blood sugar. A diabetic person's body either fails to use insulin properly or fails to produce it at all. People with diabetes must, therefore, limit their sugar intake or take insulin. Uncontrolled or unregulated diabetes resulting in hyperglycemia or hypoglycemia can create a life-threatening situation. Onset of the symptoms of this disease is so gradual that many are not even aware they have it for a long time. Diabetics develop a number of complications that can include cardiovascular disease, vision problems, kidney failure, and nerve damage that can lead to amputations in serious cases.

There are two types of diabetes, Type 1 and Type 2. In Type 1 diabetes, traditionally diagnosed in children and young adults, the body does not produce enough insulin. In Type 2, which accounts for about 95% of cases, body's cells resist insulin's attempt to transport sugar. This type is most common in people who are overweight or obese, 60 or older, and members of minority groups such as American Indian and Alaska Natives, blacks, and Hispanics. In 2009, 9% of adults 18 years of age and over had been told by a doctor that they had diabetes. The CDC estimates that 1 in 10 adults has diabetes now, but the number could grow to 1 in 5 or even 1 in 3 by the year 2050 if current trends continue (Auslander & Freedenthal, 2006; Barnes, Adams, & Powell-Griner, 2010; Stobbe, 2010; Vital and Health Statistics, 2010).

Obesity correlates with excess mortality, and the obese are at risk of heart disease, stroke, diabetes, gallbladder disease, hypertension, osteoarthritis, and some cancers. Among children and adolescents, being overweight increases the risk of hypertension, high cholesterol, orthopedic disorders, sleep apnea, diabetes, and low self-esteem. In 2009, based on their body mass index (BMI), 35% of Americans were overweight (BMI between 25 and 29.9), and 27% were obese (BMI equal to or greater than 30). Compared with 29% of women, 42% of men were overweight.

Obesity percentages were similar for men and women. Compared with 32% of Hispanic adults and 26% of white adults, 38% of black adults were obese. Compared with 31% of Hispanic women and 24% of white women, 43% of black women were obese. Of Hispanic men, 33% were obese, compared with 32% of black men and 27% of white men. The percentage of adults 20 to 74 years of age has more than doubled from 15% in 1976 to 1980 to 35% in 2005 to 2006. Similarly, there has been an increasing prevalence of overweight children since 1976 to 1980. In 2005 to 2006, 15% to 18% of school-age children and adolescents were overweight. The percentage of preschool-age children (2–5 years of age) who were overweight doubled from 1976 to 1980 (climbing to 5%). The trend is obvious. Diet, physical activity, genetic factors, environment, and health conditions contribute to overweight and obesity (National Center for Health Statistics, 2010a; Vital and Health Statistics, 2010). "Weight loss can be an extremely difficult process. Time commitments, the cost of healthy foods, limited opportunities for physical activity, and lack of awareness of the negative effects of obesity can all be barriers to weight loss" (Barnes, Rogers, & Tran, 2007, p. 328).

Mental Disorders

Mental disorders will continue to afflict Americans. A national survey involving the most comprehensive look at the mental health of U.S. citizens to date found that far more people suffer from mental disorders than previously assumed. This survey used interviews with a nationally representative sample of 8,098 people aged 15 to 54 and employed the latest official psychiatric diagnoses. Its major findings were that (a) nearly one in two adults experienced a mental disorder at some time in his or her life, (b) almost one in three suffered from a mental disorder during the previous year, and (c) roughly one sixth of the population grappled with three or more mental disorders over the course of their lives (Bower, 1994).

The Genetic Threat

In addition to the diseases associated with unhealthy lifestyles and the emotional problems of living, there is the genetic threat. Advances in medical care will result in the survival of more and more people who have congenital illnesses and disabilities. This already is happening on a smaller scale. As these people live longer—long enough to reproduce—they will increase the genetic burden on the society of the future. The future will witness a race between genetic illnesses and genetic engineering. At the same time, the psychosocial needs of those who have such illnesses will need to be attended to. "Genetic diagnoses touch on intimate, deeply personal areas of life: sexuality, decisions to conceive, and decisions to terminate pregnancy for genetic reasons. A genetic diagnosis also may reveal family secrets, such as incest or adultery" (Rauch, 1988, p. 393).

New and Old Diseases

As hinted earlier, the future health care scene will show the appearance of diseases different in marked ways from those known today as well as the reappearance of some of those that had been conquered and were thought to be obliterated. Ullman (1988) included among the new diseases of the future (a) diseases of the immune system—in addition to AIDS—resulting from the deficiency or overactivity of the immune system; (b) newer viral conditions incurable with known therapies; (c) more bacterial infections resistant to available antibiotics; and (d) allergies to foods and common substances.

Researchers at Washington University in St. Louis have discovered a new lung disease that they have labeled "reactive airway dysfunction syndrome," or RADS. RADS is brought on after an unusually short exposure to a toxic substance; its effects continue to disable patients long after their exposure ("Suddenly Breathless," 1990). More than 90% of staphylococcus strains now resist treatment with penicillin and related antibiotics. The organisms that cause pneumonia, ear infections in children, and tuberculosis are becoming harder to kill. Researchers at the CDC estimate that infections resistant to antibiotics already add $4 billion per year to health care costs (American Society for Microbiology, 1995). We have forecast that the future will see an AIDS vaccine, as well as a cure, but that is not likely to happen soon enough. Even though the growth rate of the disease is declining, AIDS will continue to take its toll in terms of the suffering of its victims and their families, the helplessness of the service community, and the strain on U.S. health and social welfare resources.

Some of the old diseases also will stage a comeback. Neville, Bromberg, Ronk, Hanna, and Rom (1994) observed a striking increase in multidrug-resistant tuberculosis among patients admitted to the Chest Service of Bellevue Hospital in New York. These researchers reviewed the laboratory susceptibility test results of 4,681 tuberculosis cases over a 20-year period, from 1971 to 1991, and found that combined resistance to the drugs isoniazid and rifampin increased from 2.5% in 1971 to 16% in 1991, with higher rates noted for individual drugs. George E. Schreiner, an epidemiologist, considers the hantavirus a potentially serious threat to public health that may turn out to be more devastating than AIDS. The hantavirus causes hemorrhagic fever, which carries a mortality rate of greater than 70% (Smirnow, 1994).

Medicalized Social Problems

Alcohol and Drug Abuse

Alcohol and drug abuse will continue to challenge the health care community and society at large despite improved knowledge about pharmacological treatment of substance abuse and development or refinement of other therapeutic approaches, such as rational recovery (Galanter, Egelko, & Edwards, 1993), cognitive therapy (Wright, Beck, Newman, & Liese, 1993), and behavioral therapy (Leukefeld, Godlaski, Clark, Brown, & Hays, 2000). The 2009 National Health Interview Survey data show that last year, overall, 52% of adults 18 years of age and over were current regular drinkers and 13% were current infrequent drinkers. Compared with 43% of women, 61% of men were current regular drinkers. As age increased, the percentage of current regular drinkers decreased. Educational attainment and family income were positively associated with current regular drinking status. Compared with 42% of Hispanic adults and 39% of black adults, 58% of white adults were current regular drinkers. Gender- and race-related differences were as follows: 66% of white men were regular drinkers compared with 56% of Hispanic men and 50% of black men; 51% of white women were current regular drinkers compared with 31% of black women and 28% of Hispanic women (Pleis, Ward, & Lucas, 2010). The formidability of the alcohol abuse problem is not likely to lessen in the future.

The drug abuse scene also is not likely to change significantly in the future, despite more research showing the damage done by drugs. Drubach, Kelly, Winslow, and Flynn (1993) explored the effects of substance abuse on the cause, severity, and recurrence of traumatic brain injury in 322 admissions to a large rehabilitation inpatient facility. They found that patients tended to be young and predominantly male and that although motor vehicle crashes were the most common cause of injury, those reporting drug or drug and alcohol abuse were more likely to have sustained violent injuries, such as gunshot wounds. Drug abuse also is a common cause of stroke in young patients (Kokkinos & Levine, 1993). The National Transportation Safety Board, in collaboration with the National Institute on Drug Abuse, investigated fatal-to-the-driver trucking accidents in eight states over a 1-year period. The study found that one or more drugs were detected in 67% of drivers and that 33% of them had detectable blood concentrations of psychoactive drugs or alcohol (Crouch et al., 1993). Drugs (and drinking) not only kill and maim users but also contribute to many other problems. In the future, new chemical entities will be invented to combat drug abuse, and such alternatives to drug abuse as "virtual reality" will be created. Virtual reality is a computer program that takes the user to an illusional world of three-dimensional structures—an experience as powerful as any psychedelic drug but without any associated physical addictions or psychotic behavior (McNally, 1990). The drug abuse problem will persist, however.

Smoking

Smoking continues to be the leading cause of premature and preventable death. During 2000 to 2004, about 443,000 premature deaths each year were attributed to cigarette smoking. Smoking causes death from heart disease, stroke, lung and other types of cancer, and chronic lung diseases. New research shows that chemicals in cigarettes can harm the body from the moment they enter the mouth by attacking tissues as smoke travels to the lungs. Smoking also causes DNA damage and weakens the immune system's ability to prevent damaged DNA from causing cancer (Peterson, 2010). Exposure to secondhand smoke causes premature death and disease in children and adults who do not smoke. Smoking during pregnancy is linked to poor pregnancy outcomes. Educational attainment is closely linked to cigarette use. In 2007, adults with less than a high school education were three times as likely to smoke as those with a bachelor's degree or more education. Adults with at least a bachelor's degree were less likely than other adults to be current smokers and more likely to never have smoked.

In 2009, 21% of adults 18 years of age and older were cigarette smokers; 23% of men compared with 18% of women were current smokers. There were differences based on race as well: 25% of white men were current smokers compared with 23% of black men and 18% of Hispanic men. Among women, 21% of white women were current smokers compared with 19% of black women and 9% of Hispanic women. In 2007, 20% of high school students in grades 9 through 12 had smoked cigarettes in the past month. Female high school students were equally as likely to smoke as male students. Of all high school students, 14% had smoked cigars and 8% had used smokeless tobacco in the past month (National Center for Health Statistics, 2010a; Vital and Health Statistics, 2010).

The new law has given the Federal Drug Administration power to restrict marketing of tobacco products and has banned companies from adding flavors such as clove or strawberry to cigarettes (Peterson, 2010). Smoking will loosen some of its grip in the future but will continue to be a danger to the health of Americans. Researchers will learn about the many ill effects of smoking not before realized. Besides the generally known fact that smoking is the single most important cause of cancer (e.g., lung cancer, breast cancer, oral cancer), recent studies have revealed its other harmful effects as well. For example, Morgado, Chen, Patel, Herbert, and Kohner (1994) studied the effect of smoking on retinal blood flow and autoregulation in subjects with and without diabetes. They found that smoking caused a significant decrease in retinal blood flow and the ability of retinal vessels to autoregulate hyperoxia in both groups. Thus, smoking has a detrimental effect on vision. A study by Howard and associates (1994) not only confirmed the strong relationship between active smoking and increased thickness of the carotid artery wall but also found that even exposure to passive smoking is related to greater carotid artery thickness.

Another study (Sharara, Beatse, Leonardi, Navot, & Scott, 1994) found that women who smoke have an accelerated development of clinically detectable diminished ovarian reserve, which may be a principal mechanism reducing fertility in this group. Smoking also is associated with many periodontal diseases (Mandel, 1994). Czeizel, Kodaj, and Lenz (1994) found that smoking by pregnant women raised the relative odds for congenital limb deficiency in their offspring. Other studies also have found a relationship between maternal smoking during pregnancy and intellectual impairment in children (Olds, Henderson, & Tatelbaum, 1994), maternal smoking during pregnancy and problem behaviors in children in middle childhood (Fergusson, Horwood, & Lynskey, 1993), and tobacco smoke in the home and children's cognitive development (Johnson et al., 1993). Researchers also are finding that even secondhand smoke can adversely affect the physical health of children (Marx, 1993) and that youngsters who smoke are much more likely to use alcohol and illicit substances (Gray, 1993; Torabi, Bailey, & Majd-Jabbari, 1993). A dynamic combination of complex pharmacologic, psychological, and sociocultural factors, however, makes cigarette smoking an extremely difficult problem to deal with (Christen & Christen, 1994). The complexity of the situation will continue to challenge our ingenuity and resources.

Social Problems

Poverty

Poverty can be considered the parent of many problems. It affects its victims in numerous ways and has a special affinity with illness. Research studies point to a causative link between poverty and ill health (McMahon, 1993). As Wilkinson and Marmot (2003) put it, "People further down the social ladder usually run at least twice the risk of serious illness and premature death as those near the top" (p. 10). Poverty forces the poor to live in environments that create conditions and encourage lifestyles inimical to their health. The poor not only live in dangerous and unhealthy environments but also have poor nutritional habits and detrimental lifestyles that leave them in poor health with multiple disease conditions. Because of the lack of resources, they cannot obtain health care adequate for their needs. If race (being black) is used as a proxy for poverty, its effect on health is reflected in the black infant mortality rate of 13.4%, which continues to be more than twice the white infant mortality rate of 5.6% (Mathews & MacDorman, 2010).

A look at the quality of care for cancer patients who are poor provides another example of how poverty affects not only health but also health care. U.S. society has a special sensitivity, concern, and consideration for victims of cancer, but the poor tend to receive poor cancer care. This inadequacy is highlighted by several studies. Berkman and Sampson (1993) found that poor people are more likely to be diagnosed with cancer when the disease is advanced and treatment options are significantly more limited. Limited access to medical care carries the additional risk of denied access to community resources, which often require referrals from the health care system. Underwood, Hoskins, Cummins, and Williams (1994) discovered the following characteristics of cancer care for the economically disadvantaged: (a) Care was deferred because of costs; (b) care was described as "fragmented," "impersonal," and "symptomatic"; (c) patients were discouraged from worrying about bodily changes; (d) patients were discouraged from seeking state-of-the-art care; (e) patients experienced difficulty communicating their needs and concerns; and (f) poverty interfered with efforts to participate in volunteer activities.

A study of posthospitalization care of low-income, urban-dwelling, black cancer patients in the Philadelphia area (O'Hare, Malone, Lusk, & McCorkle, 1993) found that the poor had significantly greater symptom distress related to frequency of nausea, intensity of pain, and difficulty in breathing and that their personal care and home activity needs were not being met adequately. Byrd and Clayton (1993) called the state of care for black cancer patients the "African-American cancer crisis."

The problem of poverty, with all its sordidness, will persist in the future. In 2007, 12.5% of Americans lived in poverty. The faces of poverty also will remain essentially the same. At all ages, a higher percentage of Hispanic and black persons than of white are poor. The poor include a disproportionate percentage of children. In 2007, children represented 35.7% of all Americans living in poverty. More than 13 million children (18%) lived in poverty, and another 15.7 million (21.2%) were classified as near poor with family income between 100% and 200% of the poverty level (National Center for Health Statistics, 2010a). The

infant mortality rate—the risk of death during
the first year of life—in the United States is
worse than in other industrialized nations.
Furthermore, large disparities exist among the
various groups of the American population.
During 1995 to 2006, the infant mortality rate
was consistently highest for infants of black
mothers. The rate also was high among infants of
American Indian or Alaska Native mothers and
Puerto Rican mothers (National Center for
Health Statistics, 2010a).

Low-income children are at significantly
higher risk for psychological, emotional, and
learning disorders, as well as chronic physical
conditions such as hearing and speech impairments. They also are more exposed to unhealthy
and violent environments. A study (Durkin,
Davidson, Kuhn, O'Connor, & Barlow, 1994)
investigated the relationship between socioeconomic disadvantage and the incidence of severe
childhood injury resulting in hospitalization or
death. The study was conducted in New York and
covered the 9-year period from 1983 to 1991. The
average annual incidence of all causes of severe
pediatric injury was 72.5 per 10,000 children, and
the case-fatality rate was 2.6%. Among the socioeconomic factors considered, low income was the
most important predictor of all injuries. Compared
with children living in areas with few low-income
households, children living in areas with predominantly low-income households were more
than twice as likely to receive injuries from all
causes and four and a half times as likely to
receive assault injuries. The effect of neighborhood income disparities on injury risk persisted
after race was controlled.

Homelessness

Homelessness is another manifestation of
poverty. The number of homeless has been rising
constantly and significantly. According to the
most recent statistics from the National Law
Center on Homelessness and Poverty, 3.5 million
Americans are homeless. On any given night,
several hundred thousand are living and sleeping
on the streets, in parks, and in shelters. Today's
homeless are younger, more ethnically diverse,

and more likely to be members of families than
in the past. They include higher proportions of
women and minorities and a growing number of
people with full-time jobs. Among all the homeless, 17% are women. They often are victims of
domestic violence and sexual abuse who lack
education, affordable housing, affordable child
care, and medical care. A study by Richards,
Garland, Bumphus, and Thompson (2010) has
proposed that a dual nature of victimization (personal and political) is responsible for the increasing number of female homeless.

Children under age 18, usually part of a family
headed by a mother, are among the fastest growing homeless groups (Institute of Medicine,
1988b). The National Center on Family Homelessness estimates that as many as 1 in 50 U.S.
children (1.5 million) are homeless or "precariously housed." Physical and mental health problems are much more prevalent among homeless
youth. They also are more likely to be exposed to
violence and drug use at an early age (Cohen,
2009). Rukmana (2008) investigated where
homeless children and youths came from. The
study identified 545 homeless children and youths
in 219 homeless families. Their residential origins
were not heavily concentrated in poor neighborhoods but also were in less-poor neighborhoods.
The study revealed that domestic violence, which
knows no socioeconomic boundaries, explains
the spatial distribution of the residential origins of
homeless children and youths.

Factors associated with homelessness, such as
exposure to adverse weather, trauma, and crime;
overcrowding in shelters, often resulting in unusual
sleeping accommodations; poor hygiene and nutritional status; alcoholism; drug abuse; and psychiatric illness, have clear health implications. But
homelessness may not be merely associated with
illness; it may be the breeder of illness. Abdul
Hamid, Wykes, and Stansfeld (1993) reviewed the
literature on homelessness and concluded that the
psychiatric needs of many of the homeless may be
a direct result of poverty and homelessness.
Nevertheless, health problems commonly seen in
homeless adults include skin ailments; respiratory
infections; chronic gastrointestinal, vascular, dental, and neurological disorders; and traumatic

injuries. Homeless children may have respiratory and ear and skin diseases, as well as special problems such as failure to thrive, developmental delay, neglect, and abuse (Usatine, Gelberg, Smith, & Lesser, 1994). While discussing the health care needs of homeless adolescents, Morey and Friedman (1993) concluded that these teenagers are at risk for sexually transmitted diseases including HIV infection, hepatitis, tuberculosis, accidents, and trauma. Mental health issues of depression, low self-esteem, suicidal behavior or ideation, and hostility—often compounded by drug abuse—also are common. A study of 336 homeless people aged 18 and older found that a substantial minority claimed to have health problems and that 47% of these did not receive needed medical care (Piliavin, Westerfelt, Yin-Ling, & Afflerbach, 1994).

The problem of homelessness is going to persist in the future because homelessness is now seen as an acceptable feature of American life. Conservative political forces are asserting that either homelessness is not much of a problem after all or such problems flow from the personal and moral failures of those who are homeless (Blasi, 1994).

Violence

The United States seems to thrive on violence and has accepted it as part of its culture and—more frightening—as part of its entertainment. During his or her lifetime, a child of 12 will see more than 200,000 acts of violence on television, and many will witness more than 40,000 murders on television (Thomas, 1992). The reality is not less frightening. The picture of crime and violence can be imagined by the following crime clock statistics: In 2009, one violent crime occurred every 23.9 seconds and one property crime every 3.4 seconds. These crimes took the forms of murders, rapes, assaults, robberies, burglaries, and thefts. The country experienced one murder every 34.5 minutes, one forcible rape every 6 minutes, one robbery every 1.3 minutes, one aggravated assault every 39.1 seconds, one burglary every 14.3 seconds, one larceny-theft every 5 seconds, and one motor vehicle theft every 39.7 seconds

(U.S. Department of Justice, 2010). More and more people are at risk of personally experiencing acts of violence.

The crime situation is not likely to improve significantly in the foreseeable future. Certain conditions associated with crime, such as "increasing heterogeneity of populations, greater cultural pluralism, higher immigration, realignment of national borders, democratization of governments, greater economic growth, improving communications and computerization, and the rise of anomie—lack of accepted social norms" (Stephens, 1994, p. 22), plus the proliferation of violent media that reinforce all forms of violence, will continue to set the stage for enactment of crime.

People experience violence not only at the hands of strangers but also at the hands of their own parents, spouses, and children. Health care professionals see, in emergency room trauma cases, the obvious results of violence in the streets. They also are required to see and recognize not-so-obvious cases of domestic violence. These cases of violence take the form of (a) child abuse—children may be physically abused, sexually abused and exploited, physically neglected, or emotionally abused and deprived; (b) spousal abuse, or IPV (intimate personal violence)—violence against women may also take the form of physical, sexual, and emotional abuse; and (c) elder abuse—which similarly encompasses physical, psychological, financial, and social abuse. The incidence and prevalence of all these types of abuse are on the rise.

Child Abuse

Child abuse is a social problem that has no boundaries. It occurs among all socioeconomic groups and in all locations—rural, urban, and suburban—and in all settings—children's homes, foster homes, child-care centers, and residential institutions. Information from the Administration of Children and Families (U.S. Department of Health and Human Services) and Child Welfare Information Gateway shows that during the federal fiscal year 2006, nearly 3.6 million cases of suspected child abuse were investigated, 905,000 children were victims of maltreatment, and an estimated 1,530 children died as a result of abuse or neglect. This number probably is not reflective of the true picture, as child fatalities are believed to be underreported. Besides the major types of abuse mentioned above, other types of maltreatment include abandonment and congenital drug addiction. Although victims are categorized on the basis of the prominent symptoms of maltreatment, children experience a combination of various types of abuse. A physically abused child is emotionally abused as well, and a sexually abused child also may be neglected.

Child abuse and neglect can adversely affect a child's physical, intellectual, social, and psychological growth and development. In the words of Green and Roberts (2008),

> The effects of child sexual abuse may include fear, anxiety, depression, anger, hostility, inappropriate sexual behavior, poor self-esteem, substance abuse, and difficulty with close relationships. Effects of physical child abuse can include the immediate effects of bruises, burns, lacerations, and broken bones as well as longer-lasting effects such as brain damage, hemorrhages, and permanent disabilities. Physical trauma and abuse can also affect children's physical, social, emotional, and cognitive development. Emotional abuse, also known as psychological maltreatment, can seriously interfere with a child's cognitive, emotional, psychological, or social development. The effects of emotional abuse may include insecurity, poor self-esteem, destructive behavior, withdrawal, poor development of basic skills, alcohol or drug abuse, suicide, difficulty forming relationships, and unstable job histories. (p. 79)

In their paper titled "The Neurobiological Toll of Child Abuse and Neglect," Neigh, Gillespie, and Nemeroff (2009) say that abuse may cause alterations in the hypothalamic-pituitary-adrenal axis—a major mediating pathway of stress response—which in turn may contribute to longstanding effects of early life trauma. In addition, the effects of abuse may extend beyond the victim into subsequent generations as a consequence of epigenetic effects transmitted directly to offspring and/or behavioral changes in affected individuals.

Spouse Abuse

Spouse abuse is now called *intimate personal violence* (IPV), a term recommended by the CDC, which defines it as violence committed by a spouse, ex-spouse, current or former partner (of the same or opposite sex) in any of the following four forms: physical, sexual, threats of physical or sexual violence, or psychological/emotional abuse. There are other, more elaborate definitions of IPV, such as the following:

> [IPV is a] pattern of assaultive and coercive behaviors that may include inflicted physical injury, psychological abuse, sexual assault, progressive social isolation, stalking, deprivation, intimidation, and threats. These behaviors are perpetrated by someone who is, was, or wishes to be involved in an intimate or dating relationship with an adult or adolescent, and are aimed at establishing control by one partner over the other. (Family Violence Prevention Fund, 2002)

Nearly 5.3 million intimate partner victimizations occur each year among American women aged 18 and older (National Center for Injury Prevention and Control, 2003).

Elder Abuse

Elder abuse, as hinted above, includes several different types: (1) physical abuse, (2) sexual abuse, (3) emotional abuse, (4) financial exploitation, (5) neglect, (6) self-neglect, and (7) abandonment. Wolf (2000) captured the reality of elder abuse in the following words:

> Unlike some child abuse, which focuses solely on the child and parent (or surrogate parent), and relationship or spouse abuse, which deals with intimate partner relationships, elder abuse covers a wide range involving adult children, intimate partners, more distant relatives, friends, neighbors, caregivers, and other people in whom the older person has placed his or her trust. In addition to multiple relationships, each with its specific set of interpersonal dynamics, elder abuse has a financial component too not associated with either children or battered women. Pensions, social security, and home

ownership have made elders easy prey for unscrupulous caregivers, business service personnel, and even family members. (pp. x–xi)

The National Elder Abuse Incidence Study (National Center on Elder Abuse, 1998) found that about 450,000 elderly in domestic settings were abused or neglected during 1996. When elderly persons who experienced self-neglect are added, the number increases to about 551,000 in 1996. That study also confirmed the "iceberg" theory of elder abuse and neglect, which holds that for every abused and neglected elder reported and substantiated, there are five additional abused and neglected elders who are not reported.

SIGNIFICANCE OF THE CHANGING HEALTH CARE SCENE FOR SOCIAL WORK

We have discussed major changes within the health care system and in society at large that will challenge that system in the future. These changes have the potential to create social work opportunities of immense importance. The anticipated demographic and other sociological changes, the persistence of major social problems, and society's expectations from health care establishments and health professionals will bring into bold relief the inadequacies of the dominant health care professions for dealing with the situation.

At this point in its history, social work seems to be losing ground in U.S. hospitals, and although it has increased its presence in ambulatory care and other nonhospital health care settings, it has done an inadequate job of marketing its image and importance. Social workers must turn the challenges of the future changes into opportunities of unprecedented professional significance. From an account of the anticipated changes in society and the health care system, we identify several major themes and discuss the relevance of social work to them. The "how" of future social work contributions is woven into the material for the subsequent chapters. These themes are (a) the

needs of the chronically ill, both the elderly and others with disabilities; (b) the needs of the victims of major social problems such as poverty, homelessness, violence, AIDS, and substance abuse; (c) the need of the public to change its views of health and illness and its health-related behaviors; (d) the need of health care providers to change their attitudes and behaviors for providing family-centered care that treats the patient as a partner; and (e) the need of the health care community—professionals and organizations—to know how to resolve ethical issues involved in the application of technology to health care and to make decisions about who should benefit from new technologies. The concept of "quality of life" will pervade all these themes.

1. *Chronic illness* in the elderly, as well as in others with disabilities, will be the greatest challenge for the health care system of the future. In 2005, 54.4 million Americans (18.7%) reported some level of disability. Of those, 34.9 million (12%) reported severe disability. As age increases, so does the prevalence of disability. Disabling conditions interfere with the everyday lives of the disabled and also adversely affect their economic status. Among those aged 25 to 64 with a severe disability, 27.1% were in poverty, and the poverty rate for those aged 65 and older with a severe disability was 10.1% (Brault, 2008). The bulk of the current health care system is structured and rewarded for acute care. Acute illness is of short duration and generally ends in either full recovery or death. There is no full recovery in chronic illness. Lorber's (1975) observation still may have an element of truth: Physicians and nurses cannot cure the chronically ill; they feel frustrated, often secretly wish the patient away, and are then burdened with guilt.

Most of the chronically ill are cared for in their own homes, personal care homes, domiciliary homes, boarding homes, foster homes, and nursing homes with assistance from such agencies as outpatient clinics, mental health centers, adult and child day-care centers, hospices, and home-care agencies. Most of these are social service programs planned, directed, and staffed by social workers who have, over the years, developed some practice principles, models of service, strategies, and techniques for effective intervention with the chronically ill. Their experience can be a significant asset to the health care system of tomorrow.

2. *Social problems* such as poverty and homelessness, violence and person abuse, AIDS, and substance abuse defy easy solutions and are beyond the resources of any profession. The health care community is ill-equipped to deal adequately with even the health consequences of these problems. The need is for multipronged, multidisciplinary, comprehensive, and well-coordinated approaches. Social workers are perhaps the only professionals who have closely observed the lives of the victims of these problems. They understand the realities of these victims, know how to relate to them and intervene in their lives, and deal sometimes with the problems and at other times with the consequences of those problems. Their knowledge, sensitivity, and skills in relating to and motivating these people and in mobilizing resources on their behalf are some contributions social workers can make to future plans and programs for these populations.

3. *The attitudes and behaviors of the public* about illness and wellness need to change, not only for people's own physical and mental health but also because the changed public attitudes and expectations will in turn force health care providers to change their attitudes and behaviors. Bringing about such change, however, is difficult because people see things from frames of reference they are familiar with, and those patterns of perception determine their behavior. Traditionally, the health care system has rewarded people for passive and unquestioning attitudes and blindly obedient behaviors. Social work macro practice involves, among other things, educating people, organizing communities, and lobbying policymakers. Public attitudes and behaviors change as a result of education, as well as in response to public laws. Social workers have more skills appropriate for these purposes than do other health care professionals.

4. *Attitudes and behaviors of health care professionals* must change to meet the challenges of the future effectively. The needed change will involve (a) a more holistic view of people and their problems; (b) a proactive stance involving a wellness orientation and the prevention and early detection of problems; (c) willingness to treat the patient as a partner; (d) interprofessional collaboration in substance as well as in form; and (e) a commitment to the idea of quality of life, rather than mere quality of services. Despite Ferguson's (1992) claim that many of his physician colleagues will welcome the chance to climb down off their pedestals and encourage patients to get up off their knees, these changes in position will be difficult because (a) habits die hard; (b) health care professionals in the future will function in many alternative delivery systems, quite different from those of today; (c) they will be required to coexist and collaborate with many more diverse health care providers; (d) professional boundaries will be much more blurred than at present; (e) consumers of health care will themselves judge the quality of services provided to them; and (f) the continued advances in health care technology will pull professionals in the opposite direction. Tension is bound to exist within and among the various professional groups.

The central focus of social work is on the person in his or her life situation, which demands simultaneous attention to the individual and the environment. Social workers are trained to look at the total picture, to consider the relevant larger societal forces—malignant as well as benevolent— while dealing with the private problems of individuals, and to keep in mind the suffering of the individual while dealing with public issues. This perspective compels them to collaborate with all those who can contribute to problem solutions. Their unique perspective and professional expertise, particularly their mediation skills, are important assets. The ethical principles that guide social work practice can help health care providers learn how to treat patients as partners.

5. *Ethical challenges* will multiply as a result of (a) the increased cultural diversity of the U.S. population, (b) the high cost of life-expanding

medical technology, (c) issues of the appropriateness of that technology's use, (d) questions of equity in the availability of that technology, (e) divergent views about the quality of life, and (f) issues of professional authority and patient autonomy. Referring to the major ethical issues faced in the health care world, Friedman (1991) said,

> It is extremely painful to seek answers to questions of care (or non-care) of the dying; prolongation of the lives of fragile, doomed newborns; euthanasia; institutional survival versus community need; confidentiality of sensitive or dangerous information; meaningful informed consent; and how patients and providers can better relate to and trust each other. (p. 44)

Situations generating such questions will increase manifold in the future. Social work experience in respecting the client's right to self-determination and the practice principles and techniques relevant to that experience can contribute to the resolution of ethical conflicts and dilemmas.

Social Work Assets for Future Roles in Health Care

London (1988) identified the following four conditions that can help in dealing with change and mitigating risk: (a) respect for the past, (b) ability to adapt, (c) confidence in the future, and (d) recognition of the inevitability of change itself. Ample evidence suggests that these conditions already exist in social work and can be further strengthened easily.

Respect for the Past

Social work in health care has an impressive, proud, and rich past. In the 19th century, social workers were in the forefront of the movement for reforms in labor, housing, relief, sanitation, and health care (Wallace, Goldberg, & Slaby, 1984). They participated in the prevention, case finding, and treatment of tuberculosis, venereal disease, and maternal and child health problems (Mantell, 1984). A social worker, Edward Devine, formed the National Tuberculosis Association and led the war against tuberculosis (Lewis, 1971; Quam, 2008). Social workers opened or were instrumental in the opening of free dispensaries for the poor in many cities. The roots of social medicine are to be found in organized social work (Rosen, 1974). Their response to the epidemics of influenza, polio, tuberculosis, and venereal disease in the first quarter of the 20th century was exemplary. During and after World War I, they worked as employees of the armed services with injured soldiers, families of those gone to war, veterans, the Red Cross, and the Department of Veterans Affairs. Throughout the 20th century, social workers have contributed their commitment and skills to health care settings of every type—hospitals, medical clinics, nursing homes, rehabilitation centers, hospices, home health agencies, and health departments. Social workers should have no difficulty in respecting this past.

Ability to Adapt

Social workers do not lack in adaptability. An example of the ability of social workers to adapt is the way they responded to the restructuring of financing and provision of services in hospitals under the DRG system. That system imposed a rigid time frame for accomplishing all medical and social objectives pertaining to a patient's admission. A psychosocial assessment had to be completed, problems identified, interventions planned and carried out, and the patient's family and community readied for his or her return home within the time limit set for his or her DRG.

Within a remarkably short period, however, health care social workers rallied and prepared themselves for the delivery of needed services under vastly different circumstances. Social work departments were reorganized, priorities reordered, roles redefined and sometimes reassigned, and staffing patterns reviewed. Sometimes the results were positive and social work departments expanded; at other times, the results were negative and departments contracted; and in some cases, they were eliminated altogether. More significant in the long run, however, was the way health social workers reconceptualized their practice to assess client needs earlier and more rapidly to continue effectively providing the best social work services within the new time constraints (Carlton, 1989, pp. 228–229).

Social workers are adopting computer technology to demonstrate the efficacy of their services. Kossman, Lamb, O'Brien, Predmore, and Prescher (2008) have described how Mayo Clinic's Section of Medical Social Services created a computer program with many capabilities that have resulted in numerous benefits, including accountability, use as a clinical tool, ease of use, protection of patient confidentiality, time efficiency, and trend identification. They were able to measure productivity of social workers and justify a 38% increase in staffing from 1997 to 2002.

Confidence in the Future

Social workers must have confidence in the future in view of the very nature of anticipated future changes. Whether it is the emphasis on wellness rather than illness, the need for comprehensive approaches to problems rather than piecemeal tinkering (done today), or treating the patient as a partner rather than a grateful and obedient recipient of services (as expected in the past), the entire health care community can benefit from social work philosophy and practice principles. Knowing *what* social workers can give to that community and *how* their values and skills can set them apart as potential leaders should enable social workers to anticipate the future with confidence.

Recognition of the Inevitability of Change

Recognition of the inevitability of change is a condition that any profession desirous of increasing its respectability and societal approval must fulfill. It has taken social work practically the

whole of the 20th century to secure legal status through licensing laws in all 50 states. Much more remains to be accomplished, and social workers must accept the inevitability of change. They must become proactive enough to give change the desired direction.

In terms of the professional wherewithal necessary for effective contributions to the health care world of tomorrow, social workers' basic philosophy, knowledge, and skills provide a foundation strong enough to build newer models of practice. The remainder of this book is devoted to understanding the needs of the different health care sectors and to discussing social work knowledge and strategies appropriate for meeting those needs.

Critical Thinking Questions

1. Contrary to our forecast, imagine that the Patient Protection and Affordable Care Act of 2010 ceases to be the law of the land. Will that affect social work roles in the different sectors of health care recommended in this book? If yes, how? If no, why not?

2. The elderly will make up an increasingly larger proportion of the American population. Their claims to societal resources for health care and social services are likely to create intergenerational friction. How should social work deal with that problem at the policy and program levels?

NOTES

1. More than 26,000 patients underwent successful organ transplantations in 2006. The survival rates of those transplanted with organs are consistently improving. One-year graft survival rates in 2006 were as follows: 96.2% for kidneys from living donors, 90.8% for kidneys from deceased donors, 87.5% for hearts, 85.9% for livers from living donors, 83.2% for livers from deceased donors, 83.6% for lungs, 76.3% for pancreases, 70.8% for hearts/lungs, and 69.6% for intestines (Organ Procurement and Transplantation Network, 2010). The survival rates beyond 1 year are impressive as well.

2. For example, at the Planetree Model Hospital Unit in San Francisco's Pacific Presbyterian Medical Center, patients wear their own robes and pajamas, sleep on flowered sheets, sleep as late as they like, and have visitors at all times; their family members cook for them in a special patients' kitchen and are trained to serve as active care partners; and all things are arranged at the convenience of the patient, rather than at the convenience of the medical staff. The results of this pilot program so far show that it is working. "The Planetree unit consistently runs at 85% occupancy and has a waiting list. More than 300 Pacific Presbyterian doctors have voluntarily affiliated with the unit for patient referrals, up from an initial 75. The unit has handled every type of med-surg case, and with no more nursing staff than comparable units" (Coile, 1990, p. 270).

3. HIPPA is the Health Insurance Portability and Accountability Act of 1996. The Accountability part of the act deals with the problem of preserving the privacy of medical information. The *standards for Privacy of Individually Identifiable Health Information* called the *Privacy Rule* established under this law address: (1) the use and disclosure of individuals' health information (called *Protected Health information*) by organizations subject to the Privacy Rule (called *Covered Entities*), and (2) individuals' right to understand and control how that information is used. The Office of Civil Rights within the Department of Health and Human Services is responsible for enforcing the Privacy Rule. The Covered Entities are essentially all health care providers and those working with health plans (all public and private health insurers). *Protected Health Information* under the Privacy Rule refers to information that identifies the individual and individually identifiable health information that is maintained or transmitted by health care providers. Under HIPPA, disclosure of Protected Health Information (PHI) by a covered entity is allowed only as (1) required by the Privacy Rule, (2) permitted by the Privacy Rule, and (3) authorized by the individual who is the subject of the information.

(1) *Required Disclosures.* A covered entity must disclose protected health information in only two situations: (1) to individuals (or their personal representatives) when they request access to or an accounting of disclosures of the PHI, and (2) to the Department of Health and Human Services when conducting an investigation.

(2) *Permitted Disclosures.* A covered entity is permitted to disclose PHI without the individual's authorization for treatment, coordination and management of services, payment, and health care operations (i.e. quality assessment and improvement activities, medical reviews, audits and compliance-related legal services, and specified insurance functions).

(3) *Disclosure authorized by the individual:* An individual may authorize the release of his/her Protected Health Information, but the authorization must contain the following elements to be valid.

Core elements: (i) a description of the information to be used or disclosed, (ii) the name and other specific identification of the person/s authorized to make the disclosure, (iii) the name and other specific identification of the person/s to whom the covered entity may make the disclosure, (iv) a description of the purpose of the requested use or disclosure, (v) an expiration data that relates to the purpose of the use or disclosure, and (vi) signature of the individual and date.

Required statements adequate to place the individual on notice of (i) the individual's right to revoke the authorization; (ii) ability or inability to condition treatment, payment, enrollment, or eligibility for benefits on the authorization; and (iii) the potential for the disclosed information to re-disclosure by the recipient.

Plain language: The authorization must be written in plain language.

Copy to the individual: The covered entity must provide the individual with a copy of the signed authorization.

Main sources of the above information are Olinde and McCard (2005) and U.S. Department of Health and Human Services (2003).

2

HEALTH CARE SETTINGS

Their Past

To help the reader adequately understand and prepare for the anticipated changes in the health care world, we present a brief history of the main health care settings. These include acute care, ambulatory care, preventive care, and long-term care settings. The importance of some of these will wax, and that of others will wane. These changes will, in turn, create different needs for these settings. This chapter is aimed at putting the changing conditions and emerging needs of these settings into a historical perspective because organizations, like people, cannot escape their pasts; they affect their ability to influence the future. Social workers have played significant roles in the history of all these settings. Because of space limitations in this book, however, their place in these histories has not been pointed out. Their contributions are incorporated into discussions of future, setting-specific social work roles and responsibilities in subsequent chapters.

ACUTE CARE SETTINGS

Hospitals are essentially the settings for acute care. The hospital, an age-old institution for the custodial care of the infirm poor, slowly has

evolved as the center of the medical world. Although the history of the modern hospital can be traced back to hospital-like institutions in the ancient world, the modern hospital's recognizable predecessor is an institution of the same name found in medieval Europe. In the absence of commercial inns, lodging houses called hospitals—run by religious organizations—were set up for people going on religious pilgrimages. The travelers were expected to stay in these hospitals just for the night. In time, the local homeless also were allowed to stay and for longer periods. Because many of the homeless were physically ill, nursing care was necessary, and in time, medical consultation was sought (Goldwater, 1943).

During colonial days in the United States, almshouses served as hospitals. They housed the physically ill, along with the homeless, criminals, orphans, and those with mental illness. Prior to the establishment of the first almshouse in Philadelphia in 1713, "the only hospitals in America were temporary structures erected in seaport towns to contain the spread of contagious disease" (Wallace, Goldberg, & Slaby, 1984, p. 3). As the cause of infectious diseases was identified as communicable, infected patients were isolated in special wards or facilities. That was the beginning of the hospital independent of almshouses.

Conditions of these hospitals were usually abominable: Persons with acute and chronic medical and psychological problems were mixed together and were cared for by those who had little training or equipment (Altman & Henderson, 1989). "The true public hospital evolved during the latter half of the 19th century, stimulated by the Civil War when huge general hospitals were constructed in the major American cities" (Blaisdell, 1994, p. 761). The image of the hospital as an asylum for the poor and the destitute, however, persisted.

The rise of modern medicine around the beginning of the 20th century changed the nature and functions of the hospital. It not only led to an improvement in the quality of *caring* through highly skilled nursing but also transformed the hospital into a place for *curing* through the use of scientific medicine. Physicians needed more precise control of patient care and treatment than was possible in the home.

> Precise and elaborate rituals of aseptic surgery could be observed more easily in a special wing of a special building than in a hurriedly rearranged bedroom or domestic kitchen. When aseptic methods made it safe for the surgeon to open the abdomen and other body cavities, there was a rapid increase in the number and complexity of operations, which he dared perform. This resulted in such a great increase in the number and complexity of surgical instruments that transporting them became a problem. During the past 50 years, clinical applications of research discoveries such as X-ray, the measurement of basal metabolism, the electrocardiograph, and radioactive isotopes necessitated the development of costly and bulky equipment. Laboratory examinations were becoming increasingly important in patient care and could be made available more promptly and efficiently when the patients were gathered under one roof than when they were scattered through resident areas. (Burling, Lentz, & Wilson, 1956, p. 5)

Major changes occurred after World War II. The U.S. government actively subsidized medical education, research, and the building of new hospitals. The advent and spread of private health insurance through employment also stimulated the growth of hospitals. After 1965, when the federal and state governments greatly expanded their participation in the financing and delivery of health care services, hospitals were the major beneficiaries. They continued as centers of increasingly more specialized and technologically sophisticated medical care. During the 1970s and 1980s, hospital-based care became progressively more expensive and moved beyond the reach of more and more people. Now the need for accessible and affordable health care is stimulating the search for other approaches to the provision of health services. Hospitals are joining that search and exploring ways of expanding their presence beyond their boundaries.

The hospital's purpose, source of origin, and relationship with the community have varied regionally. Along the Atlantic seacoast, hospitals were founded by wealthy citizens as charitable institutions for the care of the poor. In the South, hospitals were founded by a local surgeon as a workshop for his use and convenience. In the far West, hospitals often were subsidized by the local community and operated on a pay-as-you-go basis (Burling et al., 1956). Hence, voluntary nonprofit hospitals have a stronger tradition in the Northeast, and for-profit hospitals long have been more strongly established in the South and West. Besides these regional differences, hospitals also have reflected the pluralism of U.S. society.

> By 1900, the United States was dotted with hospitals run by hundreds of different private groups, including Roman Catholics, Lutherans, Methodists, Episcopalians, Southern Baptists, Jews, blacks, Swedes, and Germans, depending on the power structures of local populations. The patterns have also varied geographically, both within states and between regions. (Stevens, 1989, p. 8)

Although by 1900 hospitals had been transformed from asylums for the poor into modern scientific institutions, they had not completely disassociated themselves from their past in terms of the original purpose for their being, their relationship with physicians, and their place in the community. Overall, they have symbolized

American ideals, "combining as they do science, philanthropy, and social obligation with technological innovation and power of the purse" (Stevens, 1989, p. 351). Governments also have had a tremendous effect on hospitals. Many private hospitals were built with governmental money acquired through the federal Hill-Burton program and local funding sources, as well as subsidies via tax-exempt bond financing. The major sources of payment for medical services are the federal Medicare and Medicaid programs and employment-based health benefits, which are subsidized by the government, as these are not taxed as income to employees. Also, "health care is subject to extensive governmental regulation by way of licensure requirements, reimbursement rules, and the various conditions of participation that apply to organizations that wish to seek or maintain eligibility for government funding" (Gray, 1991, p. 2). At the same time, government's part in the actual delivery of health care services is limited. Military and Department of Veterans Affairs hospitals, state psychiatric hospitals, and county and municipal hospitals are the only major public health care systems. Most individuals and organizations providing medical services are in the private, nongovernmental sector. The nonprofit hospitals dominate the scene and provide 70% of nonfederal short-term beds. Ownership of a hospital, however, is less important as an indicator of what the hospital does than the clients it serves and the management policies it pursues. Nonprofit hospitals are income-maximizing institutions managed as businesses, and for-profit hospitals are instruments of social policy. Hospitals use conflicting models of service that overlap both public and private domains:

> On one side is a model of hospitals as supply-driven, technological systems, analogous to an electrification system or a system producing military aircraft. Hospitals produce surgery, procedures, X-rays, expertise, even babies. On the other is a model of hospitals as community services, with lingering religious, humanitarian, and egalitarian goals, more analogous to a system of schools. (Stevens, 1989, p. 6)

U.S. hospitals have tried to "meet American ideals of technology, science, expertise, charity, voluntarism, equity, efficiency, community, and the privilege of class all at once, to everybody's satisfaction" (p. 355) and, understandably, have not succeeded in reaching so many and such ambiguous goals.

Hospitals may be classified on several bases. They may be seen as big or small, urban or rural, rich or poor, for-profit or nonprofit, public or private, and research or nonresearch. Until the late 1960s, the typical hospital could be described fairly as an independent, nonprofit, proprietary institution. Nonindependent hospitals owned by government or by religious organizations were exceptions. Over the past 40 years, a new entity, resulting from mergers of hospitals into or takeover by multi-institutional systems, has appeared on the health care scene.

> Local control declined as large numbers of independent hospitals became part of multi-institutional systems (both for-profit and nonprofit). Ownership of institutions by publicly traded, investor-owned companies began and grew rapidly. Various kinds of new, mostly for-profit health care organizations—ranging from ambulatory care centers to HMOs [health maintenance organizations]—emerged without the traditional voluntary ethos. Some of the diagnostic, treatment, and rehabilitation centers are locally owned by entrepreneurs (often physicians) or hospitals. But there is also representation by investor-owned companies operating multiple facilities. (Gray, 1991, p. 4)

Therefore, current hospitals can be viewed more realistically as belonging to three major categories: (a) community hospitals, (b) hospitals as parts of larger multi-institutional systems, and (c) academic medical centers. Each of these has a different set of purposes, priorities, and organizational setups. Nevertheless, they all share, in varying degrees, such common characteristics as segmentation, social stratification, money standard, technological identification, division between physicians and hospitals, and an authoritative role for university medicine (Stevens, 1989).

1. *Segmentation.* We already have mentioned the diversity and pluralism of U.S. hospitals. Even within the broad categories suggested above, the variety of hospitals, in terms of their affiliation, ownership, and size, is remarkable. The following statistics highlight that diversity. There are 5,795 registered hospitals in the country. Of these, 5,008 are community hospitals, which include nongovernment not-for-profit (2,918), investor-owned for-profit (998), and state and local government hospitals (1,092). The remaining are federal government hospitals (211), nonfederal psychiatric hospitals (444), nonfederal long-term care hospitals (117), and other (e.g., prison) hospitals (15; American Hospital Association, 2009b). Of the community hospitals, 1,997 are rural hospitals and the remaining 3,011 are urban. Of all the hospitals, almost a quarter (23.5%) have fewer than 50 beds, 23.7% have 50 to 99 beds, 24.8% have 100 to 199 beds, and 28% have more than 200 beds (American Hospital Association, 2009b).

2. *Social stratification.* U.S. hospitals continue to serve as vehicles for defining social class and race. Urban public hospitals such as Bellevue and Kings County in New York, Philadelphia General, Cook County in Chicago, and San Francisco General—many of these being the descendants of the late 18th-century workhouses or almshouses—remain primarily for the poor.

Even as these hospitals, like other hospitals, were "medicalized" in accordance with progressive, scientific ideas in the late 19th and early 20th centuries—and, indeed, many became major teaching centers—they continued to attract a relatively large proportion of the poorest Americans and of racial and ethnic minorities. The poor, in turn, became the medical schools' "teaching material." These patterns continue today in the large proportion of Medicaid (welfare) patients treated in academic centers (Stevens, 1989, pp. 9–10).

3. *Money standard.* All aspects of hospital operations are infused by the money standard of success. Hospitals attract paying patients by presenting themselves as having something valuable to sell. Appealing to upper-class patients involves show, unnecessary extras, and even waste. The pay nexus influences decisions about services so that resources are concentrated in areas of maximum profit. People have tended to think of health care as an economic as well as a social good and have preferred the economic dimension (Eisdorfer & Maddox, 1988). Hospitals have reflected that societal preference. The language of hospital administration is filled with the jargon of economics and management, not of medicine (Alper, 1984). The hospital's obsession with cost control has overshadowed the concern about needs for medical care. While comparing the hospital priorities of the 1960s with those of the 1980s, Kane (1988) found that they had shifted from ACCESS, QUALITY, and cost to COST, quality, and access. This continues to be true.

4. *Technological identification.* Hospitals have focused on acute care and technology, particularly surgery, which is the mainstay of the short-stay hospital. This focus has had diverse consequences. In the words of Stevens (1989),

> The modern physician, associated with the new hospitals, was—and is—a master engineer, a hero in the American mode, fighting disease with 20th-century tools. But the early emphasis on surgery has focused hospitals, in turn, around technical spaces such as operating rooms. Generation after generation has characterized the 20th-century hospital in industrial terms as a factory or workshop. The success and visibility of the hospital in providing acute, specialized care has also obscured its relatively limited role in the overall picture of health and disease. (p. 12)

5. *Division between physicians and hospital.* Physicians have considered the hospital an extension of their private practice of medicine, and physicians and hospitals cooperate closely. Physicians, however, do not belong to the hospital; they are officially its guests and are given "privileges" of admitting and treating its patients. Physicians are essential for hospitals, but the goals and service agendas of the two are often different—thus, a built-in tension exists between hospitals and the medical profession. The following trends are further complicating the situation.

Nearly 90% of the 4,300 ambulatory surgery centers, which have cropped up in the past 25 years, are owned by physicians. Physicians also own about 100 specialty hospitals. "Specialists are bailing out of hospitals to found, manage, and own their facilities" (Reece, 2007, p. 124). These entities are competing successfully with hospitals. On the other hand, despite the general resistance of hospitals, there are a few examples of physician-hospital joint ventures, where hospitals and physicians are sharing revenues and responsibilities. "In Nashville, a group of entrepreneurial neurosurgeons struck a deal 'piggybacking' an 18-bed specialty hospital, featuring six operating rooms doing 250 procedures a month, upon St. Thomas Hospital's 683-bed hospital" (Reece, 2007, p. 124). Then, some physicians are approaching hospitals to become hospitalists, doctors who are employees of the hospital and who practice exclusively within the hospital.

6. *Authoritative role for university medicine.* Medical schools have a strong but informal influence on hospitals. Although only a minority of hospitals has formal affiliation with medical schools, teaching hospitals are the most powerful. They have been the centers of research, generators of new knowledge and skills, and upgraders of medical and surgical practices. The combination of medical schools and associated hospitals created academic medical centers, which are important parts of the hospital scene. These not only train medical residents and other health care professionals and conduct research but also provide health care to patients and offer nonhospital services such as health screening, community outreach, health fairs, health information centers, patient education centers, and support groups. These hospitals also have been affected by managed care. Lee and Mongan (2009) described that effect as follows:

> Boston's teaching hospitals found that they were having difficulty with three of their missions: patient care, teaching, and research. Stand-alone hospitals could not offer the range of care that patients needed, gave medical students only a fleeting glimpse of the sickest patients, and provided a narrow base for medical research. The result was that the traditional academic medical center risked becoming less relevant to its patient community and constituents. (p. 121)

These centers have used different approaches to survive and retain their eminence.

Overall, hospitals are powerful social institutions:

> They are affirming and defining mirrors of the culture in which we live, beaming back to us, through the scope and style of the buildings, the organizational "personality" of the institution, and the underlying meaning of the whole enterprise, the values we impute to medicine, technology, wealth, class, and social welfare. (Stevens, 1989, p. 14)

They also are sensitive to messages from their environment and have been adaptive and pragmatic organizations.

In the olden days, hospitals attempted to alleviate a broad range of human ills—poverty and hopelessness, as well as disease—but gradually narrowed their focus to bodily disease. That focus continued to narrow so that hospitals in the second half of the 20th century were treating only acute physical illness. Now that trend has been reversed.

In the future, hospitals will turn around and widen their scope to cover all types of services, from acute tertiary care on the one extreme to health promotion on the other. The forecast is that demographic and other sociological changes will place new demands on the health care system, that technological advances will make it possible to treat many illnesses that require hospitalization today on an ambulatory basis in the future, and that a more holistic approach to health and illness will emphasize wellness. These changes will significantly alter the purpose, function, and organization of hospitals. The new functions of future hospitals will justify another classification based on the type and level of health care they provide. Some hospitals will become the nucleus of primary care activities, others will provide predominantly secondary care, and still others will become centers of tertiary care. The commitment to the concept of "comprehensiveness of care" will, however, compel most hospitals to incorporate elements of other levels of care into the level in which they specialize. Even within each level of care, variations will exist among hospitals, as their past characteristics will continue to affect their future characteristics.

AMBULATORY CARE SETTINGS

Ambulatory care is where the patient first comes into contact with the health care system and continues in order to stay in the system. Ambulatory care has no universally accepted definition. The diversity of care providers, settings, and services makes it difficult to define. The easiest way to deal with this difficulty is to stick with the literal meaning of the word *ambulatory* and call ambulatory care the care provided to the *walking* patient, irrespective of who provides that care, where it is provided, and the level of care provided. This care would, thus, encompass all services provided to noninstitutionalized patients (Williams, 1991).

A physician serving the walking patient is variously called an ambulatory care physician, a primary care physician, or a general practitioner, but he or she also may be a pediatrician, an obstetrician, or a surgeon. The service provider may not even be a physician; he or she may be a nurse practitioner or a physician assistant. The setting may be the private office of a physician in solo practice, offices of physicians in group practice, a free-standing clinic, a neighborhood health center, a public health clinic, a hospital outpatient department, an ambulatory surgery center, an urgent care center, or a hospital emergency room. Roemer (1986) identified the following eight types of organized ambulatory health care on the basis of their sponsorship: (a) hospital outpatient departments, (b) public health agency clinics, (c) industrial health service units, (d) school health clinics, (e) voluntary clinics, (f) private-group medical practices, (g) health

centers of other public agencies, and (h) health maintenance organizations (HMOs).

The services provided in ambulatory care settings may cover the whole gamut and include (a) preventive services such as screening for diseases, immunization and vaccination, and health education; (b) routine care services, including diagnostic, counseling, follow-up, and therapeutic care; and (c) more complex services involving specialized tests, procedures, and facilities (Williams, 1991). These services also can be classified as primary, secondary, and tertiary care. Although primary health services include preventive measures that may be environmental, educational, or personal and first-encounter-with-a-provider care, in this chapter, the meaning of prevention in primary care is restricted to personal prevention. "Common forms of personal preventive measures are immunization, surveillance of expectant mothers and babies, and adult examinations for detection of chronic diseases" (Roemer, 1986, p. 29).

Primary care relates to the well, the "worried well," the presymptomatic patient, and the patient with disease in early symptomatic stages. The secondary care function relates to patients with symptomatic states of diseases. . . . The tertiary care function encompasses levels of disease which are seriously threatening the health of the individual. (Reynolds, 1975, p. 893)

Primary, secondary, and tertiary care represent stages in the continuum of care from the least to the most intensified. There is room for variance, however, in the judgment about where one stage ends and the other begins. Although most of the services provided in ambulatory care settings would fall under essentially primary and to a lesser extent secondary care categories, the services rendered in ambulatory surgery centers and emergency rooms require specialized skills and sophisticated equipment. Although such settings increasingly are vying with hospitals as sites of medical miracles, we include emergency medical services under ambulatory care because their focus is on the walking patient. The needs of patients using emergency rooms for emergency and nonemergency problems are different in their nature, intensity, and urgency from those of patients seen in other ambulatory settings. Nevertheless, the emergency room serves as the primary physician, as well as the acute and emergency care facility, for the poor and multiproblem patient (Clement & Durgin, 1987). The increasing use of the emergency room for primary care has a long-term trend (Williams, 1991).

Ambulatory care has a long history. As pointed out above, until 1900, hospitals were asylums for the poor and the destitute and hospital-based care was dreaded and stigmatized. Ambulatory care was the preferred mode of service. In those days, the physician did not have much to give. His or her role as a healer was "predominantly one of patient supporter, occasionally providing palliative therapy and very occasionally providing effective curative therapy" (Williams, 1991, p. 4), and these services could be provided easily and equally well in the physician's office or the patient's home. Virtually no technology supplemented the art of medicine, and a physician could carry all his or her tools in a "little black bag." Moreover, "a vision of the hospital as morally stigmatizing and possibly dangerous underlined a very positive function for outpatient charity medicine" (Rosenberg, 1989, p. 2). In towns and rural areas, most municipalities and counties paid local physicians to treat the poor in their homes. Dispensaries were the places to which the urban poor turned for health care. Dispensaries where private physicians treated the needy patients free of charge originally were set up in England and France in the 17th century; the Philadelphia Dispensary was the first to be established in the United States in 1786. It was followed by similar dispensaries in New York in 1791 and Boston in 1796 (Rosenfeld, 1971). Hospitals and almshouses also provided outpatient care in the form of prescriptions. The Philadelphia Hospital, founded in 1751, opened the first hospital outpatient department in 1786 (Pascarelli, 1982).

Dispensaries, however, were the major source of health care for those who could not afford a physician's services privately. By the beginning of the last quarter of the 19th century, 29 dispensaries had been founded in New York and 33 in Philadelphia. These dispensaries treated increasingly larger numbers of patients. For example, whereas in 1860, 134,069 patients were treated at New York City's dispensaries, the corresponding number for the year 1900 was 876,000. These dispensaries increased not only in number but also in diversity. Ambitious would-be specialists among physicians were instrumental in opening new dispensaries and reorganizing old ones on specialty lines (Rosenberg, 1989).

Dispensaries reached their highest point in the decade before World War I. They were everywhere. Whereas some were devoted to providing care and curative services, others—the majority—were dedicated to the prevention of such diseases as tuberculosis and syphilis.

> Only a handful of medical graduates could find house officerships in urban hospitals; such positions were limited to a small minority of the fortunate. However, a far greater number of physicians could and did volunteer to serve in outpatient units as they accumulated clinical skills. (Rosenberg, 1989, p. 2)

In the last decade of the 19th century, clinics were established at teaching institutions such as Johns Hopkins and Massachusetts General Hospital, as well as at a few hospitals unaffiliated with medical schools. By 1900, about 150 such clinics had been founded, two thirds affiliated with medical schools (Rosenfeld, 1971).

The advent of scientific medicine brought the hospital and inpatient care into prominence. Whereas in 1873, only 178 hospitals (including mental hospitals) were available throughout the country, the number of general hospitals increased to nearly 4,400 by 1910 (Roemer, 1986). This rise in the number and prominence of hospitals eclipsed the importance of ambulatory care. Many general dispensaries gradually were subsumed into hospital emergency rooms and outpatient specialized clinics, whereas the functions of the preventive dispensaries were performed by community health centers. They also lost their importance for medical training. By the 1920s, internship and residency had become a required aspect of every physician's training, and the importance of voluntary outpatient work declined. Unlike the hospital, outpatient medicine's history of association with the poor continued to affect the status of ambulatory care.

> Outpatient medicine bore the burden of its welfare origins. Never a part of normal fee-for-service medicine, and marked by an often casual and routine quality, it has always been regarded with a touch of disdain—tolerated rather than aspired to by the majority of physicians. (Rosenberg, 1989, p. 4)

Many changes, particularly since World War II, have had significant effects on ambulatory care. The federal government actively subsidized medical education, research, and the building of new hospitals, and stimulated numerous medical discoveries. After 1965, the federal and state governments greatly expanded their participation in the financing and delivery of health care services. The two major approaches to governmental involvement can be characterized as an individual-based (or insurance or entitlement) approach and an institution-based (or provider or grant program/direct service) approach (Davis & Millman, 1983). The Medicare and Medicaid programs are examples of the former; Veterans Affairs hospitals, National Health Service Corps, and community health centers are examples of the latter. Although theoretically distinct, in reality, the two approaches interact a great deal. The growth of hospitals, developments in health care technology, and insurance programs—both governmental and private—entitling more and more people to sophisticated inpatient treatment made hospital care attractive as well as expensive. Gradually, the cost of health care—of which inpatient care accounts for a major chunk—became a major concern.

Ambulatory care now is seen as a significant part of the solution to the problem of high cost. The current picture of ambulatory care includes many entities, such as (a) physicians in solo practice; (b) health care providers in group practice—both fee-for-service and prepaid types; (c) hospital-based outpatient departments; (d) health centers and clinics—government financed and/or operated, as well as private and voluntary; and (e) emergency care centers—hospital-based and free-standing. The following are the highlights of the history of these entities.

Solo Practice

Most ambulatory care traditionally has been provided by physicians in office-based solo practice. These physicians provide what can be called routine care, follow-up or ongoing care for relatively simple primary care problems (Williams, 1991). These physicians may not all be general practitioners—that is, family physicians, general internists, and general pediatricians—because a significant portion of women receive all their medical care from obstetricians during their childbearing years and because many patients with single-organ-system diseases receive their primary care from specialists (Petersdorf, 1993). Moreover, the number of generalists has been decreasing progressively. In 1931, only 17% of physicians specialized in a single branch of medicine, but by 1970, that number had risen to 80%, correspondingly reducing the availability of primary care physicians significantly (Pascarelli, 1982). To reverse this trend, the Comprehensive Health Manpower Training Act of 1971 authorized grants to hospitals for residency training in family practice, and the 1976 Title VII of the Health Professions Education Assistance Act broadened the federal incentive to cover the development of undergraduate as well as residency training not only in family practice but also in general pediatrics and general internal medicine. Despite about $50 million in Title VII grants going to medical schools annually between 1977 and 1985, the percentage of medical graduates planning certification in these generalist disciplines actually declined during those years—in family medicine, from 17.8% to 13.3%; in general internal medicine, from 27.9% to 10.7%; and in general pediatrics, from 8.8% to 5.8% (Greer, Bhak, & Zenker, 1994). That trend has continued. In the words of Reece (2007),

> Multiple reasons exist for this decline: fragmentation from too many scattered small practices, inadequate reimbursement, insufficient capital, operational inefficiencies, poor business practices, too little prestige, low morale, too few doctors entering primary care specialties, competence from nurse practitioners and retail clinics, patients choosing alternative practitioners, and too many doctors leaving with resulting stresses on those who remain. (p. 21)

In Chapter 1, we referred to the efforts of the Association of American Medical Colleges and others to increase the proportion of medical graduates entering generalist practice. The consensus seems to be that, to meet U.S. health care needs, the appropriate mix of specialist and generalist physicians should be 50% of each group (Schroeder, 1993). Raising the proportion of generalist physicians to 50% will involve changing the admission policies of medical schools, reorienting their preclinical and clinical curricula, reconfiguring graduate medical education, and retraining physicians originally trained as specialists. According to Schroeder's calculation, not until the year 2040 would 50% of all physicians be generalist. This picture of the current and projected availability of medical personnel for ambulatory care has relevance for the group practice as well.

Physicians in solo practice are a diminishing group. The solo practice model made those physicians solely responsible for all their patients 24 hours a day, 7 days a week, every day of the year. Today, their lifestyle demands a balance between their personal and professional responsibilities. Furthermore, in the olden days, they normally provided all the medical care required by their patients. That is not possible now because of the rapidly advancing knowledge in every field of medicine and resulting specializations. The cost of malpractice insurance began to rise in the 1970s, and inflation raised the office lease and rental expenses. Before the introduction of Medicare,

Medicaid, and other government programs, physicians received payment for their services from patients or from Blue Cross/Shield and a small number of other private insurance carriers. Billing and collection were simple (Sultz & Young, 2001).

> For the private physician's office, regulation, record maintenance, and billing requirements burgeoned overnight in complexity and volume. Solo-practice office administration, once the province of the physicians themselves, with possibly a receptionist and a part-time bookkeeper, began to require an increased level of sophistication and a great deal more time. (p. 114)

Furthermore, in view of the ever-more-expensive technologically sophisticated medical equipment, the cost of establishing a practice is becoming prohibitive (Williams, 1991). In an insightful discussion of the politics of ambulatory care, Bellin (1982) listed a number of problems a solo practitioner is likely to experience in establishing and managing his or her practice, coexisting with other physicians in the area, and maintaining staff privileges at local hospitals. From a consumer-satisfaction perspective, Coile (1990) said, "No doctor can take patients' loyalty for granted today. To maintain high rates of return business, physicians are turning to customer relations programs that go beyond 'charm school' for physician office staff" (p. 13). Many solo practitioners cannot afford marketing services; they opt for group practice. The following scenario may not be far-fetched in the future: The nonaligned physicians are either "superstars" whose talents are so in demand that they hold privileges at several competing hospitals or "lone wolves" who subsist on the few remaining fee-for-service patients or work for a temporary-physician personnel agency (p. 239).

Group Practice

Group medical practice has experienced a more rapid growth than any other type of organized ambulatory care. This practice also represents a form of managed care, which is seen as a solution to the problem of steeply rising health care costs. The growing popularity of group practice is in total contrast to the opposition it received from other individual physicians and their societies in the early days of its history. Pascarelli (1982) traced the history of group practice to the 1870s, when the Homestake Mining Company established a medical group for its workers in South Dakota. The Northern Pacific Railroad did likewise in 1883. The first nonindustrial group practice, the famous Mayo Clinic in Rochester, Minnesota, was established in 1887, demonstrating that this type of practice was feasible in the private sector as well and "represented a reputable model for group practice in a national atmosphere of fierce independence, where group practice was viewed with skepticism and distrust" (Williams, 1991, p. 14).

Skepticism had, at times, taken the form of open opposition by the American Medical Association and local medical societies. Physicians in group practice often were denied privileges in local hospitals, and patients referred by them were refused treatment by community-based specialists. Group practice also had legal constraints. In such a hostile atmosphere, group practice had difficulty growing and prospering. "The early development of group practice occurred principally in the Midwest and West and in smaller communities that lacked hospitals. The pivotal physician was often someone who had trained at the Mayo Clinic" (Pascarelli, 1982, p. 8). By the early 1930s, medical groups had grown to about 150 throughout the United States. In 1931, a national committee established to assess medical care needs and costs suggested that (a) group practice play a major role in the provision of medical care, (b) these groups be associated with hospitals for comprehensive care, and (c) all services be prepaid (Committee on Cost of Medical Care, 1932). The American Medical Association condemned the report and declared that group and salaried physicians were unethical (Sultz & Young, 2001).

Parallel to the development of group practice was the development of medical care insurance.

Taking roots in scattered communities throughout the country in the last half of the 19th century, and under a wide variety of auspices, the principle of pooling risks and resources to budget and pay for the costs of medical care gradually spread. (Rosenfeld, 1971, p. I-14)

Groups for mutual protection that organized primarily to provide medical care, such as La Societe de Bienfaisance Mutuelle de San Francisco (which built its own hospital in 1852), the German Benevolent Society of San Francisco, and the French Mutual Benefit Society of Los Angeles, began appearing in the 1850s. The first major prepayment programs were organized by the Southern Pacific Railroad of Sacramento, California, in 1868, the Missouri Pacific Hospital Association in 1872, and the Northern Pacific Beneficial Association in 1882. Other entities that developed group practices were unions in industries, such as the Iron Molders Union (in 1859) and the Brotherhood of Locomotive Firemen and Engineermen (in 1873). The International Ladies Garment Workers' Union organized a health center in New York in 1918. In the same year, the Endicott-Johnson Corporation developed a program that combined the organization of financing and services. A group practice plan organized and financed by the Farmers' Union Cooperative Hospital Association was established in Elk City, Oklahoma, in 1929 under the leadership of Michael A. Shadid, an immigrant physician. The members owned shares in the community hospital, and services were provided by a group of five physicians and two dentists. At about the same time, two physicians—Donald E. Ross and H. Clifford Loos of Los Angeles—organized a partnership of physicians and contracted with the city's water and power department for providing medical services to employees on a prepayment basis. One side effect of the Depression on hospitals was the birth of the Blue Cross program in 1933, which was followed by Blue Shield in 1939, sponsored by state medical societies (Rosenfeld, 1971).

The prepaid group practice, the prototype of the present-day HMO, was first organized in the late 1920s and 1930s. The Kaiser Permanente Foundation Plan, originating in California; the Group Health Cooperative of Puget Sound (Seattle),

Washington; the Group Health Plan of Minnesota; and the Group Health Association (GHA) of Washington, D.C., were the earliest HMOs. The establishment in 1937 of the GHA, a nonprofit membership corporation of federal employees, was a significant development. The American Medical Association held that the plan (Group Health Insurance) offered by the GHA was unethical and expelled GHA-salaried physicians (Sultz & Young, 2001). In 1938, the GHA took the American Medical Association to court. It claimed that the Sherman Anti-Trust Act was being violated because the group's medical staff were denied membership in the district medical society and appointment to a hospital staff. In 1943, the U.S. Supreme Court found the American Medical Association to be in violation of the law. This decision paved the way for the further development of prepaid groups, particularly during the years following World War II (Pascarelli, 1982).

Many labor unions and community organizations established programs of group practice prepayment after World War II. Prepaid groups were criticized as "socialized medicine practices" in which patients did not have free choice of physicians and physicians did not have any incentive to practice good medicine (Watters, 1961). HMOs did constitute a departure from free-market dynamics.

> The HMO is basically a strategy for complete removal from the orbit of the market of a population of patients and health care providers. Buyers and sellers make an agreement, a fixed-price contract, for future delivery (usually for 1 year) of needed medical care. (Roemer, 1986, p. 111)

This was viewed as the first step in a broader assault on the medical market. Such opposition and restrictive state laws inhibited the growth of HMOs (Bracht, 1978). The situation gradually changed. The number of group practices began to rise after World War II. These practices were found to be providing excellent care while effectively controlling the cost escalation of the free medical market. This finding led to the enactment of federal legislation in 1973 for the promotion of prepaid group health organizations. In order to sell the public and Congress on this model of care, the Nixon administration referred to prepaid group practices as *health maintenance organizations* (Bodenheimer & Grumbach, 2002).

Advantages of group practice from the perspective of the provider include the following: no heavy initial investment, shared operation of practice, centralized administrative function (performed by professional management in large groups), lesser burden of operating cost, sharing of patient-care responsibilities that results in greater flexibility of working hours and more time for vacation and continuing education, greater opportunity for formal and informal peer review and continuing education, and greater earnings (Bodenheimer & Grumbach, 2002; Owens, 1988; Williams, 1991). Lee and Mongan (2009) pointed out another benefit of what they call "groupness":

> Larger organizations have visible and sometimes conspicuous roles in society, so they must confront issues that are easily overlooked by small physician practices—issues like care for the uninsured, conflicts of interest, and identification of physicians whose ability to practice has been impaired by mental or other health problems. (p. 175)

Most group practices are legal entities unto themselves, while others are part of larger organizations such as hospitals. A group practice can be organized legally in a number of ways: (a) a sole proprietorship in which one individual is the owner and others are his or her employees; (b) a partnership in which all members of the group share ownership and liability; (c) a professional corporation in which stock is issued and the stockholders, usually members of the group, own the corporation; and (d) other forms, including associations and foundations. Most groups are partnerships or professional corporations (Williams, 1991). In prepaid groups, such as Kaiser Foundation Health Plan, most principles of group practice are incorporated but physicians and other providers usually are salaried.

As an instrument of managed care, all models of group practice—HMO, PPO (preferred provider organization), and its variant, EPA (exclusive provider arrangement)—grew. Historically, the managed care movement was dominated by HMOs, but starting in 1986, PPO enrollment not only achieved parity with HMOs when both reached 25 million but outstripped them (Richman, 1987). However, boundaries between HMOs and PPOs blurred. The fastest-growing kind of HMO was the "open-ended HMO," which works like a PPO. By the turn of the century, these managed organizations started to decline. For example, in 2000, HMO enrollment dropped by 400,000 from 1999, and by 2001, of the 6 million Medicare recipients enrolled in HMOs, 1.5 million were forced to find other insurance arrangements as their HMOs pulled out of the Medicare program due to monetary losses. Risk-bearing physician groups and individual practice associations fared even worse. Concerns that many plans were more interested in profits than patient care created disenchantment with managed care (Bodenheimer & Grumbach, 2002).

Hospital-Based Outpatient Departments

In 1875, the United States had fewer than 200 hospitals. Most of the health care was provided in either physicians' offices or patients' homes. Poor people received care through dispensaries. The growing population of the country—from 9 million in 1820 to 105 million by 1920 (Pascarelli, 1982)—necessitated more health care resources. To the other settings of health care were added more hospitals and hospital outpatient departments. By 1909, the number of hospitals had grown to 4,359 with a total bed capacity of 421,000. Hospitals, particularly local government hospitals, began to establish outpatient departments that were used mostly by the poor. Teaching hospitals also provided ambulatory care to children and youth under federal grants (under 1965 Social Security Amendments and the Child Health Act of 1967).

Outpatient departments, however, were of low priority for hospitals (both public and private) and their medical staff. The purpose of hospital-based ambulatory services was to provide health care to the sick poor and to provide training for medical students and residents, the former often becoming a means for the latter. "They [outpatient clinics] were most often staffed by medical students, who were mandated to serve there, and by the hospital-affiliated physicians of lowest tenure and rank, who agreed to see patients in return for admitting privileges" (Sultz & Young, 2001, p. 117). Understandingly, the quality of services was uneven. These clinics typically are classified by medical specialties and were held at specified times each week. Most patients could not pay high out-of-pocket fees. The fees for hospital-based ambulatory care usually were paid from public sources and were fixed at a rate that did not cover costs. On the other hand, reimbursement often was at cost rather than at a fixed fee (Zavodnick, Katz, Markezin, & Mitchell, 1982). Hence, these departments were not moneymakers, and, therefore, hospitals or physicians had no financial incentive to take an active interest in them.

This situation has been changing over the past three decades. The drive to reduce health care costs, the growing proportion of elderly in the population, and the push toward preventive medicine started giving ambulatory care special significance, and hospital-based outpatient services were bound to gain unprecedented importance. The quality of outpatient services also received needed attention. In 1973, the Joint Commission on Accreditation of Hospitals adopted its first set of outpatient standards. These standards defined hospital-based ambulatory care service and dealt with its various dimensions, such as sponsorship of services and staffing, education and training of service providers, written policies and procedures, facility design and equipment, medical records, and audits and evaluation. These standards forced the hospital boards, administrators, and staff to start viewing ambulatory care favorably.

While ambulatory services typically compose the minority share of the revenues of larger hospitals, their revenue and growth potential are explosive in comparison with inpatient services (Zismer, as quoted in Reece, 2007). Coile (1990) observed that a few small and well-diversified hospitals were beginning to experience a 50:50 ratio of inpatient revenue to ambulatory revenue. Ambulatory care had cut the umbilical cord that tied it to inpatient care. The growth of ambulatory care was no longer dependent on shifting inpatient procedures to an ambulatory basis. Most inpatient procedures already had been shifted by changing medical practice and payer policies. That picture was truer of urban hospitals than of their rural counterparts for some time. While discussing strategies for survival of rural hospitals and focusing on the needs of the elderly, Buada, Pomeranz, and Rosenberg (1986) said that because, historically, the hospital has been the most highly organized form of health care delivery for the elderly, it should use that strength to become the dominant provider of long-term care services. Hospitals have been heeding that advice.

Moreover, the adoption of diagnosis-related–group hospital reimbursement methodology, which emphasizes decreased lengths of stay, has added to the importance of outpatient clinics.

> Facing declining inpatient revenue, increasing influence of managed care, and shifting medical education emphasis on primary medicine, hospitals initiated reorganization and expansion plans for outpatient clinic services that focused heavily on primary care areas. Teaching hospitals planned jointly with their affiliated medical schools, and nonteaching facilities followed suit to pursue expansion of both the volume and array of outpatient services with primary care as the core. (Sultz & Young, 2001, p. 119)

Now, hospital outpatient clinics are organized like those of private physician group practices and are aesthetically pleasant, well equipped, and customer oriented (Sultz & Young, 2001). In the future, hospitals will organize and deliver multispecialty ambulatory care in clinics far removed from their brick-and-mortar settings (Reece, 2007).

Health Centers and Clinics

Health centers and clinics compose a large group and include many ambulatory care settings, such as public health department clinics, community health care centers, ambulatory surgery centers, clinics of other public agencies (e.g., the Department of Veterans Affairs, military services, Indian Health Service), industrial health units, school health clinics, prison health centers, voluntary disease-specific clinics (e.g., cancer-screening clinics), and general health clinics established by voluntary agencies. In the sections that follow, we look at the first three of these in some detail.

Public Health Department Clinics

Public health department clinics have been around for more than 100 years. They have their origin in the health center movement of the late 19th and early 20th centuries. Public health campaigns aimed at controlling smallpox, tuberculosis, venereal disease, infant and child mortality, mental illness, and other problems were the order of the day. In 1904, the first clinic for the treatment of communicable pulmonary disease was established in New York City. This clinic pioneered the use of public health nurses for controlling tuberculosis and provided prevention, early case detection, and treatment services. A rapid growth of public health departments occurred during the years 1900 to 1920. These departments organized a variety of special clinics oriented to the prevention of disease. During the Depression, when so many people could not afford to pay for health care privately, the idea of providing comprehensive care through public health centers became attractive, and the Public Works Administration made funds available for building health centers. Later, in the 1940s, additional funds were provided under the Hill-Burton legislation for building health centers in rural and urban areas (Pascarelli, 1982).

Health districts were modeled after school districts, and they sought to interest local people in the health centers. "Neighborhood residents were involved in the programs of these centers in an effort to achieve a 100% participation in the services of the center. Household surveys were conducted by block representatives, and patients were recruited by resident 'aides'" (Rosenfeld, 1971, pp. 1–10). They did not attain the prominence of school districts, however. Health centers were blamed for not providing comprehensive health services, and organized medicine opposed the public approach to medical care. For these and other reasons, these districts failed to involve their communities in the health center movement and other health care concerns. "Unlike school districts, health districts were kept firmly in the hands of municipal officials and public health officers, with little if any participation by the community. The typical board of health consisted primarily of providers" (Pascarelli, 1982, p. 6). Health districts established around health centers, however, have survived and served as an important element of ambulatory health care. Besides a state health department in each state, there are 3,000 county, city, and other municipal health departments in the country (Wall, 1998).

> As the provision of personal health services evolved under health department auspices, so did the opposition of organized medicine, based on the contention that government was competing with private practice medicine for patients. The influence of organized medicine's opposition was largely successful in limiting the health departments' personal health services to providing care for patients only in the lowest income population groups and to offering other types of care in which private physicians had little interest. (Sultz & Young, 2001, p. 131)

The focus of public health department clinics has continued to be on prevention and early detection. They did broaden the scope of their services to include family-planning services (birth control), prenatal care and childhood immunizations, chronic disease detection, and general primary care for economically disadvantaged families (Breslow & Fielding, 2007; Roemer, 1986).

Public health agencies have suffered all along from inadequate resources. The fascination of the public and professionals with dramatic, high-technology diagnostic and therapeutic medicine also affects the allocation of U.S. health resources. Less than 1 percent of the almost $1 trillion spent annually for health care is allocated to government public health activities. State and local governments struggling with large deficits often sacrifice the personnel and services of their public health agencies (Sultz & Young, 2001).

Community Health Care Centers

Community health care centers, also known as neighborhood health centers, were products of the 1960s. They appeared in poor urban neighborhoods dominated by minority populations. Some of these were started by youth groups who were not satisfied with the services of hospital outpatient departments or public health clinics. "The young people would raise money for renting an empty store and purchasing drugs, while professional services were solicited and obtained on a voluntary basis from doctors, nurses, pharmacists, and others" (Roemer, 1986, p. 44). Others emerged out of the antipoverty programs. "The Great Society of the Lyndon Johnson era stressed the right to health care and community participation in decisions and stirred the emotions, hopes, and imagination of ambulatory care professionals" (Pascarelli, 1982, p. 9). Sponsored by the newly created Office of Economic Opportunity, these health centers set out to accomplish more than the provision of comprehensive primary care services. They operated with multiple goals, many of which were not directly related to health service delivery.

> Health was defined very broadly, as including physical, mental, social, economic, environmental, and political aspects. Thus, improved housing, better sewer and water systems, employment, job training, community economic development, counseling, advocacy with other social services and, perhaps most important, personal and minority group power building were all major goals of neighborhood health programs. (Davis & Millman, 1983, pp. 25–26)

Most of these clinics did not last beyond the 1970s; fiscal woes began to afflict them. The Johnson administration was followed by Republican presidencies, and the Office of Economic Opportunity was dismantled. Initially, these centers were prohibited from serving insured or paying patients, and later they were expected to become self-sufficient by billing and collecting for their services. For Medicaid purposes, most states refused to recognize health centers as institutional providers like hospital outpatient departments, and the centers could be encompassed under no other legal entity. Thus, most centers had to rely on billing at private physician rates, using one or more of their medical staff for billing purposes. Private physician rates were generally too low to support even solo practice physicians, much less the cost of a health center (Davis & Millman, 1983, p. 28). They also suffered from other problems, such as a lack of integration with other health care providers (their physicians finding it difficult to obtain admitting privileges at local hospitals), difficulty recruiting and retaining professional personnel, heavy involvement of community boards in personnel issues, and poor planning and coordination. Most of these centers failed to survive.

These clinics serve patients from minority communities, women of childbearing age, infants, HIV-infected persons, substance abusers, and the homeless. Besides providing primary and preventive care services, these clinics assist in linking their patients with health, social, and welfare programs. Now they receive funding under the Public Health Service Act with grants administered by the Bureau of Primary Care, Health Resources and Services Administration of the Department of Health and Human Services. Some of these are organized under the aegis of local health departments, others as parts of human service organizations, and still others as stand-alone, not-for-profit organizations (Sultz & Young, 2001). In 1999, 900 community health centers at 3,000 sites were serving 1,000 million people (Bodenheimer & Grumbach, 2002).

Ambulatory Surgery Centers

Ambulatory surgery centers are another entity to join the group of ambulatory care settings. These are both hospital units and freestanding facilities. The first freestanding ambulatory surgery center was the Dudley Street Ambulatory Surgical Center in Providence, Rhode Island, opened in 1968 by a group of five physicians. The Surgicenter

established by Wallace Reed and John Fox in Phoenix, Arizona, in 1970 has become a model for other developing freestanding facilities (O'Donovan, 1976). Now, nearly 90% of the 4,300 ambulatory surgery centers are freestanding and owned by physicians (Reece, 2007).

Such centers are proliferating all over and are sources of a wide range of primary care as well as an answer to urgent problems. The speed of their growth is reflected in the number and variety of procedures performed in these centers. Ambulatory surgeries increased from 35% of all surgeries performed in September of 1995 to about 75% in April of 1998 (Lee & Mongan, 2009). Several factors are responsible for this phenomenon. Sultz and Young (2001) have identified the following causes: (1) the development of general anesthetics that resolve so safely and quickly that patients can return to normal functioning within hours of surgery; (2) advancements in surgical equipment, materials, and techniques that eliminate or reduce the invasive nature of many procedures and their accompanying complications and risks; (3) pressures to reduce costs of care from Medicare, insurance companies, and managed care organizations; (4) encouragement by Medicare for ambulatory surgical procedures—between 1991 and 1998, the number of Medicare-covered procedures rose from 1,200 to 2,200 (when an approved procedure is performed on an ambulatory basis, Medicare pays 100% of "reasonable charges" instead of the usual 80% (Coile, 1990); and (5) happiness of both physicians and patients—the former do not have to contend with the complexity of operating room scheduling and staff and equipment availability in a hospital setting, and the latter find the ambulatory surgery centers easier to get to, less complex, and more user-friendly and responsive to their needs than hospitals. These centers are likely to grow further in the future.

Emergency Care Centers

Emergency care centers have been a part of the health care scene for quite some time.

Traditionally, most hospitals found it easy to justify the establishment of emergency services in contrast to outpatient departments. This type of treatment was not available in physicians' private offices, and for many hospitals it constituted a good source of inpatients. (Pascarelli, 1982, p. 10)

Emergency departments of teaching hospitals deployed medical interns and residents. Their coverage of the emergency room was considered a part of their training.

Often, to earn extra income, residents would contract to "moonlight" extra hours for their assigned hospital or for other hospital emergency departments. Nonteaching hospitals also hired residents on a contracted basis to cover the emergency department or required attending staff to provide rotating coverage. (Sultz & Young, 2001, p. 122)

More than 90% of community hospitals provide emergency services 24 hours a day, 7 days a week. From 1993 to 2003, the U.S. population grew by 12% but emergency room visits grew 27%, from 90 million to 114 million (Reece, 2007). Now, these services are provided by specialty personnel in sophisticated facilities equipped with advanced technology. These services also have increased in their (a) complexity, (b) range, and (c) integration with other community resources, such as alcohol and drug treatment programs, mental health centers, and social services.

These changes are the result of several factors. In 1966, the National Academy of Sciences produced the document *Accidental Death and Disability: The Neglected Disease of Modern Society.* It highlighted the need for improvement in emergency medical care and provided the blueprint for subsequent work, which culminated in a federal law. The Emergency Medical Services Systems Act of 1973 and its amendments in 1976 and 1979 provided mechanisms and funds for communities to establish emergency medical services systems aimed at reducing death and disability rates from all types of emergency illnesses (Boyd, 1982). The law mandated that emergency medical care programs must address, plan, and implement a "systems approach" to the provision of services and specified a number of requirements to assist planners, coordinators, and operators in establishing comprehensive programs

(U.S. Department of Health, Education, and Welfare, 1975). That led to the development of a new specialty—emergency medicine. Since 1979, emergency medicine has been recognized as a medical specialty requiring physicians to receive extended specialty training and experience to attain board certified status, as in other specialty fields (Sultz & Young, 2001).

The number of patients using hospital emergency room services has been rising steadily, although most patients use these services for nonurgent reasons (Roemer, 1986; Sultz & Young, 2001; Williams, 1991). Of the millions who enter the emergency medical service system each year, at least 80% cannot be considered "true" emergencies (Boyd, 1982). The diversity of patients seen in emergency rooms may include "patients with severe trauma or a sore throat, patients who are intoxicated or psychotic, transients looking for a warm place to stay, and elderly people who are merely confused" (Clement & Durgin, 1987, p. 500). Many of the patients with nonemergency conditions do have legitimate health needs. Many come because they interpret their symptoms to be serious enough to require emergency care. Others come because their private physician is either not available or has directed them to go to an emergency center. Others are directed by their physician to the emergency department of their affiliated hospital for examinations or tests requiring special equipment the physician does not have in his or her office. Many come because they have no private physician and appropriate outpatient clinics have no concurrent hours.

A study of the access of Medicaid recipients to outpatient care (Medicaid Access Study Group, 1994) found that these patients had limited access to ambulatory care outside hospital emergency departments. Still others come because they cannot afford the care they need and have nowhere else to go when they are ill (Sultz & Young, 2001). The law (COBRA, 1986) requires that all emergency department patients be treated, regardless of their ability to pay. About 14% of emergency room patients are uninsured, 16% are covered by Medicaid, and 21% by Medicare. More than half of hospitals lose money in providing emergency services (Reece, 2007).

Under the new law, availability of ambulatory care through health care centers will ease some of the pressure on emergency care departments. Nevertheless, the importance of the emergency room as a site for ambulatory care is likely to continue.

Urgent Care Centers

Urgent care centers are a welcome alternative to hospital emergency rooms for non-life-threatening illnesses for patients who carry health insurance or can self-pay for care. The first urgent care center was established in 1973, and now there are more than 2,000 such centers in the country. These centers fill gaps in the health care delivery system caused by difficulties scheduling appointments with private physicians, nonavailability of those physicians during nonbusiness hours, unfamiliarity with the local health care system for individuals new to a community, and lack of appropriate service between a physician's office or an outpatient clinic and an emergency room. Patients can walk in without an appointment. These centers are located in highly visible and easy to access commercial areas (Sultz & Young, 2001). Urgent care centers are staffed and equipped to serve a broad spectrum of illness, injury, and disease. They are open 7 days a week for several hours a day.

ILLNESS PREVENTION AND HEALTH PROMOTION AGENCIES

To understand the past of the major organizations involved in illness prevention and health promotion, we look at (a) the significant worldwide events to which these organizations can trace their origins, (b) the significant ideas that have guided their philosophy, and (c) the history of public health in the United States.

Significant Events

According to Taylor, Denham, and Ureda (1982), the history of health care can be divided into three eras: era of disease treatment, era of preventive medicine, and era of health promotion. The *era of disease treatment* goes back to the 35th century BC, when evil spirits were exorcised, war-wounded limbs were cauterized or amputated, and various minerals, plants, and animal parts were used to treat the ill. Later centuries added to these therapies of disease treatment. The 18th and 19th centuries saw a shift of thinking from treatment to prevention.

Widespread implementation of smallpox vaccination was followed by Pasteur's discovery that attenuated chicken cholera organisms could bring protection against virulent bacteria, setting the stage for the many vaccines later developed. In 1901, Walter Reed in Havana confirmed that the *Aedes aegypti* mosquito was the vector of yellow fever; subsequent public health measures confirmed that malaria could be prevented by mosquito control. In 1914, Dr. Joseph Goldberger discovered that pellagra was caused by a dietary deficiency and that it could be prevented by consuming foods containing a "pellagra-preventive" factor, which we now know as niacin. Public health efforts to ensure safe water and milk supplies reduced morbidity and mortality due to typhoid fever. Diphtheria, pertussis, and tetanus vaccines were developed during the 1930s and 1940s. Then came the Salk polio vaccine in 1952 and the Sabin oral polio vaccine in 1960. Measles, mumps, and rubella vaccines were introduced in 1958, 1967, and 1969, respectively. Efforts to develop safe, effective vaccines for a broad variety of diseases continue in laboratories across the country. (p. 4)

The past few decades have witnessed, on the one hand, changes in the patterns of morbidity and mortality—with infectious diseases no longer topping the list of major disablers and killers—and, on the other hand, a concern with the quality of life. More and more people are now willing to take responsibility for their health. Factors that have contributed to the emergence of this era include the following.

1. *Worldwide inflation was reflected, in the United States most vividly, in the ever-rising costs of medical treatment and rehabilitation without corresponding gains in health and mental*

health. This reality was highlighted by uninspiring outcome studies of health and mental treatments. These, in turn, generated cost-containment concerns and efforts in the 1970s and 1980s.

2. *The returns on investments in medical care and communicable disease control were diminishing.* This, plus the rapid diffusion of scientific evidence linking lifestyle and chronic disease, and the development of skills and techniques for behavioral and lifestyle changes led to selected efforts of health, hospital, and industrial groups to redirect medical care funds toward prevention-oriented programs.

3. *The community development and mass communications movements and technologies of the 1950s and 1960s were beginning to affect large segments of the population.* Recognition was growing that prevention was easier and less costly than treatment and that many people were suffering from preventable illnesses and problems. This was happening in the midst of a growing disillusionment with conventional medical approaches and the appearance of imaginative concepts encompassing social, mental, and spiritual qualities of life. A shift to an emphasis on holistic health resulted in changes in cultural norms about health and fitness among large groups of the population.

4. *The inequality in the availability and quality of treatment for people of different social classes, cultures, and races was documented.* This came at the time of the civil rights and women's movements. On the one hand, these movements demanded transfer of authority and resources to people previously deprived of these; on the other hand, they emphasized self-help and taking charge of one's life (Bloom, 1987; Bracht, 1987; Green & Raeburn, 1990).

In short, the country seemed to be ready for the challenge of what Terris (1983) called the "second epidemiological revolution"—the fight against chronic diseases. Alternative health interventions that were appearing also fit in with the consumer movement and were empowering. "Self-help is empowering, anti-expert, anti-authority, choice-oriented, and it increasingly questions the external world-view" (Riessman, 1994, p. 54). A new era had begun, the era of health promotion.

More than the other two eras, the era of health promotion has been ushered in as a social movement, and much of its impetus has arisen from persons and institutions outside the medical mainstream: joggers, weight control groups, Alcoholics Anonymous, tobacco opponents, and others. (Taylor et al., 1982, p. 5)

Significant Ideas

Although the importance of health promotion was recognized as early as the first quarter of the 20th century, the concept was narrowly defined and operationalized as primary prevention activities. Even the scope of primary prevention activities remained narrow. It covered only the prevention and early detection of specific diseases. That scope gradually widened. The term *health promotion* was used more than 60 years ago by a medical historian, Sigerist (1946), when he defined the four major tasks of medicine as (a) promotion of health, (b) prevention of illness, (c) restoration of the sick, and (d) rehabilitation. He spelled out the conditions for health promotion—a decent standard of living, good labor conditions, education, physical culture, means of rest and recreation—and called for the coordinated efforts of politicians, labor, industry, educators, and physicians to ensure these conditions. Kelly, Charlton, and Hanlon (1993) identified four levels of health promotion—environmental, social, organizational, and individual—and urged that all four be understood and integrated for successful health promotion. It has taken several decades for health professionals to appreciate the richness of the concept of "health promotion."

Back in 1920, C. E. A. Winslow's definition of *public health* not only captured the changing scope of public health but also reflected the direction of that change:

Public health is the science and art of (1) preventing disease, (2) prolonging life, and (3) organizing community efforts for (a) the sanitation of the environment, (b) the control of community infections, (c) the education of the individual in personal hygiene, (d) the organization of medical and nursing services for the early diagnosis and preventive treatment of diseases, and (e) the development of social machinery to insure to everyone a standard of living adequate for the maintenance of health, so organizing these benefits as to enable every citizen to realize his birthright of health and longevity. (Winslow, as quoted in Hanlon & Pickett, 1984)

The terms *public* and *health* provide the themes for what public health is all about. *Public* does not refer to the auspices under which a health program is carried out but, rather, to the public it serves (Rice, 1957). The agency providing services may be governmental (federal, state, and local) or voluntary and private. *Public* also involves organized community effort. Individual effort is important but must be augmented by communitywide work, because "neither treatment of lung disease nor exhorting individuals to avoid smoking could have achieved the reduction of smoking in public places made possible by organized community effort to adopt laws and regulations restricting smoking" (Institute of Medicine, 1988a, p. 39). Public health is also public in terms of its long-range goal of optimal health for the whole community. Beauchamp (1976) saw the mission of public health as social justice and the protection of all human life. Similar to the concept of "public," "health" has been variously defined. The World Health Organization (WHO) definition of *health* as "physical, mental, and social well-being, not merely the absence of disease or infirmity" widens the scope of public health work [1].

Until 1960, the *infectious disease model* guided the public health approach and activities. This model views the disease process as the interaction between host, agent, and environment and focuses on one agent—a microbe or traumatic event that precipitates the disease process.

By the 1960s, it was realized that infectious diseases were no longer a threat to the public's health. Chronic diseases had become the major culprits. Attention shifted to dealing with chronic diseases in whose etiologies a single cause or agent could not be identified. Hence, the *chronic disease model* was created, emphasizing processes that would identify factors associated with a specific health problem. By the 1970s, questions about the appropriateness of these models were raised (e.g., see Terris, 1975). It was suggested that the disease orientation of public health efforts should be replaced by a wellness orientation and that public health approaches should be strength oriented. By the 1980s, a broadened view of primary prevention appeared that not only included *health promotion* but also gave it a place of prominence.

A related concept is *wellness,* which is defined as "the process and state of a quest for maximum human functioning that involves the body, mind, and spirit" (Archer, Probert, & Gage, 1987, p. 311). Several models of wellness have been proposed. For example, Ardell (1988) described eight dimensions of wellness: psychological, spiritual, physical fitness, job satisfaction, relationships, family life, leisure time, and stress management. Earlier, Hettler (1984) had proposed a six-dimensional model containing intellectual, emotional, physical, social, occupational, and spiritual wellness. All these models of wellness seek to describe the "whole" or "total" person. Witmer and Sweeney (1992) tried to trace the origin of this idea of wholeness to the writings of Adler, Jung, and Maslow and proposed a holistic model for wellness and prevention over the life span: "The characteristics of wellness are expressed through the five life tasks of spirituality, self-regulation, work, love, and friendship. These life tasks dynamically interact with the life forces of family, community, religion, education, government, media, and business/industry" (p. 140). The concept of "wellness" is akin to the WHO definition of health as a state of complete physical, mental, and social well-being, and not merely the absence of disease or infirmity. "The definition viewed health as a multidimensional (holistic) phenomenon, with multiple determinants, one that can be defined by its positive (well-being) rather than negative aspects" (Green & Raeburn, 1990, p. 33). The concepts that have guided the wellness movement in the United States include self-responsibility for personal health, physical fitness, nutritional awareness, and stress management. The future will find health workers building on these ideas as the field of health promotion and wellness grows.

History of Public Health

Organizationally, public health is a system of programs, policies, and personnel whose goal is to prevent disease, prolong life, and promote better health (Barker, 2003). It has been a part of the impressive work in disease prevention, and "were it not for the organized public health efforts, our nation would not be as stable, as successful, or as livable as it is" (Raffel & Raffel, 1989, p. 273).

If public health is broadly defined as conscious efforts by an authority to protect the health of the community, the history of public health can be traced back to ancient times:

> Crete, Egypt, Greece, and Rome, all, at some time, built model towns and had finely developed sanitary systems. In Rome, public baths were available to everyone; here the workers went in the evening "to wash and to undo the fatigues of the day." Inoculation against smallpox was practiced in India and China before the Christian era. Rome built leprosaria and, like Greece, sought to regulate prostitution. The latrine and the flush closet were invented not as some have said during the European Renaissance, but in Crete 3,000 years before, or earlier. The Arabic civilization carried on where Rome and Greece left off; Cordoba and other Arabian cities had health departments with sanitary inspectors. (Brockington, 1975, p. 1)

If defined as efforts to apply social, scientific, and medical knowledge to the protection of the community's health, however, public health is a modern phenomenon. Before the 18th century, although there were sporadic public efforts to protect people from epidemics such as plague, cholera, and smallpox through isolation of the ill and quarantine of travelers, these diseases often were considered a sign of poor moral and spiritual condition, to be corrected by prayer and piety (Goudsblom, 1986). By the 18th century, isolation of the ill and quarantine of the exposed became an accepted method of containing contagious

diseases. In 1701, Massachusetts passed laws for that purpose. Prior to the 19th century, however, diseases were largely undifferentiated and unclassified, and no records of births and deaths were kept. Environmental hygiene as conducted from the ancient days had little scientific basis except in the practice of inoculation against smallpox. The 19th century witnessed the identification of filth as responsible for the cause and spread of diseases, and of cleanliness as the answer:

> Illness came to be seen as an indicator of poor social and environmental conditions, as well as poor moral and spiritual conditions. Cleanliness was embraced as a path both to physical and moral health. Cleanliness, piety, and isolation were seen to be compatible and mutually reinforcing measures to help the public resist disease. (Institute of Medicine, 1988a, p. 58)

The efforts of Edwin Chadwick, secretary of the Poor Law Commission in Britain in 1838, greatly influenced the sanitary reform movement. The commission conducted studies of the life and health of the working class of the entire country. The findings of those studies led to the passage of the Public Health Act of 1848, which "must forever be a landmark in the history of world public health" (Brockington, 1975, p. 4). Chadwick's ideas emphasizing environmental aspects of hygiene also influenced developments in North America. Local sanitation surveys were conducted in several American cities. A report of the Massachusetts Sanitary Commission based on a survey done by Lemual Shattuck led to the creation of the state board of health in 1869. Many of the principles and activities, including the maintenance of records and vital statistics, proposed by Shattuck later came to be considered fundamental to public health (Rosenkrantz, 1972). By the end of the 19th century, scientific knowledge about causes and prevention of many diseases had advanced significantly. As pointed out earlier, bacteriologic agents of such diseases as tuberculosis, diphtheria, typhoid, and yellow fever were discovered, and it was learned that both people and the environment could be agents of disease (Institute of Medicine, 1988a).

Thus, public health began in the United States in the 19th century with the need to control such communicable diseases as smallpox, typhoid, and diphtheria. The first public health activities were in large cities, and their focus was on improving sanitation. Local boards of health were formed for this purpose.

> They developed ordinances regarding waste disposal, street drainage, removal of filth, drainage of swamps, and other measures that would improve the sanitary environment. Quarantine of homes and ships, and much later immunizations, were also important functions of local boards of health aimed at preventing the spread of infectious diseases. (Raffel & Raffel, 1989, p. 263)

The first state board of health was formed in Massachusetts in 1869, and by 1900, all states had boards of health. These boards were concerned with the statewide control of communicable diseases. Departments of public health with full-time staffs evolved to carry out the functions of boards of health. These functions gradually expanded to include (a) environmental sanitation surveillance, (b) school health and immunization, (c) maternal and child health care, (d) limited care for indigent patients, and (e) screening for and control of such diseases as tuberculosis and venereal diseases (Bracht, 1978). Their thrust was illness prevention.

Each state is sovereign in its authority and responsibility for protecting the health of its citizens. Not only are the power and authority of local governments regarding health derived from the state, but the powers of the federal government in the field of health also are delegated by the states (Grant, 1987). In reality, all levels of government—state, local, and federal—as well as many nongovernmental agencies are involved in public health work.

State Public Health Departments

State health departments vary significantly in their organization. Raffel and Raffel (1989) found three basic models of organization operating. In the *first,* a board of health (typically appointed

by the governor and approved by the state senate) has policy or administrative functions. These boards either appoint or strongly influence the appointment of key department personnel. They have authority over not only the overall direction of the department but also the enforcement of public health laws

> by holding hearings on violations, hearing appeals on health officer actions, and by issuance of board orders for compliance with the laws. Board orders must be enforced by law enforcement agencies, although the recipient of a board health order can, of course, appeal it in the state courts. (p. 266)

These boards function well when the professionalism of their members prevails over their political agendas.

In the *second* model, the department is headed by a secretary or commissioner of health appointed by the governor. The success of this model also depends on the quality of both the appointed official and the governor who appoints him or her.

> If a governor avoids tough issues, if a governor tends to appoint incompetents or political hacks, then the board system might be preferred. If, on the other hand, there is an unprogressive board, then a strong governor with a competent secretary of health would be preferred. (Raffel & Raffel, 1989, p. 267)

In the *third* model, an umbrella organization such as a department of human resources is created that includes health along with other agencies such as mental health, education, and welfare. This department is headed by a secretary. The state health officer reports to that person. Improved coordination of services provided by related agencies is the rationale for this model, but the organization of the department alone does not necessarily result in improved coordination. Many other variables come into play.

Beitsch, Brooks, Menachemi, and Libbey (2006) combined and analyzed the data from two 2005 surveys conducted by the Association of State and Territorial Health Officials (ASTHO) and the National Association of County and City

Health Officials (NACCHO). Their findings confirm the diversity of the structures and governance of state public health agencies. Of all state health departments, 29 (58%) are freestanding (independent), whereas the other 21 (42%) are a part of an umbrella agency. Of all the states, 24 (48%) have a state board of health while the other 26 (52%) do not. Of those 24 state boards of health, 18 (75%) have policy-making and regulatory power; the others do not. The state health officer is appointed by the governor in 33 (66%) states, by secretary of health and human services in 12 (24%) states, by the board of health in 4 (8%) states, and by the governor and secretary in 1 (2%) state.

Miller and associates (1977) analyzed state public health laws and identified 44 areas as the responsibility of state health departments. These included (1) communicable disease, venereal disease, chronic disease, alcohol and drug addiction, rabies, and air and water pollution control; (2) food, housing, and health facilities inspection; (3) health personnel registration and facilities licensure; (4) dental, home, maternal/child, mental, occupational, and school health; (5) compulsory hospitalization and quarantines; (6) care of the indigent, ambulance, and emergency medical services; and (7) vital statistics. Some of the health programs (particularly state tuberculosis, mental health, and mental retardation hospitals, and licensure of health personnel, hospitals, nursing homes, and other health care facilities) are operated directly by the state health department, while the operation of others is shared with the local health agencies, with the state health department setting the standards of performance for the local agencies and providing state funds to supplement the local resources.

In the world since September 11, anthrax, SARS (severe acute respiratory syndrome), flu vaccine shortage, fear of avian flu, and Hurricane Katrina, all state public health departments also are required to be prepared for dealing with man-made and natural disasters. Thus, the scope of state public health department programs and functions is vast, ranging from disease monitoring and data collection to environmental regulation and Medicaid administration (Beitsch et al., 2006). The Committee for the Study of the Future of Public Health had found that whereas some state health departments are active and well equipped, others perform fewer functions and have meager resources (Institute of Medicine, 1988a). Further,

states are organized for public health in ways that might fragment instead of uniting environmental or mental health with other components, that under-emphasize and underfund one or another of the essential services of public health, and that provide little if any subsidy to the local public health infra-structure. (Tilson & Berkowitz, 2006, p. 904)

Local Public Health Departments

The degree of autonomy enjoyed by local public health agencies varies greatly among states. Their organizational pattern also varies greatly.

In New England, local departments tend to be on a city or town basis, county government being weak or nonexistent. In the South, local departments tend to be organized on a county basis. And there are in-between arrangements, as in Pennsylvania, in which there is a provision for county health departments (but very few in existence), local government (sub-county, town, borough, etc.) units with largely environmental responsibilities, as well as regional state health department offices. In some parts of the country, we find metropolitan and other kinds of multijurisdictional departments, that is, multicounty or combined city-county departments. (Raffel & Raffel, 1989, p. 273)

Results of the 2005 surveys reported by Beitsch et al. (2006) confirm this variance in the jurisdiction of local health agencies. County is the jurisdiction of 1,348 (58.7%); city and town/township of 366 (5.9%); city/county and multicounty/district of 551 (23.9%); and other of the remaining 32 (1.4%) local public health departments.

Some of these departments are technically sophisticated and provide impressive services, whereas others' ability and quality of services are questionable. The 1985 study by the Institute of Medicine of the National Academy of Sciences revealed that in many localities, "there is no health department. Perhaps the area is visited occasionally by a 'circuit-riding' public health nurse—and perhaps not" (Institute of Medicine, 1988a, p. 3). Similarly, a local health department profile prepared by the National Association of County Health Officials in 1985 showed that there were 2,932 organized local health units in the United States, most of them too small to receive adequate funds from limited local tax bases (Koplin, 1993).

These departments also vary in their relationships with other local health care agencies and private care providers. The situation has changed since the beginning of 2002, when federal funds became available for improving public health and medical emergency preparedness. However, the proportion of funds distributed to local health departments has varied greatly across states (Salinsky & Gursky, 2006).

Federal Public Health Service

Over the years, the federal government has acquired tremendous power in the field of health. Although the federal government has no constitutional authority to provide direct health services, it does provide some; mostly, it buys the action it wants by providing money to state and local governments and nongovernmental agencies. The "Powers of Congress" portion of the U.S. Constitution gives the federal government authority to (a) raise and support armies, provide and maintain a navy, and make all laws "necessary and proper" to carry out those powers and (b) regulate foreign and interstate commerce. These powers have been used to establish and operate military, naval, air force, and veterans' hospitals and services, as well as to regulate foods, drugs, product and occupational safety, and some environmental health activities.

> The power to control federal lands, along with the presidential power to make treaties (with the advice and consent of the Senate) are the source of federal activity in providing health services for Native Americans and Eskimos. Other direct service activities also rely on these clauses for legitimization. (Raffel & Raffel, 1989, p. 285)

The federal government also was helped by the Supreme Court decision in *McCulloch v. Maryland* (1819), which set out the doctrine of implied powers—powers beyond those specifically delegated in the Constitution but reasonably implied by the delegated powers (Institute of Medicine, 1988a).

The mission of the federal government's Public Health Service is to protect and advance the health of Americans by (a) preventing and controlling disease, identifying health hazards, and promoting a healthy lifestyle for the nation's citizens; (b) assisting in the delivery of health care services to medically underserved populations and other groups with special health needs; (c) administering block grants to the states for preventive and health services; alcohol, drug abuse, and mental health services; maternal and child health services; and primary health care; (d) ensuring that drugs and medical devices are safe and effective and protecting the public from unsafe foods and unnecessary exposure to human-made radiation; (e) conducting and supporting biomedical and behavioral research and communicating results to health professionals and the public; (f) monitoring the adequacy of health workers and facilities available to serve the nation's needs; and (g) working with other nations on global health problems (Public Health Service, 1980).

The Public Health Service began in 1798 when a law was passed to provide for the relief of sick and disabled seamen. This law led to the establishment of what later came to be known as Public Health Service hospitals. The establishment of a one-room laboratory at the Marine Hospital in Staten Island, New York, in 1887 was the beginning of the current National Institutes of Health. The functions of the Public Health Service broadened after the passage of the Social Security Act, which authorized annual grants to the states for the investigation of disease and problems of sanitation (Raffel & Raffel, 1989). A significant milestone in the history of the federal government's involvement in health is the Public Health Service Act of 1944, which broadened the scope of previously established Public Health Service functions and reshaped it to meet the requirements not only of the day but also of the future. It authorized the Public Health Service to make grants and contracts (leading to the growth of extramural programs) and to work with and support the efforts of state health departments; strengthened and expanded its Commissioned Corps (to include nurses, sanitarians, and other specialists); and expanded the office of its surgeon general, "which has proved to be such a bully pulpit for educating our people in good health habits" (Lee, 1994, p. 466). The Public Health Service is now a part of the U.S. Department of Health and Human Services and operates the following six agencies:

1. Alcohol, Drug Abuse, and Mental Health Administration

2. Centers for Disease Control and Prevention

3. Agency for Toxic Substances and Disease Registry

4. Food and Drug Administration

5. Health Resources and Services Administration

6. National Institutes of Health

The federal Public Health Service has been active in the following components of national leadership in public health: (a) identifying and speaking out on specific health problems, (b) allocating funds for national public health objectives, (c) building constituencies to support action on those objectives, and (d) supporting the development of knowledge and databases. The federal government sometimes has bypassed the state and local agencies in carrying out federal health priorities, however, at other times, it has reduced federal funds earmarked for public health activities by turning over more public health decision making to the states (Institute of Medicine, 1988a).

Public health policy coordination and proposals for federal oversight emerge from the Association of State and Territorial Health Officials (ASTHO) and its professional affiliates. Federal responsibilities for public health rest in the several agencies of the U.S. Department of Health and Human Services (HHS), although health programs are also operated by the Departments of Defense, Veterans Affairs, and Agriculture and the Environmental Protection Agency. (Tilson & Berkowitz, 2006, p. 904)

Which federal agency is in charge of the health security part of the public health function is unclear. The creation of the Department of Homeland Security (DHS) has complicated relationships between the federal and state governments.

The role of the DHS relative to that of HHS continues to evolve and is not entirely clear to outside observers. State and local public health officials are perplexed by questions of funding streams and governance as the DHS and HHS continue to synchronize and harmonize their roles. The responsibilities of the Department of Defense (DoD) and the National Guard add complexity to the federal public health preparedness and response apparatus. (Salinsky & Gursky, 2006, p. 1021)

Nongovernmental Organizations in Public Health

The other element of the illness prevention and health promotion picture is made up of numerous private, nongovernmental entities. These include health-related agencies and private physicians and their organizations. The line between public and private responsibilities for public health never has been hard and clear; it has shifted and blurred over the years. When public health activities were essentially matters of sanitary engineering and environmental hygiene, private physicians were active participants in the joint public and private efforts.

With the discovery of bacteria and the development of immunization techniques, however, disease prevention could no longer be so easily defined solely as a communitywide affair. The line between prevention and treatment began to fade, and the domains of public health and private medicine could no longer be easily separated. This development created a certain amount of tension between the two that has never fully been resolved. (Institute of Medicine, 1988a, p. 51)

Of the nongovernmental agencies involved in public health work, some are quite old, whereas others are comparatively new; some are generic in their activities and scope, whereas others are concerned with the prevention and treatment of specific diseases. The following is a partial list of prominent agencies:

American Cancer Society

American Diabetes Association

American Heart Association

Epilepsy Foundation of America

March of Dimes

National Association for Mental Health

National Council on Alcoholism

National Easter Seal Society for Crippled Children and Adults

National Kidney Foundation

National Society for the Prevention of Blindness

National Tuberculosis and Respiratory Disease Association

Planned Parenthood

United Cerebral Palsy Association

There is a general lack of collaboration among the various agencies—government and nongovernment—engaged in public health work.

The United States is in the era of health promotion, and the factors that gave birth to this era still prevail. They will continue as forces encouraging the health promotion and wellness movement in the future. However, there is a long way to go. Many people in communities all over the country do not have access to the benefits of illness prevention and health promotion activities and programs. Threats to public health not only persist but also are increasing. These threats include enduring problems, such as injuries and chronic illness; impending crises foreshadowed by such developments as the toxic byproducts of a modern economy; reemergence of old killers, such as tuberculosis; and bioterrorism and other attacks.

Based on its 1985 study, the Institute of Medicine (1988a) concluded that the country "has lost sight of its public health goals and has allowed the system of public health activities to fall into disarray" (p. 1). Its findings highlighted the need for improvement in all aspects of public health in the United States. A significant reason for the sorry state of the country's public health system is misplaced priorities and resources. More than 75% of federal health care dollars are spent on the care of people with chronic illnesses such as cancer, heart disease, and stroke, whereas less than 0.5% is spent on preventing those same diseases. According to Beitsch et al. (2006), the spending of state and local public health agencies constitutes less than 2.5% of the overall U.S. health care spending.

Tilson and Berkowitz (2006) are of the opinion that the situation has improved since 1988. They and others who share this opinion give the following as evidence of improvement:

1. The federal government has "instituted alignment of reforms of federal funding to local areas, recognizing the need to identify and build a viable local agency system instead of bypassing it" (p. 902).

2. The federal government has provided $5 billion to states to revitalize the public health sector. This is leading to (a) increased capacity and testing capability of public health laboratories, (b) improvements in technology, (c) purchase of communication equipment, (d) employment of more personnel, (e) preparedness training, (f) new partnerships with other government and volunteer agencies, and (g) some organizational changes (Lurie, Wasserman, & Nelson, 2006).

3. The Robert Wood Johnson Foundation funded the Turning Point Initiative, which has supported 21 states in "creating considerable innovation in collaboration, increased capacity for policy development, and a new or strengthened structure for improving the public's health" (Tilson & Berkowitz, 2006, p. 902).

4. The Public Health Functions Work Group of the American Public Health Association has developed and adopted the concept of "10 essential services for public health" (p. 905).

5. ASTHO, NACCHO, and the Centers for Disease Control and Prevention are collaboratively exploring the possibility of a national accreditation program for public health agencies (Salinsky & Gursky, 2006).

6. NACCHO has initiated highlighting activities of local public health departments for special recognition in its Model Practices Database (Salinsky & Gursky, 2006).

On the other hand, there are those who see a much less optimistic picture. Their assessment of the state of public health in the country is based on the following factors:

1. As the authority for public health resides with state governments, each state health department crafts policy and entrusts the local health departments to implement it.

The result is a nationally fragmented public health enterprise characterized by diverse practices across 3,000 local agencies charged with meeting various missions under 50 health departments. The patchwork of capabilities, agency sizes, lines of authority, and workforce training impedes public health's interoperability and surge capacity with and across states (Salinsky & Gursky, 2006, p. 1018).

2. There are no educational or training standards for the public health workforce. Public health agencies need personnel with expertise in informatics, epidemiology, logistics, and risk communications, and basic training in the tenets of public health practice and disease control. A disconnect persists between the public health practice community and educational institutions. There is a need for "more work to determine the ideal mix in the public health workforce and the training standards and credentialing mechanism to ensure competency" (Salinsky & Gursky, 2006, p. 1024).

3. Outdated staffing models are prevailing in public health departments. "Government rarely remunerates highly skilled public health employees and, in recent years, has filled public health positions with contract or soft-money slots rather than career positions. Dedicated but often marginally prepared people function through on-the-job training" (Salinsky & Gursky, 2006, p. 1018).

4. Public health departments are struggling to recover from years of being under-resourced. Historically, states emphasized patient care by their public health departments (which were increasingly funded by federal government) and reduced funding for their population-based services (Beitsch et al., 2006; Salinsky & Gursky, 2006).

5. The $5 billion transfer of federal money to states to improve public health was directionless funding because it was an effort to bolster the existing infrastructure. "Congress did not design the grant programs to reform the structure and orientation of public health" (Salinsky & Gursky, 2006, p. 1019).

6. Given the nature of new threats to public health, regionalization is needed in planning for public health preparedness. A regional approach will result in the effective and efficient use of resources and in the reduction of fragmentation of the organizations and assets of government and private agencies (Salinsky & Gursky, 2006). However, regionalization is hard to attain because of the sovereignty of states.

We end this section with a quote from Beitsch et al. (2006):

We are asking public health to be on call around the clock with the same workforce that was numerically insufficient for the daunting tasks it faced before bioterrorism and Hurricane Katrina. Moreover, funding often flows in rigid categorical streams, which must be spent in specific ways, thereby reducing flexibility and efficiency. (p. 920)

LONG-TERM CARE SETTINGS

Long-term care seems to have no boundaries in terms of settings of care, types of services, diversity of service recipients, and variety of service providers. Kane (2011) has divided long-term care into two groups: postacute care and long-term care. Under the former, he has included (1) inpatient rehabilitation facilities, (2) skilled nursing homes, (3) long-term care hospitals, (4) home health care, (5) outpatient rehabilitation, and (6) hospice/palliative care. The latter group includes (1) nursing homes, (2) assisted living care, (3) adult foster care, (4) independent living, (5) continuing care retirement communities, (6) board and care, (7) home care/personal care, and (8) day care or adult day health centers. Others (e.g., Sultz & Young, 2001) have included among long-term care facilities (1) nursing homes, (2) assisted living, (3) home care, (4) hospice care, (5) respite care, (6) adult day care, (7) aging-in-place programs, and (8) continuing care retirement and life care communities. According to the calculations of Kaye, Harrington, and LaPlante (2010), 10 million to 11 million community-dwelling Americans need help with life's daily activities, and about 1.5 million are in nursing homes. Adding the two to determine the country's long-term care population yields about 12 million. That is roughly 4% of the total population.

Smith and Feng (2010) have traced the evolution of long-term care over the past 100 years and divided that history into the following five phases or cycles of development.

1. *Controlling indigent care costs: The Indoor Relief solution (1910–1930).* The organization of long-term care in this period reflected the desire of communities to minimize the cost of maintaining the indigent. It was based on the belief that making relief punitive and stigmatizing would discourage people from seeking assistance. Only the most desperate would have to be cared for. Care was provided through "outdoor relief" in the form of cash assistance, "indoor relief" in the form of poorhouses or poor farms, or through an "auction system" under which the indigent person became the ward of the lowest bidder. Most counties and municipalities created poorhouses or poor farms. In 1930, roughly 2% of the elderly population was housed in either local poorhouses or state mental hospitals. Lodges and fraternal orders rose to rescue poorhouse

residents. Voluntary homes for the elderly were established, which later evolved into nonprofit nursing homes.

2. *Eliminating poorhouses: The old-age income security solution (1930–1950).* The Great Depression and the massive increase in the indigent population made extending indoor relief to all the needy impossible. The notion of punishing people for indolence also changed. Under Title I of the Social Security Act of 1935, the federal government provided matching funds to states for cash payments to low-income elderly. That law specified that no federal aid be given to people cared for in public institutions.

> Local officials, eager to reduce the financial burden on local government, relocated their public charges to private boarding homes where they would be eligible for federal Old Age Assistance, then proceeded to shut down their poorhouses and poor farms. (Smith & Feng, 2010, p. 31)

Private boarding homes evolved into for-profit nursing homes.

3. *Assuring access to affordable medical services: Health insurance for the elderly (1950–1970).* Medicare and Medicaid legislation (Social Security Act Amendments of 1965) combined the Social Security model of universal entitlement (Medicare) and the Old Age Assistance model (Medicaid). These led to the elimination of many disparities in hospital and physician use but distorted the evolving long-term care system in two ways: First, they increased the medicalization and institutionalization of care. Second, Medicaid emerged as the default payer of long-term care, resulting in the segregation of long-term care from mainstream medical services.

4. *Controlling provider abuses: Strengthening state and federal enforcement (1970–1990).* During the mid-1970s, financial and patient care scandals in the Medicaid nursing home system produced a backlash against nursing homes. National nursing home reform legislation (a part of the Omnibus Budget Reconciliation Act of 1987) created standards of care in nursing homes

certified to receive Medicare and Medicaid funds. Medicare and many state Medicaid programs adopted prospective payment methods, which created disincentives for nursing home care for less medically complex patients. Occupancy rates of nursing homes started declining. The market for alternatives to nursing home care grew.

5. *Providing long-term care that people actually want: Market reform (1990–2010).* Developers of residential living arrangements for those who need long-term care appeared on the scene, and providers of health care and social services in and near people's homes proliferated. State Medicaid programs took advantage of home- and community-based waivers to fund services that would enable nursing home-eligible persons to live at home or in other less expensive settings. The Supreme Court's 1999 *Olmstead* decision that services should be provided in the most integrated setting appropriate for the person also helped in the shift to home- and community-based care.

We have categorized long-term care into three major groups: (a) nursing homes as representatives of institution-based long-term care, (b) community residential care settings as representatives of "quasi-institution"-based care, and (c) home-based/near home-based care provided in recipients' homes or within their easy reach.

Nursing Homes

Despite the risk of repeating some of the material presented above, we provide another perspective on the history of nursing homes. County homes and almshouses can be viewed as the predecessors of present-day nursing homes. Those institutions were society's response to the needs of people who could not care for themselves and had no family to care for them. These people included "the disabled, handicapped, aged, widows with children, orphans, the feebleminded, the deranged, the chronically ill, and the unemployed" (Brody, 1977, p. 31). With the exception of a few of these categories, such as widows with children and the unemployed, today's nursing homes care for persons who would have had to live in almshouses and county homes in the 19th and early 20th centuries.

By the 1920s, nonprofit homes for the aged, caring for the indigent "well aged," appeared under sectarian auspices. Almshouses, county homes, and mental hospitals were the facilities for those with physical and mental impairments. Social Security legislation in the 1930s led to the creation of the nursing home as the successor of the almshouse. The law prohibited those living in government-supported institutions from receiving Social Security. Nursing homes appeared as the answer to this problem. These were private businesses that provided custodial care for the elderly who did not have their own homes and families (Clark, 1971) and were too frail to be cared for in the community. The federal government's main concern at the time was with the poor old (and the need to remove them from almshouses) and not the frail old.

> As it turned out, many of these poor elders were also frail and required supportive care. The combination of cash income and need for care led not to home care, but to the birth of modern proprietary nursing homes. . . . Then as now, some form of home care would have been the preferred alternative of many frail old. But the manifest concern was poverty, not frailty, so the issue and alternative solutions were never joined. Thus, nursing homes grew up over the ensuing 20-year period addressed to the frail old. (Hudson, 1990, p. 273)

Other factors also contributed to this growth. Interest in old people was growing, as exemplified by the first National Conference on Aging in 1950. The Hill-Burton Act (1946) provided financial aid, the Small Business Act and Small Business Investment Act (1958) provided loans, and the 1959 amendment to the National Housing Act provided mortgage insurance to facilitate the construction and equipment of nursing homes. The passage of Medicare and Medicaid in 1965 made federal funds available for purchasing long-term care (Clark, 1971).

In the 1960s, states had started discharging the elderly from mental hospitals and into the community. Community services were not adequate for the increased demand, and many of the discharged patients needed round-the-clock care. Many of these patients went to nursing homes. The power of the nursing home lobby also helped the expansion of the nursing home industry (Vladeck, 1980). A contrast between the number of nursing home beds in 1939 and 1970 illustrates the dramatic growth of nursing homes. It is estimated that 25,000 nursing home beds were available in 1939. In three decades, that number jumped to almost 1 million in 1970 (Brody, 1977). Over the past 25 years, nursing homes' share of the long-term care market has been declining. Now, there are 16,100 nursing homes with 1.7 million beds. At an occupancy rate of 86%, there are 1.5 million nursing home residents (Jones, Dwyer, Bercovitz, & Strahan, 2009).

All nursing homes provide four basic types of services: (a) nursing care, (b) personal care, (c) residential services, and (d) medical care. *Nursing care* includes giving medicines orally and by injection, tube feeding, catheterization, and wound care, and may also involve physical, occupational, and speech therapy services. *Personal care* includes help in walking, bathing, dressing, and eating. *Residential services* encompass provision of a protective environment, supervision, and appropriate social services. *Medical care* includes visits by a physician who orders and monitors medications, special diets, and restorative and rehabilitative procedures.

Nursing homes perform a social function, and they receive public money through several channels. Medicaid and Medicare programs are the major sources of payment for their services. Not-for-profit nursing homes are also publicly subsidized through tax exemptions and tax-exempt capital financing; therefore, they are subject to governmental regulation and scrutiny. With government financing of nursing home care came regulation of the nursing home industry by both federal and state governments. However, it did not ensure a high level of quality of care throughout the industry. Material pointing to abuses of basic human rights of nursing home residents started appearing in both lay and professional literature. The litany of nursing home abuses included (1) care that disregarded patients' right to human dignity, (2) lack of activities for patients, (3) lack of dental and psychiatric care, (4) overmedication and under-medication of patients, (5) inadequate and untrained staff, (6) unsanitary conditions, (7) theft of residents' belongings, (8) inadequate safety precautions, (9) unauthorized and unnecessary restraints, (10) failure to act on complaints in a timely manner, (11) reprisals against those who complained, (12) negligence resulting in injury and death, (13) discrimination against patients from minority groups, (14) reimbursement fraud, and (15) ineffective inspection and nonenforcement of laws (Sultz & Young, 2001).

Exposés on the deficiencies of nursing homes led to congressional hearings on the state of nursing home care and public outcry. These resulted in

1. strict enforcement of Medicare and Medicaid guidelines,

2. increased enforcement of nursing home licensure requirements,

3. more active accreditation procedures by the Joint Commission on Accreditation of Health Care Organizations,

4. laws related to elder abuse reporting,

5. enforcement of federal guidelines for the use of physical restraints, and

6. establishment of ombudsman programs.

Former Senator Claude Pepper (1986), who devoted most of his political career to championing the cause of the elderly, articulated the rights of the institutionalized as follows: (a) the right to complain and seek redress of grievances; (b) the right to make basic personal choices; (c) the right to privacy; (d) the right to maintain personal possessions; (e) the right to freedom from verbal abuse; (f) the right to adequate and appropriate medical and nursing care; (g) the right to freedom of movement; (h) the right to a clean and safe living environment; (i) the right to freedom of speech, assembly, and religion; and (j) the right to freedom from physical and sexual abuse.

The Centers for Medicare and Medicaid Services have started publishing the Nursing Home Compare report cards, and a few studies of their effect on the quality of nursing home care have appeared in the literature. Mukamel and associates (2007) reported the results of a survey of a random sample of nursing home administrators. Among survey respondents, 59% were reviewing the quality scores of their facilities regularly and many were taking specific actions to improve quality. Another study (Mukamel, Weimer, Spector, & Zinn, 2008) sought information on 20 specific actions taken by nursing homes in response to the publication of the report card. Two of the five quality measures showed improvement following publication of the report card. Several specific actions were associated with those improvements. The researchers concluded that report cards may motivate providers to improve quality but also raised questions as to why this approach was effective in only some and not all dimensions of care.

Despite the above measures, the quality of care provided by nursing homes continues to vary greatly. On the one hand, some nursing homes go beyond the quality of care and endeavor to improve their residents' quality of life by incorporating organizational and architectural changes, pets, plants, community involvement, and self-directed work teams into the nursing home experience (Coleman et al., 2002). These efforts reflect the culture change in nursing homes that we referred to in Chapter 1. On the other hand, some nursing homes lack the personnel and wherewithal to maintain even the minimal standards of required care. Over the years, many research studies have looked for the reasons for such variance [2].

A shift away from nursing home-based care and toward home- and community-based long-term care started and is being helped substantially by government. In the 1980s, Congress gave states Medicaid waivers to use for keeping patients out of nursing homes or for moving those in nursing homes to other long-term care programs. States have used Medicaid waivers for both upstream and downstream approaches. The upstream approach, known as "nursing home diversion" involves helping people with long-term care needs in receiving home and community-based services so they can avoid nursing home placement. The downstream approach, known as "nursing home transition" helps nursing home residents return home with appropriate support services.

A few states are leaders of the upstream approach. They have crafted Medicaid policies that put community-based long-term care on an equal footing with nursing home care and, thus, have removed the "institutional bias" of Medicaid. Most states have not yet established such policies, and Medicaid institutional care bias prevails at both federal and states levels. Other states, such as Texas, are advocates of the downstream approach. They coined the phrase, "Money follows the person." Their efforts led to the passage of the Deficit Reduction Act of 2005, which authorized a national Money Follows the Person Rebalancing Demonstration program (Reinhard, 2010).

In 2007, 30 states were awarded $1.4 billion in grants to pay for 12 months of services for people who have spent at least 6 months in a long-term care institution. States receiving grant funds are eligible for a higher percentage of federal matching dollars to cover the cost for people moving out of institutions and into community settings. (p. 45)

In 2007, the U.S. Administration on Aging launched a Community Living Program that will strengthen states' capacity to reach older adults and their families before they make a decision for nursing home placement.

Nevertheless, nursing homes will continue as an important element of long-term care in the future. A person who survives to age 65 has a 40% chance of spending some time in a nursing home before his or her death, and that risk increases with age (Spillman & Lubitz, as quoted in Kane, 2011). Nursing homes have a long way to go to improve both their services and their public image.

Community Residential Care Settings

Long-term care in noninstitutional settings takes many forms. Although the advent of Social Security led to the creation of nursing homes, it also encouraged several other more informal arrangements for the nonsick homeless elderly. According to Wilson (2007), the various kinds of boarding homes for the aged (variously known as adult care homes, board-and-care homes, convalescent homes, domiciliary care homes, rest homes, and retirement homes) that did not convert to nursing homes continued to grow. Some of these were for the well-to-do, while others were for the poor. Facilities for the well-to-do include retirement homes and continuing care retirement and life-care communities. Wilson reserved the term *residential care facilities* for settings that served low-income elders. Over the past 20 years, a new term that has come into vogue is *assisted living facilities*. This term defies definition and is used for any facility that falls between independent living and nursing home. We discuss assisted living at some length later in this section.

The origin of a residential arrangement within a private home—a sort of adult foster care—has been traced back to AD 600, and such foster homes have been used in the United States for almost 100 years for the care of those with mental illness (McCoin, 1983). Application of the "foster care" concept to the elderly and persons with mental retardation is a recent phenomenon. The formal beginning of the use of foster homes for the care of the elderly can be traced to 1967, when a demonstration program was authorized by the Department of Health, Education, and Welfare in Washington State to provide foster home care for the elderly (Fenske & Roecker, 1971). This type of care for the elderly has room for further growth. Foster family care came to be recognized as a viable and cost-efficient approach to the residential care of people with mental retardation (Best-Sigford, Bruininks, Lakin, Hill, & Heal, 1982). This type of care, nevertheless, still lacks a precise definition.

Adult foster care is a community-based living arrangement in which an individual who is not fully capable of self-care is taken into the home of a nonrelative, often referred to as a provider, operator, or caretaker. In this setting, the client receives room, board, daily care, and supervision as needed. The provider, in turn, is compensated for his or her duties. (Brockett, 1981, pp. 4–5)

The family-like environment is the major characteristic of this type of care. Originally, the arrangement between the resident and the care provider was private and informal even though the resident's method of payment was usually government financed. This arrangement gradually changed. Several factors influenced the development of the concept of "foster care" and its many operationalizations.

The legislative response to the deinstitutionalization movement provided for community mental health centers for outpatient supervision and follow-up of patients discharged from mental hospitals. Communities were not ready for the housing and other needs of these patients. Many hospitals, state mental health departments, and cities began establishing foster care programs for the deinstitutionalized population (Fenske & Roecker, 1971). Creation of the Supplemental Security Income (SSI) program theoretically made possible the national-level oversight of SSI recipients' quality of life. Later, the concern with the quality of these and other living arrangements led to the enactment of the Keyes legislation, which mandated that states set standards for SSI recipients living in foster homes (Sutherland & Oktay, 1987). No federal role was established, however, to review standards or to enforce the legislation (Oktay & Palley, 1988).

These noninstitutional living arrangements include small homes caring for one to six residents, board-and-care homes, domiciliary care homes, sheltered residential facilities, and group homes. There is no consensus about how each type of care is different from the others. The number of persons cared for seems to set the types apart from one another. McCoin (1995) viewed many of these as representing a continuum of community-based (noninstitutional) care for adults and covered them under the umbrella term *adult residential care.* Notwithstanding the importance of the care component of foster care homes, we label all these as quasi-institutional because they must maintain a minimum standard of care and are subject to the monitoring and accountability mechanisms of some governmental agency. The degree of regulation of and support provided to these sources of long-term care varies greatly despite the fact that most recipients of this type of care are vulnerable. They have mental impairment, developmental disability, and/or are frail elders. Most studies of this type of care fall into two groups—one concentrating on the homes caring for veterans and the other investigating homes caring for residents from the general population.

The Department of Veterans Affairs (VA) has the most experience in establishing, fostering, regulating, and supervising foster care homes. Haber (1983) described the VA Community Residential Care program. These VA homes are carefully evaluated and inspected, their care providers (called sponsors) are trained and given ongoing advice and assistance, and the veterans placed there are visited regularly by social workers. Linn, Caffey, Klett, and Hogarty (1977) conducted an extensive study of five VA residential care programs and found these homes to be a viable family substitute and a stepping stone to other community life. Sickman and Dhooper (1991) studied 46 sponsors providing residential care to veterans in Kentucky and found a vast majority of them doing an admirable job of caring for veterans living under their roofs. Studies of nonveterans in foster home care have investigated the socioeconomic characteristics of home operators, their reasons for taking on this responsibility, the degree of integration of residents in the family life of the operators, and the extent of their acceptance in the community (e.g., see Blaustein & Veik, 1987; Bradshaw, Vonderharr, Keeney, Tyler, & Harris, 1976; Thompson et al., 1989).

Oktay and Volland (1987) described the startup of a hospital-based community care program for frail elderly and evaluated it as a viable alternative to nursing home care. These homes are largely free from the abuses of patients' rights and other negatives generally associated with nursing homes. They do provide a more family-like environment and add to the choices of those who cannot live independently and want to avoid nursing home placement. The degree of "family-like" atmosphere in these homes varies, however. Dhooper, Royse, and Rihm (1989) studied 50 adults with mild and moderate mental retardation living in four types of community residential settings and found that type of setting is associated with the subjects' perception of the extent to which their needs are being met and the degree of choice they exercise in everyday activities. Setting also has an influence on the other objectives of placement. Willer and Intagliata (1982) compared deinstitutionalized adults with mental retardation in two residential alternatives—family care and group homes—in terms of the improvement in their self-care, social, and community living skills. Those in the family care home were significantly more likely to improve their maladaptive behavior, whereas those in the group home were more likely to improve community living skills. Residents in both settings displayed essentially no improvement in self-care skills. All these homes need to do a better job of working toward greater community integration of those in their care. Their importance is likely to increase in the future.

As pointed out above, there is no agreement on what a typical assisted living facility is, what minimal services it provides, and where it fits in the continuum of long-term care. Most consumers view it as a residential and care alternative when they cannot continue living independently in their homes or apartments (Stone & Reinhard, 2007). Wilson (2007) described the origin and growth of assisted living facilities and identified three essential components of assisted living: (1) a *residential environment* that provides for a resident's private space as well as public community spaces shared by all residents; (2) an *operating philosophy* that emphasizes a resident's choices and normal lifestyle; and (3) a *service capacity* that delivers routine services as well as specialized health-related services. She described four models of assisted living facilities:

1. *Hybrid model:* So called because it incorporated the characteristics of facilities as they evolved on the East and West coasts. These emphasized residential-style settings, variable service capacity, and a philosophy of resident autonomy.

2. *Hospitality model:* So called because it was developed by hoteliers-turned-housing-providers and focused on "concierge-type services such as housekeeping, laundry, meals, activities, and transportation. Direct provision of personal care and health-related services was viewed with reluctance" (p. 15).

3. *Housing model:* So called because its advocates were concerned about the aging population living in settings with limited access to services. They were also attracted to the concept of a service coordinator who could function as a case manager. Early adopters of this model were nonprofit organizations and continuing care retirement community providers.

4. *Health care model:* So called because it evolved from nursing homes engaged in vertical integration. Some added independent housing units to their campuses. These followed the traditional care approaches and had strict move-in and move-out criteria. They defined assisted living as a distinct stage between independent living and nursing home and viewed it as a stop on the way to nursing home.

Stone and Reinhard (2007) listed the following models of assisted living:

1. *Independent housing with services model:* This model is characterized by low-cost or subsidized residential settings and residents' access to home care, personal care, and health-related services. Most of these facilities employ full- or part-time service coordinators, and many have developed comprehensive programs that integrate services of health care providers and aging services agencies for their residents. Funds for these come from a variety of sources.

2. *Freestanding market-rate assisted living:* These facilities created by mostly for-profit developers are essentially for the well-to-do, with the average monthly cost ranging between $2,100 and $2,900 in 2004. These may provide personal care, medication reminders, and some nursing care in house or through contracts with outside agencies.

3. *Freestanding low-income assisted living:* The Coming Home Program, funded by the Robert Wood Johnson Foundation (Jenkins, Carder, & Maher, 2004), and Connecticut's Assisted Living Demonstration Project (Sheehan & Oakes, 2004) are two examples of this model. These facilities are for moderate- to low-income seniors. Their development and operation require subsidies for both the real estate and service costs as well as the coordinated effort of several government agencies. Their viability is unclear.

4. *Nursing expansion into assistant living:* Some nursing homes have converted one or more of their floors or wings into assisted living facilities. Others have built assisted living facilities on or close to their campuses. These are a tool for diversification, marketing, and financial survival for nursing homes; however, they also provide those who can pay to live in these facilities another choice of residential environment when they no longer can live in their own homes.

5. *Continuing care retirement communities:* These include independent living apartments or cottages; facilities for services such as housekeeping, meals, social services, wellness, home health care, and access to medical services; and nursing homes. These are almost exclusively private-pay organizations. This model explicitly recognizes assisted living as a residential and care setting for those who cannot live independently. Some of these are bringing in hospice services to enable residents to die in their apartments rather than having to enter a skilled nursing center.

6. *Comprehensive health and long-term care models:* Some vertically integrated hospitals and health care systems have developed assisted living facilities to coordinate services for the elderly and disabled in their communities. Those provide examples of these models. Assisted living is viewed as a residential setting for those who need only personal care and oversight.

"It is important to note, however, that comprehensive hospital, health, and long-term care systems that achieve administrative integration do not always achieve good service integration" (Stone & Reinhard, 2007, p. 28).

Almost all models of assisted living use government funds. Most states are including assisted living in their Medicaid waivers. States license and regulate assisted living facilities and, in the process, create different types of these facilities. For example, Florida has four different licensure types related to the kind and intensity of care provided: (1) standard, (2) limited nursing services, (3) extended congregate care, and (4) limited mental health (Zimmerman & Sloan, 2007). Standard-licensed assisted living facilities serve the elderly (mostly white women) with physical care needs. Assisted living facilities that hold specialty licenses (limited nursing services and extended congregate care) offer extra physical care and serve the elderly who are more physically frail. Assisted living facilities with limited mental health licenses serve younger and ethnically diverse clients who are more likely to be single men (Street, Burge, & Quadagno, 2009). Even within a state, actual practices may differ from regulations.

Payment rules and incentives, state planning and licensing laws, quality oversight processes, and state long-term care policy goals provide incentives and disincentives for making assisted living a substitute for other forms of care, such as nursing homes and home care. (Stone & Reinhard, 2007, p. 28)

Home-Based/
Near Home-Based Care

The category home-based/near home-based care is used broadly to include care provided in the home of the person, as well as care within his or her easy reach. The recipient of this community-based care usually is called a "client" and not a patient. *In-home* care includes "a very complex and varying series of services, responsibilities, costs, and relationships" (Williams, 1990, p. ix).

The services may be aimed at improving, restoring, or maintaining the person's functioning and independence. These may be directed toward the person and/or his or her family caregiver and may be provided by formal caregivers from health and human services professions and organizations and/or informal caregivers from the person's own social network.

Home care can either be long-term provision of supportive care and services to chronically ill clients to avoid institutionalization, or short-term intermittent care of clients following acute illness and hospitalization until clients are able to return to an independent level of functioning. (Sultz & Young, 2001, p. 290)

Most of the organizations providing *in-home* care are home health care agencies, homecare aide agencies, and hospices. *Near-home* services may be provided through health clinics, mental health centers, and social service agencies. The degree of comprehensiveness and coordination of the services provided varies greatly.

The history of most of these services can be traced clearly to different laws providing for the needs of different population groups, even though the home care industry has existed in the country since the 1880s. The Federal Vocational Rehabilitation Act of 1920 focused on the vocational retraining and job placement of disabled service personnel; its amendment (the Barden-Follette Amendment), in the early days of World War II, extended the provisions to civilians. The Vocational Rehabilitation Act of 1954 provided for additional services. The Rehabilitation Act of 1973 represents the most significant societal mandate for the civil rights of individuals with disabilities (Hirschwald, 1984), and the 1978 amendments to that act expanded the meaning and scope of services. The Older Americans Act of 1965 has been the cornerstone of federal involvement in a number of community services for older persons. The Older Americans Act, Title III, provides for funding for congregate meal sites, senior citizens' centers, home care, home-delivered meals, transportation, chore services, telephone reassurance, home visits, and the

Nursing Home Ombudsman Advocacy Program (U.S. Senate Special Committee on Aging, 1991). Medicare and Medicaid (Titles XVIII and XIX of the Social Security Act) also have been major sources of funds for many long-term care services for the aged and those with disabilities, both old and young. Title XX of the Social Security Act funds a variety of social services, including adult day care, adult foster care, protective services, homemaker services, transportation, and home-delivered meals. In 1983, federal government realized the importance of hospice care from both financial and quality-of-life perspectives and decided to include hospice care as a part of Medicare benefits. That change became effective in 1987. When a patient chooses hospice care, Medicare becomes the primary insurer.

> The Hospice Medicare benefits cover services related to the terminal illness, including physician visits and services, nursing care, medical equipment, medical supplies, drugs for symptom control and pain relief, short-term in-patient and respite care, home health aide and homemaker services, physical and other therapies, social work services, and grief support and counseling. (Raymer & Reese, 2008)

The growth of community-based services, particularly in the home care industry, is also a societal response to such demographic and economic factors as these:

1. The number of older persons is increasing, and they desire to live in their own homes in familiar communities. An AARP survey (Bayer & Harper, 2000) found that 90% of adults aged 65 and older prefer to stay in their homes as long as possible.

2. The number of informal caregivers available to care for their relatives is decreasing. Female family members, who have traditionally been informal caregivers, are now a part of the workforce along with men.

3. Innovations in high-technology home care are expanding the categories of diseases and chronic conditions that can be cared for effectively in the home setting.

4. Medicare and Medicaid reimbursement has become a stable source of income (for in-home care providers), and these programs have been allowing for expanded coverage (Sultz & Young, 2007). Medicare is the largest single payer of home health services. In 2009, Medicare spending accounted for about 41% of home health expenditures. Medicaid payments for home care are divided into three main categories: the traditional home health benefit, personal care option, and community-based waivers. Other public funding sources include the Older Americans Act, Title XX Social Services Block Grants, Veterans Affairs, and Civilian Health and Medical Program of the Uniformed Services (National Association for Home Care & Hospice, 2010).

5. The increasing cost of health care is highlighting the need to find less-expensive substitutes to institution-based health care.

Several research studies have shown that home- and community-based services are (1) cost-effective and helpful to persons recuperating from a hospital stay; (2) effective in reducing hospital admissions, lengths of stay, and readmission of psychiatric patients; and (3) protective of the physical and mental health of frail and disabled elderly. These services also reduce their risk for placement in nursing homes (Burr, Mutchler, & Warren, 2005; Gaugler, Kane, Kane, & Newcomer, 2005; Howell, Silberberg, Quinn, & Lucas, 2007; Hughes et al., 1997; Pande, Laditka, Laditka, & Davis, 2007; Sheldon & Bender, 1994).

In the case of infants, toddlers, and children with disabilities, the need for home-based services gradually decreases as the venue of care shifts to schools and other outside-the-home settings such as sheltered workshops. In the case of older persons with disabilities, failing health, and increasing self-care limitations, the need gradually increases. Thus, the need for home-based care occurs more commonly among older adults. The services they need may range from assistance with activities of daily living to high-tech medical care to maintaining their homes as viable settings for care. An ample description of home care services would include medical diagnosis and treatment; nursing care; medication; physical, occupational, and speech therapy; mental health care; provision of medical supplies and equipment; personal care; health aide and homemaker assistance; home repair and maintenance service; adult day care; respite care; and even social companionship (Kane & Kane, 1987). Hospice programs provide state-of-the-art palliative care and supportive services to patients who are at the end of their lives and to their significant others around the clock, 7 days a week, in both the patient's home and facility-based settings. An interdisciplinary team made up of professionals and volunteers provides physical, social, spiritual, and emotional care. Assistance also is offered to the patient's family during the bereavement period (Raymer & Reese, 2008).

Home-based formal care is provided by professionals and paraprofessionals who are either from different service organizations working together or representing a single service agency or are self-employed. Informal care providers are unpaid relatives, friends, or neighbors.

> Home care varies in scope, intensity, and duration. Sometimes it consists of no more than a single service, delivered intermittently, for a short period of time. Alternately, home care can include many different forms of service provided around the clock for months and even years. (Caro, 1990, p. 26)

Types of home care services can be classified in several ways, such as the goal and focus, nature of service, degree of technology used, level of professional expertise, variety of personnel needed, and so on. In terms of specific services, "home care encompasses a potential list of 101 services" (Handy, 1995, p. 49). Focus on the nature of care yields two major models of care: one emphasizing *home health* services and the other *personal assistance/personal care* services. In the home health model, the treatment of health conditions is the primary concern and self-care limitations are of secondary importance.

Aging in place is a program espoused by gerontologists, providers of geriatric services, and government. The following assumptions and facts support it:

1. Most people prefer to remain actively engaged in their own care to the full extent of their ability, in their own residence and within the context of their own family.

2. Longevity and quality of life are enhanced when older people are able to remain in their own homes.

3. Programs that encourage aging in place and the concurrent maintenance of independent living are cost-effective.

4. Moving to institutional settings tends to cause transfer trauma and relocation stress syndrome.

5. It is possible to care for people in any setting with the right planning and appropriate resources (Kane, 2011; Sultz & Young, 2001).

6. Even those who choose continuing care retirement communities to "age in place" find transitions between the three levels of care in those communities stressful and disempowering (Shippee, 2009).

A number of health and human service programs to ensure aging in place have been developed. Commercial companies are offering services to remodel homes so that the elderly can stay in their homes and maintain their independence and mobility. There is a National Aging in Place Council, and certified aging-in-place specialists are available to provide seniors the necessary help. Services provided by most aging-in-place programs frequently include (1) nursing services, (2) home care aide services, (3) homemaker services, (4) a 24-hour emergency response system, (5) home-delivered groceries and/or meals, and (6) adult day care (Sultz & Young, 2001). New technologies are being incorporated into the delivery of these services in order to increase their efficacy and efficiency. On Lok Senior Health Services in San Francisco and Programs of All-Inclusive Care for the Elderly in other parts of the country are examples of successful aging-in-place programs.

Eligibility for home-based and community-based services varies by program, age, income level, physical condition, and previous experience. The payer defines the care. For example, home health care provided by certified home health agencies is covered by Medicare. More socially oriented home care may be covered by Medicaid waivers, state programs, and programs under the Older Americans Act, or may have to be paid for by the client. Not only are the type, nature, frequency, and intensity of services varied but the arrangements for payment for those services are also numerous. With his focus on the degree of consumer control, Kapp (1990) identified the following home care delivery models:

- *Home care provision by a governmental agency model.* Care providers were government employees, the funding for whose services came from state appropriations for home care services or a combination of federal and state Medicaid dollars. The consumer (care recipient) had no choice about who provided the services.
- *Purchase of service from an agency model.* The governmental unit responsible for the home care program contracted with a private for-profit or nonprofit agency to provide the needed services on a case-by-case basis. The consumer had more control because his or her satisfaction was likely to be important to the home care agency.
- *Direct consumer contract with a home care or other agency model.* The consumer selected the service agency that was certified for Medicare and/or Medicaid participation, and the third party (Medicare, Medicaid, or an insurance company) paid for the service. The consumer's choice was constrained by the limited availability of qualified agencies.
- *Independent provider model, with government as fiscal agent.* The consumer recruited independent service providers who were not employees of a home care agency. The governmental agency responsible for the home care program paid for the services. This model gave the consumer much greater autonomy than those listed above.
- Independent provider model, with the consumer hiring, supervising, and paying the provider with money from a governmental agency. This model was the same as the independent

provider model except that the consumer paid the provider directly with money provided by the governmental agency responsible for the home care program.

Over the past decade, there has been a movement toward consumer direction in publicly financed personal care programs. Since 2001, most states have implemented at least one consumer-directed program within their Medicaid home- and community-based services. These programs make the consumer/recipient of services responsible for recruiting, hiring, training, scheduling, supervising, and paying the provider of their personal care services (Kitchner, Ng, & Harrington, 2005; Scherzer, Wong, & Newcomer, 2007). However, states have taken steps to help consumers with their new administrative and financial management responsibilities. Scherzer et al. (2007) have identified the following three models of financial and other management supports:

1. *Fiscal/Employer Agent model.* In this model, the consumer is the common-law employer and the service worker is an independent provider. The consumer hires, trains, supervises, and fires the worker. The agent, which may be a government or private organization, conducts background checks, processes hiring paperwork and timesheets, disburses paychecks, and manages federal and state employment taxes, unemployment insurance, and workers' compensation.

2. *Agency with Choice model.* In this model, the agent may be an entity such as a center for independent living or a home care or home health care agency. This agent is the common-law employer of the worker. The consumer is the "co-employer" or "managing employer" responsible for recruiting, selecting, training, and supervising the worker but may be assisted in these tasks. The agent's responsibilities are similar to those in the previous model.

3. *Public Authority model.* In this model, the agent is an independent government or quasi-government entity. The consumer is the common-law employer and hires, trains, supervises, and fires the worker. The agent supports the consumer by maintaining a worker registry and providing

training to both the consumer and worker. The fiscal tasks are handled by a third entity, usually the state or county department administering the home- and community-based program.

Little is known about how well these models are working and how well or ill each compares with the others.

In terms of the organization and overall quality of services of home care agencies, again, the variation is significant. Handy (1995) described several organizational models. That variation is understandable in view of the fact that 33,000 home care providers operate in the United States (National Association for Home Care & Hospice, 2010). Delivery of services is complex and often fragmented. Grant and Harrington (1989) listed six types of providers of home care in California: (a) licensed-only (not certified) agencies, (b) licensed and certified home health agencies, (c) nurses' registries, (d) employment agencies, (e) unlicensed and temporary personnel agencies, and (f) public contract providers. These differed in how they were regulated. State licensing standards did not go beyond the federal Medicare standards for home health care. Home care agencies could seek accreditation voluntarily from the Joint Commission on Accreditation of Health Care Organizations, the National League for Nursing, or the National Home Caring Council, but few sought accreditation—mainly because of the cost and the lack of incentives (Balinsky, 1994). Studies found that there was inadequate staff screening, supervision, and training; high rates of personnel turnover; poor coordination of services; inadequate and inappropriate care (e.g., dispensing of medications and treatment by inappropriate personnel); inadequate clinical records; use of workers with inadequate knowledge about client status and care plan; and unprofessional and criminal conduct on the part of workers, such as tardiness or absenteeism, theft and fraud, and drug or alcohol abuse(Cantor & Chichin, 1990; Grant & Harrington, 1989; MacAdam & Yee, 1990).

Throughout the 1990s, concerns about the quality of services along with the fiscal integrity of Medicare-supported home health care were voiced, and the government—the Clinton administration and Congress—responded with a pilot project, Operation Restore Trust, which was conducted in several states. The improvement measures that have been adopted since include (1) separation of Medicare funding for home health care services into two streams, one for posthospital care and the other for chronic health problems, with the intent to reduce unnecessary and inappropriate services; (2) change in the Medicare reimbursement method from a retrospective to prospective basis; (3) requirement that home health agencies conduct criminal background checks of home health aides as a condition of employment; (4) requirement that the qualification of nurse aides include completion of appropriate nurse aide training or meet the competency evaluation requirements; (5) requirement that home health agencies provide their staff continuous feedback on qualifications and performance as part of their continuous improvement programs; (6) requirement that home health agencies discuss with their patients the expected outcomes of care so that those patients can be more involved in planning their care; (7) requirement that home health agencies coordinate all care prescribed by physicians for their patients with other agencies serving those patients; (8) requirement that all home health agencies implement a standardized reporting system—the Outcome and Assessment Information Set (OASIS); and (9) requirement that new Medicare prospective payment system for home health care services be linked to OASIS data (Sultz & Young, 2001).

In-home care is a major piece of community long-term care. It also has special importance for most people because of all the "cultural associations with home—autonomy, familiarity, history, relationships, privacy, and dignity" (Kane, 2001, p. 296). This type of care allows for the preference of most elderly and others with disabilities to stay out of nursing homes. It recognizes the contributions of informal caregivers and enhances their resources. The need for home-based/near home-based services is bound to grow in the future.

Critical Thinking Questions

1. The focus of attention and health care resources is likely to shift from inpatient care to outpatient care and wellness programs. Why should social work not accept the losses experienced in the acute care sector and not cease efforts to regain the lost ground?

2. The flow of money determines the direction of change for most institutions and organizations. Appropriately funded *upstream* (helping persons with long-term care needs stay out of nursing homes) and *downstream* (helping nursing home residents return home) approaches are becoming popular. How can social workers help nursing homes thrive in this unfavorable atmosphere?

NOTES

1. The constitution of WHO begins with a set of principles, the first of which is, "Health is a state of complete physical, mental, and social well-being and not merely the absence of disease or infirmity" (WHO, 1958, p. 459).

2. Researchers have investigated whether there were differences between for-profit and not-for-profit nursing homes in terms of such dimensions as access, cost, efficiency, and quality. O'Brien, Saxberg, and Smith (1983) reviewed several of these studies and found that not-for-profit nursing homes had higher quality but lower efficiency (higher costs). On the other hand, Davis (1991) analyzed the findings of several other studies and determined that, "in light of the data, it would be premature to conclude that non-profit nursing homes provide higher quality care, *ceteris paribus*" (p. 147). A study of for-profit and not-for-profit nursing homes in Pennsylvania by Aaronson, Zinn, and Rosko (1994) found that not-for-profit nursing homes provided significantly higher quality of care to both Medicaid beneficiaries and self-pay residents than did for-profit nursing homes.

An Institute of Medicine (1986) study looked for other causes of poor quality of care in nursing homes and identified inadequate supervision of care by physicians and professional nurses as a primary reason for poor quality. Sheridan, White, and Fairchild (1992) explored human resource management factors for understanding why some nursing homes, both for-profit and not-for-profit, failed to provide adequate care. They found that staff members' job attitudes, opinions about elderly residents, and perceptions of the organizational climate varied between the successful for-profit and not-for-profit homes. Among other things, the organizational commitment was much higher in successful not-for-profit than in successful for-profit nursing homes. More recent work has focused on nursing home work practices and their effect on employees' job satisfaction. For example, a study by Bishop, Squillace, Meagher, Anderson, and Weiner (2009) found that wages, benefits, and job demands were associated with job satisfaction of nursing assistants. Their job satisfaction was greater when they felt respected and valued and had good relationships with their supervisors.

3

FUTURE NEEDS OF HEALTH CARE

This chapter brings into bold relief the important emerging needs of health care. As did the previous chapter, it focuses on settings in the four main health care sectors: acute care, ambulatory care, preventive care, and long-term care. It discusses major needs of these settings and identifies major common needs of health care providers across settings. Finally, it points out potential social work contributions for meeting those needs—for both care settings and care providers.

FUTURE NEEDS OF ACUTE CARE SETTINGS (HOSPITALS)

Although acute care hospitals will change in significant ways in the future, some of their characteristics, as discussed in Chapter 2, will persist. Those characteristics are diversity and segmentation, social stratification, the money standard, technological identification, division between physicians and hospitals, and the authoritative role of university medicine (Stevens, 1989). The diversity of hospitals will continue. Many hospitals will expand their role to become more comprehensive in their services and to improve their responsiveness to societal needs. The new law, the Patient Protection and Affordable Care Act of 2010, will allow for more expanded access to health care. The expanded role of hospitals will reduce the degree of segmentation and social stratification. At least for the next few decades, demand for medical services will exceed available resources, cost containment measures will increase, and expensive medical technology will be rationed. Patients with money will continue to hold a special appeal for hospitals that will, thus, continue to be income-maximizing institutions. Technological identification will persist but will be tempered by a shift toward a holistic approach emphasizing the concepts of "wellness" and "quality of life."

The division between physicians and hospitals over issues of finances and quality of care will persist. Hospitals will venture into ambulatory care, and physicians will perceive anything outside the hospital as their market. Hospitals and physicians will compete to provide services. Evidence of this is the growth of thousands of ambulatory surgery centers, 90% of which are owned by physicians (Reece, 2007). Although computer technology will make it possible for many more physicians and other health care professionals to participate in clinical research and although many more hospitals will provide health care to those on Medicaid and the uninsured, the authoritative role of the academic medical center will continue. On the basis of these observations, we have identified the anticipated needs of hospitals in the future. These are listed in Table 3-A below, which is then followed by a discussion of each.

Table 3-A Future Needs of Hospitals

- Venturing into new areas and activities
- Serving diverse patient populations satisfactorily
- Meeting the special needs of the elderly
- Ensuring quality of care
- Taming the computer
- Involving minorities
- Contributing to the solutions of social problems
- Retaining a position of leadership

---

1. *Venturing into new areas and activities* will be the most important need of hospitals in the next few decades. As the limelight shifts from inpatient acute care to different types of outpatient services, hospitals will diversify their missions and activities. They will try to control as many pieces of the continuum of care as possible by developing a comprehensive array of health programs and related services. Many hospitals will expand into multifaceted health care complexes. What Eisdorfer and Maddox (1988) said about community hospitals, that "many hospitals are exploring new ways of organizing care vertically and horizontally in order to supply a wide range of services to the community and to reach people not typically associated with the community hospital" (p. 6), is still true. The focus of health care in the future will be on nonacute ambulatory services emphasizing wellness, prevention of illness, and early detection and treatment. Even secondary and tertiary care hospitals will incorporate these elements into their activities for meeting the health care needs of their communities and for improving their image. The need for such change has been felt for quite some time. As a hospital director put it more than 30 years ago,

Hospitals are badly in need of image boosting. A broader look at hospitals' role in communities can do much for changing their image. One way is to consider medically underserved areas or target communities for satellite primary care facilities, as the hospitals have done in Syracuse. With appropriate community involvement and restrained public relations, the hospital may find itself in an enviable position of doing good and looking good at the same time. Primary care and decentralized hospital nonacute care services are some of the most pressing needs in high growth areas, such as many of the suburbs or small rural communities. (Yanni, 1979, p. 103)

In the opinion of a hospital president, "Perhaps more of our future than most of us ever imagined lies in this particular area" (Klima, 1992, p. 51). Specific efforts can include hospital-sponsored primary care, home care, health promotion, and wellness. The danger, however, is that while diversifying and expanding their activities, hospitals will neglect populations with special needs, such as the poor, the elderly, women, and minorities (Coile, 1990). Understanding their communities and their problems, accommodating their needs, and seeking their acceptance and recognition will be the important foci of hospitals' future planning.

2. *Serving diverse patient populations satisfactorily* will be another vital need of hospitals in the future. Most hospitals—particularly secondary and tertiary care hospitals—will continue to provide short-term, intensive, high-tech care, but that care will be more comprehensive, reflecting changes in the philosophy and nature of the hospital involvement. In Chapter 1, we described the characteristics of hospitals being built for aging boomers, hospitals designed for safety, convenience, rapid information transfer, and reflecting a culture of caring and healing. Note 2 of that chapter gives the example of the Planetree Model Hospital Unit of the Pacific Presbyterian Medical Center as a precursor of things to come. While concerned with the alleviation of the immediate medical problem, hospital care will be expected to enhance the quality of a patient's life. That will involve shifting the focus from the *problem* to the *person with the problem in his or her life situation.* That shift will lead to the conversion of the

traditionally viewed patient—a compliant but passive recipient of treatment—into an active partner in the therapeutic endeavor. The patient's life situation will be operationalized minimally as the presence and active participation of the family in his or her care and treatment. Hence, the hospital-based medical care of tomorrow will be family centered. *Family-centered care* means that care-givers (1) recognize patients' right to have those they love (their family as they define it) with them and involved in their care; (2) appreciate their family's concerns, emotions, and strengths; (3) provide the family complete and unbiased information; and (4) work for caregiver-family collaboration. That will make the patient care situation much more complex, however. Involving the family means understanding the antecedents and consequences of the patient's illness and assessing and mobilizing the family's internal and external resources. As patients become increasingly more diverse, their care also will have to be culturally sensitive. Thus, a constant need of future hospitals will be the successful provision of acute care services that (a) combine high-tech with high-touch, (b) treat patients as partners, and (c) are comprehensive.

3. *Meeting the special needs of the elderly* will be another important need of hospitals. Older patients have had a special significance for hospitals. Although those aged 65 and above composed only 12% of the U.S. population in 2006, they accounted for 43% of the total inpatient days of care and 38% of all hospital discharges (Buie, Owings, DeFrances, & Golosinksiy, 2010). Hence, hospitals can be viewed as de facto geriatric institutions and will become more so in the future (Vladeck, 1988). In Chapter 1, we forecast that a sizeable proportion of the U.S. population in the future will be made up of people aged 65 and older. The majority of them will live in the community and depend on its network of health and social work agencies. The same will be true of other, nonelderly, chronically ill members of the community. Thus, the number of older adults and others suffering from chronic illnesses will represent a substantial proportion of the population. They will require a system of

comprehensive, integrated, and continuing care that recognizes the chronic nature of their illness and their desire for functional independence. Hospitals will have to be an important part of the community's service network. For their efficiency, cost-effectiveness, and image, most secondary and tertiary care hospitals will find it necessary to (a) provide inpatient services that are medically sophisticated, organizationally well coordinated, psychosocially comprehensive, and philosophically person centered and (b) be involved in activities outside their four walls, either as sole providers of outpatient services or as collaborators with other agencies in joint service projects. How to accomplish these goals successfully will be another need of hospitals in the future.

4. *Taming the computer* will be another challenge for hospitals in the future. An increased role of computer technology is forecast for the health care of tomorrow. Already, there is computer-aided diagnosis software, electronic health records, robotic surgery, sophisticated information technology programs, and a movement toward a paperless, all-digital world (Reece, 2007). Computerization of hospital operations and records will lead to greater efficiency. Also, patients' ability to access their records will increase their involvement in diagnosis and treatment and will help in the operationalization of the "patient-as-a-partner" concept. The ease of transmitting information electronically, however, will intensify ethical concerns about the maintenance and sharing of patient data (Barzansky et al., 1993). Computer technology will aid in the standardization of patient care, which in turn may involve the risk of increased impersonalization of that care. Dealing with such concerns and guarding against the undesirable side effects of computer technology will be another major need of future hospitals.

5. *Ensuring quality of care* will continue as another important need of hospitals in the future. The concept of "quality" will have a much broader meaning. *Quality of care* will be defined as more than the quality of service in terms of the

correctness of the service procedure and appropriateness of the expertise of the service provider or even the quality of the outcome of service. It will include the quality of service and its outcome as it affects the quality of the patient's life. The push for demonstrating the quality of care thus defined will be constant. It will be necessary to quantify quality and to resolve such issues as perceived versus real quality and provider-defined versus consumer-defined quality (Friedman, 1991). Expanded access to health care will bring the issue of rationing of expensive medical technology into bold relief. Resolving ethical conflicts and dilemmas pertaining to the quality of life and rationing of care issues will be a constant challenge for hospitals of the future.

6. *Involving minorities* will become an important political necessity for hospitals in the future. Today's minorities will have grown stronger in their numbers, political activities, and claims on the sources of power and authority. Even 30 years ago, a hospital trustee expressed his caution, concern, and advice thus:

> Various community activist groups are developing nationwide, and their requests must be taken seriously and at least evaluated. A private, not-for-profit hospital in North Carolina is undergoing some very severe challenges by a group that maintains that there are not enough poor people on the hospital governing board. This same phenomenon is developing in other areas. In New Jersey, for example, a health systems agency declined to review a hospital's application because the HSA did not like the makeup of the hospital's board. These signs must be taken seriously. Hospital boards should be reviewed to ensure that they properly represent their particular communities. (Ewing, 1979, p. 12)

Hospitals of the future will have difficulty remaining noncontroversial, quiet industries as in the past. How to operate effectively in an increasingly more political environment and satisfy their constituents will be among their important needs. This need will have to be met at two levels: (a) adequate representation of the various sections of the community on the hospital's policymaking bodies and (b) satisfaction of the hospital's consumers with its practices, procedures, and services.

7. *Contributing to the solutions of social problems* will become the community responsibility of future hospitals. The health consequences of such social problems as poverty, homelessness, violence, substance abuse, and AIDS will continue to be the concern of hospitals, but the intensity of that concern will deepen. The paradox of medical success intertwined with social failure will persist.

> Hospitals signify achievements in American science and technology, but they also represent a breakdown in the public's health. In their beds lie, inter alia, victims of accidents, violence, poor nutrition, lack of knowledge, carelessness, overindulgence, poverty, and addiction, translated into damaged hearts, babies, lungs, and livers. (Stevens, 1989, p. 356)

Hospitals will be forced to examine this paradox. Hospitals have been conceived of as a high-technology system—an extended emergency service—(providing short, intensive, and acutely needed medical care) and, alternately, as a community resource for caring. Hospitals have been strictly neither a technological system nor a community-service system. Ramifications of being neither will continue to challenge the creativity and resources of hospitals. Improving the technological sophistication of hospital-based medical care will be easier in the future, but responding to the community's social health needs will be much more difficult. The idea of medicine as a "science," with hospitals as its major instrument, represented in standard definitions for prospective payment (diagnosis-related groups, or DRGs) and standard expectations about hospital use (Stevens, 1989, p. 357) has little relevance for complex social health problems, which defy such standardization. Even within the problems of health, although medical technology may have an enormous effect on the health of the individual, it has very little effect on the health of the population. How to be the instruments of medical science (a system of standardized problems and reproducible results) and also combatants of social problems, or exploring what their appropriate role in combating social problems is, will be another major need of future hospitals.

8. *Retaining a position of leadership* will be an abiding need of hospitals in the future. Hospitals have been leaders of health care organizations. In Chapters 1 and 2, we mentioned the roles played by hospitals to justify their claim to leadership. Changing societal conditions, however, are likely to challenge that claim in the future. Most hospitals will try to retain their leadership by becoming the hub of the community care system. While discussing the roles of hospitals in the community care of the aged, Eisdorfer and Maddox (1988) said, "Hospitals are already the principal gathering place for professionals, technicians, equipment, and support services that can be focused on packaging an individual's care in an infinite variety of ways" (p. 8). Hospitals are also the predominant entry points for nursing home and formal home care (Vladeck, 1988). Some marketing experts recommend that hospitals sponsor *senior membership plans* offering senior discounts, free health screenings, Medicare copayment write-offs, and the use of a senior activity center (Coile, 1990). Taking on new roles will become a necessity for the continued existence and prominence of hospitals. Deciding on the "what" and "how" of the new roles will be an important need of future hospitals.

Social workers can make significant contributions to the efforts of future hospitals in meeting each of these needs. Their professional knowledge, sensitivity, and skills give them an edge over many other health care professionals in understanding and dealing with social problems, working with diverse populations, involving minority groups, and improving the patient-centeredness of hospital care. Their values and ethical principles have relevance for dealing with

quality-of-life issues and moral dimensions of health care technology. Their experience as the bridge between the hospital and the community is an added asset for hospitals' efforts to venture into community-based activities and seek positions of leadership.

FUTURE NEEDS OF AMBULATORY CARE SETTINGS

The various entities providing ambulatory care differ in their auspices, organization, scope of service, clients they serve, and sources of funding. Some are governmental, others are voluntary, and still others are proprietary. In the scope and organization of their services, some provide general (all essential, basic) services, whereas others deliver only special services (of a single medical specialty or for a particular medical condition). General services may be comprehensive or piecemeal. In terms of the clients they serve, again, they vary greatly. Some serve all members of the community, whereas others cater to special populations, with eligibility dependent on such factors as income, age, and membership of various groups—prepayment, geographic, categorical, and others. Similarly, the sources of financing are many—both public and private and combinations thereof (Rosenfeld, 1971). Roemer (1986) attributed this complexity to three major features:

> First, since the United States is an affluent industrialized country, its health care system has abundant resources, and it spends a great deal of money. Second, since this is a federated nation, the governance of the system is highly decentralized to numerous states, counties, and communities. Third, since this nation has a free market economy, very permissive laissez-faire concepts are incorporated throughout its health care system. (p. 2)

Despite its affluence, the United States is increasingly realizing that the money spent on health care is not producing the desired results. There is much unnecessary suffering, illness, and disability. The health care system being a trillion-dollar industry, 16% of the gross national product being expended on medical and health care, and "an angle of that spending slope becoming nearly asymptotic to the vertical" (Lundberg, 1994, p. 1533) left 45 million Americans without insurance coverage for health services last year. This number became unacceptable. The new law has set in motion changes that are likely to prove significant in their consequences. Nevertheless, proceeding on the assumption that the future is never completely divorced from the past, it is safe to say that, in the future, "the heterogeneity and pluralism of the U.S. health culture will certainly not vanish" (Roemer, 1986, p. 36), but major changes will occur in the organization and patterns of health care. It is safe to predict the following changes.

Changes will occur in the organization of medical and health care practice so that (a) ambulatory services will become more popular with providers of care and hospitals will compete with other organizations for a share of the ambulatory care market, and (b) group practice will become more prominent and generalist medical practitioners will be in great demand. This prediction has started to happen already. Earlier, we talked about more and more hospitals venturing into ambulatory care and about hospital outpatient departments starting new or expanding into special programs for such patient groups as alcoholics and drug abusers, abused spouses, the elderly, and rape victims. We also discussed that more and more physicians are going into group practice, both fee-for-service and prepaid types. Even in dealing with hospitals, an increasing number of physicians are realizing that, as groups, they can negotiate with hospitals more advantageously. In the future, we will see hospital-based group practices or even physician groups contracting to run hospital services—inpatient and outpatient. "In tomorrow's dynamic health care enterprise, hospitals and physicians will create new ventures and develop new clinical and business relationships" (Coile, 1990, p. 248). The following is an example of physician-hospital joint ventures. "In Nashville, a group

of entrepreneurial neurosurgeons struck a deal 'piggybacking' an 18-bed specialty hospital, featuring six operating rooms doing 250 procedures a month, upon St. Thomas Hospital's 683-bed hospital" (Reece, 2007, p. 124). Changes will occur in the nature and pattern of health care services so that (a) comprehensiveness of services will be a necessity rather than an ideal; (b) coordination of health services within each setting, as well as between the setting and community health and social services, will become a must; (c) illness prevention and promotion of healthful lifestyles will become important parts of primary care services; and (d) it will become necessary to accommodate the special needs of major health care consumers, programmatically as well as by changing the attitudes and skills of care providers.

With the United States moving toward near-universal access to health care, those hitherto outside or on the periphery of the system will demand high-quality health care services. That will result in (a) a strain on the system's resources, (b) questions of equity, and (c) issues of quality of service.

Because the focus of health care will have shifted onto ambulatory care, the anticipated changes will make special demands on ambulatory care settings. Meeting those demands will be the greatest overall need of these settings. That need may be divided into the following three categories: (a) the need to expand their services so that some basic primary care is provided to everyone; (b) the need to provide patient-centered services marked by comprehensiveness, coordination, and continuity; and (c) the need to accommodate the special needs of hitherto-neglected groups.

1. *Expanding services:* Hospital outpatient departments, private group practice offices, health maintenance organizations, and other community-based clinics and health centers are some of the settings for ambulatory care. This diversity will persist in the future, and diversity also will increase in the scope of services provided, which may include primary care, ancillary

care, and preventive care services. Minimally, however, all these settings will be responsible for providing primary care. Some settings may have to focus on primary care and add wellness and prevention activities to their services while retaining their secondary care functions. Others, such as maternal and child health programs and public health centers, which have been essentially prevention oriented, will have to expand the scope of their services. The amendments to Titles V and XIX of the Social Security Act (Omnibus Reconciliation Budget Act of 1989) mandated that the scope of maternal and child health services be expanded from pure prevention to include primary care. Such changes are like straws in the wind, indicating the direction of change and adding weight to this prediction about the future.

Because the provision of primary care will be the most common feature of most ambulatory care settings, it is appropriate here to elaborate on the definition of primary care. *Primary care* has been defined as the care of the well, the worried well, the presymptomatic patient, and the patient with disease in early symptomatic stages. This definition tells something about the patient in relation to illness but nothing about the elements or attributes of the care. The *Journal of Public Health Policy* listed the essential elements of primary care as (a) correct diagnosis as the precondition of treatment; (b) appropriate treatment for maximum possible restoration of function; (c) relief of pain and suffering and alleviation of illness-related anxiety; (d) appropriate referral for specialized diagnostic, treatment, and rehabilitation services; (e) management responsibility for overall health of the patient; (f) preventive services, including immunization, multiphasic screening for early detection, and preventive supervision; and (g) health education and advice for health promotion, disease prevention, treatment, and rehabilitation (Milton, 1983). The Institute of Medicine (1978) defined *primary care* as accessible, comprehensive, coordinated, and continual care provided by accountable providers of health services. It thus identified accessibility, comprehensiveness, coordination,

continuity, and accountability as the attributes of good primary care. Such care will be expected to result in the care of the "whole person," not merely the treatment of an illness.

2. *Providing patient-centered comprehensive services:* All types of ambulatory settings will be expected to provide comprehensive and well-coordinated patient-centered, high-quality services. In terms of their past experience, health care organizations and providers will not have much to go on. The record of the U.S. health care system on the provision of comprehensive and coordinated services at the community level or even at the individual patient level has been far from satisfactory, despite the importance of such services. Almost 80 years ago, one major recommendation of the Committee on Cost of Medical Care (1932) was that "the study, evaluation, and coordination of medical service be considered important functions for every state and local community, that agencies be formed to exercise these functions, and that the coordination of rural with urban services receive special attention."

From time to time, coordinating councils formed at the community and state levels have focused on special problems or needs of special groups. These have had minimal impact. The Comprehensive Health Planning Act of 1966 and its follow-up law, the National Health Planning and Resource Development Act of 1974, established a nationwide network of health system agencies for assessment of community health needs, coordination of programs, and stimulation of actions to respond to unmet needs. These laws failed to achieve their objectives. Under the Reagan administration, planning efforts at the local level were "greatly eroded, leaving mainly skeleton agencies at the state level" (Roemer, 1986, p. 137). The integration of health care with other human services has remained a noble ideal.

The medical establishment's answer to the need for "total patient-oriented" basic health care has been the creation of the family practice specialty. However, as pointed out earlier, an unimpressive proportion of medical graduates are going into family practice, despite incentives and encouragement. This trend is likely to change in the future, and ambulatory care gradually will become more attractive. It will be several decades, however, before the supply of adequately trained family practitioners and other generalist physicians becomes satisfactory. "Having too few generalists means that Americans have less access to primary care, miss opportunities for prevention, and receive inappropriate, uncoordinated care when they have complex or chronic conditions" (Schroeder, 1993, p. 120). While discussing ways of correcting the imbalance in the medical workforce—the United States being flooded with specialists at the expense of generalists—Schroeder presented several possibilities, such as (a) making energetic efforts to achieve an appropriate generalist-specialist balance (50% of each), (b) increasing the generalist capability of specialists, and (c) replacing the missing generalist capability with such nonphysician substitutes as nurse practitioners and physician assistants. The goal of 50% of all physicians being generalists does not seem attainable in the foreseeable future, and the option of specialists filling in the gap will not ensure comprehensive and coordinated health care. "Many specialists who are forced to practice outside their special areas of competence will not take pleasure at straying from their fields" (p. 120). At the same time, physicians and the medical establishment will resist the idea of nurse practitioners and physician assistants replacing physicians even as primary care providers.

Even when (possibly by the middle of the century) the number of primary care ambulatory physicians is adequate, their training, orientation, and resources may not suffice to provide comprehensive services. It is forecast that families in the future will be much more varied and complex in their form and weaker in their resources, and the medical problems of major groups of patients will be intertwined with powerful social needs. For effectively providing minimally acceptable services to their clients, primary care medical personnel will have to supplement their professional resources with the resources of others.

3. *Accommodating the special needs of different groups of patients:* The elderly, nonelderly with disabilities, and victims of social problems such as homelessness, substance abuse, and violence will be the groups with special needs requiring unique consideration. These groups will be heavy users of ambulatory as well as acute care services. For identifying the needs of these major groups of consumers of ambulatory services, we look at the most often encountered situations in ambulatory care settings. We have divided all ambulatory care settings into two categories: (a) settings providing acute care and (b) settings providing nonacute care. The former include hospital emergency departments and trauma centers and freestanding emergicenters, urgent care centers, and ambulatory surgery centers. The latter include hospital outpatient departments, private group practice offices, health maintenance organizations, and public health centers and clinics. In acute care, particularly emergency care settings, the following three kinds of situations generally are encountered: (a) true medical emergencies with powerful social consequences, (b) social emergencies with vital medical dimensions, and (c) nonemergency health or social needs. Persons in each of these situations make different demands on the care setting and care providers. In nonacute care settings, chronic problems dominate, interspersed by crises that are often more social than medical. As emphasis shifts from illness management to wellness maintenance, many patients will need to be encouraged, goaded, and motivated to prevent illness and crises.

Social workers are superbly qualified to help ambulatory care settings meet their needs as discussed above. Their assets include (a) the know-how of the comprehensiveness, coordination, and integration of services; (b) a health orientation much broader than the illness focus of many other health care providers; (c) the ability to treat the total patient rather than merely the disease; (d) the understanding of the characteristics and problems of major patient groups; (e) a refined tendency to look for strengths rather than dwell on deficiencies; and (f) the skills to intervene appropriately in the lives of patients beyond the immediate medical concern.

FUTURE NEEDS OF ILLNESS PREVENTION AND HEALTH PROMOTION AGENCIES

As the wellness movement grows stronger and health care priorities shift more strongly to illness prevention and health promotion in the future, more and more agencies will appear on the scene. Hundreds of organizations, along with public health departments and health care providers, are joining a consortium for achieving the *Healthy People 2020* goals. *Healthy People* is a comprehensive framework for improving the health of Americans. It is a set of goals and objectives with 10-year targets for national health promotion and illness prevention efforts. Since 1979, *Healthy People* has set and monitored a broad range of national objectives related to meeting health needs, encouraging collaboration across sectors, and guiding individuals in making informed health decisions.

> *Healthy People* reflects the idea that setting objectives and providing science-based benchmarks to track and monitor progress can motivate and focus action. *Healthy People 2020* represents the fourth generation of this initiative, building on a foundation of three decades of work. (Department of Health and Human Services, 2010, p. 1)

Its mission is to

1. identify nationwide health improvement priorities;
2. increase public awareness and understanding of the determinants of health, disease and disability, and opportunities for progress;
3. provide measurable goals and objectives that are applicable at the national, state, and local levels;
4. engage multiple sectors in actions to strengthen policies and improve practices based on the best available evidence and knowledge; and
5. identify critical research, evaluation, and data collection needs.

The following are its overarching goals:

1. Attain high-quality, longer lives free of preventable disease, disability, injury, and premature death.
2. Achieve health equity, eliminate disparities, and improve the health of all groups.
3. Create social and physical environments that promote good health for all.
4. Promote quality of life, healthy development, and healthy behaviors across all life stages.

Healthy People 2020 covers 42 topic areas, each of which is assigned to one or more lead agencies within the federal government. Those agencies will be responsible for developing, tracking, monitoring, and reporting on the objectives pertaining to those areas (Department of Health and Human Services, 2010, pp. 2–3). Earlier *Healthy People* initiatives have been found to be worthy efforts. For example, despite the difficulty of evaluating progress toward the two overarching goals of *Healthy People 2010*—"increase the quality and years of healthy life" and "eliminate health disparities" (which subsumed 28 focus areas and 955 objectives and sub-objectives)—Sondik, Huang, Klein, and Satcher (2010) found that the leading health indicator measures suggest some progress has been made.

For conceptual clarity and with a view to include organizations that social workers are likely to be working for, we divide agencies involved in illness prevention and health promotion activities into the following three groups: (a) public health departments, which will make renewed and concerted efforts to regain prominence; (b) hospitals, which will continue to diversify their functions to include health maintenance and health promotion as important complements to their illness care activities; and (c) other organizations that will either be expanding their programs to include illness prevention and health promotion or specializing in these activities.

All these will work toward and contribute to the attainment of the goals of *Healthy People 2020* much beyond the year 2020. These three groups of agencies will provide different combinations of services related to illness prevention and health promotion. Hence, they will have some common and some unique needs. Their common needs in varying degrees will be (a) having access to adequate financial resources for their services, particularly in the next few decades; (b) knowing how best to implement the known illness prevention and health promotion approaches; and (c) developing new approaches that provide the best match between an agency's resources and the needs of individuals and groups it serves. Their unique needs will be determined by the particular constellation of such factors as purpose of the agency's activity, its client group, and its resources—both material and professional. We discuss separately the major needs of each group.

Public Health Departments

Unlike other health care organizations either already in or likely to enter the field of illness prevention and health promotion, public health establishments are the only entities whose very reason for existence has been the prevention of disease and the promotion of health. The core missions of public health are monitoring the occurrence and spread of disease, promoting infant health, immunizing children, controlling infectious diseases, conducting health education and promotion activities (Lee, 1994), and preparing for bioterrorist attacks. Although large sections of the population are becoming a part of the wellness movement, as a nation, the United States has had no commitment to the concepts of "prevention" and "health promotion." As pointed out in Chapter 2, whereas more than 75% of federal health care dollars is spent on the care of people with chronic diseases, less than 0.5% is spent on preventing those diseases, and the spending of state and local public health agencies constitutes less than 2.5% of the overall U.S. health care spending (Beitsch, Brooks, Menachemi, & Libbey, 2006).

Although the federal government can set the tone and provide the resources for health promotion efforts, action will be at the state and local levels—much more at the local than at the state level. Our focus in this discussion, therefore, is on local health departments.

That a lack of resources is affecting the ability of local health departments to address even their core functions is supported by the findings of several studies. Using a stratified random national sample of local health departments, Turnock and his associates (1994) surveyed those departments' compliance and roles with respect to 10 public health practice performance measures. These measures pertained to the three major health department practices—*assessment* (of the problems and challenges of the day), *policy development* (determining which problems to address and with what priority and tools), and *assurance* (making sure that the necessary efforts were in place to deal with the problem). They analyzed their data by focusing on (a) individual performance measures, (b) groups of measures reflecting performance in the three practice areas, and (c) the department's role as the lead agency, collaborator, or minimal. They found that very few (3%) local health departments reported compliance with all 10 of the performance measures. Overall, 31% reported compliance with seven or more performance measures, and only 19% reported compliance with the majority of performance measures for each core practice. For only one practice did more than half the departments characterize their role as the lead agency. The researchers viewed their findings in relation to the *Healthy People 2000* objective (8.14) that calls for 90% of the population to be served effectively by a local health department and concluded that extensive capacity-building efforts were necessary for that to happen by the year 2000.

In the meantime, the persistence or reappearance of communicable diseases such as AIDS and tuberculosis; the growth of noncommunicable conditions such as cancer, heart disease, and stroke; and ever-present environmental hazards continued to make added demands on these departments. Greenberg, Schneider, and Martell (1995) surveyed the local health officers of 436 Northeastern and Midwestern cities with populations between 25,000 and 500,000 about their priorities for promoting health through prevention. They also looked for differences between local health officers of the most economically stressed cities and those of the least economically stressed cities. The priority lists of the two groups were remarkably similar. The five most important public health prevention goals were (a) reducing the incidence of HIV infection and AIDS, (b) improving maternal and infant health, (c) controlling sexually transmitted diseases, (d) reducing violent and abusive behavior, and (e) immunizing against infectious diseases. The local health officers of the most stressed cities, however, were more pessimistic about achieving those goals.

Public health practitioners have not succeeded in selling the simple truths of illness prevention and health promotion. Unlike other health care issues, public health programs have lacked an effective and supportive constituency. As Gordon (1993) so aptly put it,

> Public health has always been a rocky road, as it provides no immediate gratification or feedback. It requires the ability to look to the future, which is not a commonplace trait of our political leaders who are looking to the next election rather than the status of their constituents' health in coming decades. Public health, thus far, lacks the glamour associated with hospitals, organ transplants, emergency medicine, diagnosis, treatment, and rehabilitation and does not compete well with crisis health care. (p. 263)

In the future, the logic of prevention will make more sense to the public and politicians alike, and health promotion and illness prevention will permeate and be integrated into every component of the health care system. However, this will happen slowly and gradually over several decades, and not without concerted effort on the part of public health professionals. On the one hand, overall public and professional attitudes, acute-care–oriented training of most health care professionals,

organization of health care systems, and the system of rewards for health professionals and organizations will be slow in changing. On the other hand, the self-interest of powerful economic forces will not allow them to give up their modes of making profit, even when these involve risk to people's health and lives. Roberts (1994) discussed at length how, in the matters of tobacco and smoking, car passenger safety, and guns and violence, the United States has "allowed a variety of forces to contaminate any meaningful effort to prevent the major killers of children and adults" (p. 269). This continues to be as true today as it was 17 years ago. Curbing the power of these forces to contaminate illness prevention and health promotion efforts will be an ongoing challenge. Public health professionals will need to keep reminding themselves that they must constantly "explain, promote, market, sell, interpret, propose, advocate, and communicate the need for improved public health and environmental health and protection services" (Gordon, 1993, p. 264).

In Chapter 2, it was mentioned that a majority of the 3,000 local public health units in the United States are small and do not have the financial resources to do an adequate job. They also are organized in countless ways. There is still agreement (e.g., Koplin, 1993) with Emerson (1945), who proposed that a population of about 50,000 would be optimal for one efficiently run public health unit. Hence, public health organizations at the local level can benefit from restructuring. The Institute of Medicine (1988a) report *The Future of Public Health* also found that the infrastructure of state and local health units is limited and restricts their capacity to ensure protection of the public's health. These units lack the trained personnel to coordinate the collection and analysis of data for identifying problems and setting priorities (Lee & Toomey, 1994). In the words of Tilson and Berkowitz (2006),

> The policy challenges of aligning the local infrastructure and delivering on the IOM [Institute of Medicine] vision, shared by the national leadership in public health and "owned" by NACCHO

[National Association of County and City Health Officials], include moving forward and adopting a shared organizational definition, agreed-upon parameters of function, and effective and efficient processes of measuring the performance of duties. (p. 904)

The major needs of public health departments can be summarized as follows:

1. Generating more funds for personnel and programs

2. Reorganizing for greater efficiency and effectiveness

3. Intensifying their health promotion and wellness activities

Hospitals

In the future, as the limelight shifts from inpatient acute care to other forms of health care, hospitals will diversify their activities to include illness prevention and health promotion. Their mission will become clearly the provision of comprehensive health care services. This has been happening for some time already. The American Hospital Association established the Center for Health Promotion with the purpose of encouraging and assisting hospitals to create and implement effective health promotion programs. In 1979, it published the association's policy statement on the hospital's responsibility for health promotion. That led many hospitals to rewrite their missions to strengthen their roles in maintaining and improving the health of their communities. In the words of Behrens and Longe (1987),

> Some are redefining the business that they are in, recognizing that in the past they had engaged in the "illness business" rather than the "health business." Today, these hospitals state confidently that they are in the health business—helping people in their communities regain health when they are sick or injured, helping them maintain good health when they are well, and helping them improve their health at every stage in their lives. (p. 3)

The reasons for hospitals to engage in health promotion efforts have become more prominent and compelling. These include (a) improving the health of the community, (b) improving the image of the hospital, (c) changing the hospital's service mix, (d) reducing health care costs, and (e) achieving specific financial goals for the hospital (Longe & Wolf, 1983). Behrens and Longe (1987) discussed how health promotion programs for children bring new patients to the hospital and its physicians and give it a competitive edge. Earlier, we gave some examples of how hospitals are reorganizing themselves and expanding their activities horizontally as well as vertically. Coile (1990) mentioned hospitals that are able to generate 50% of their revenues from activities other than inpatient acute care services. Many hospitals—community hospitals more than others—ventured into outpatient services. Now, their outpatient clinics are organized like those of private physician group practices and are aesthetically pleasant, well equipped, and customer oriented (Sultz & Young, 2001). This trend is sure to continue. These hospitals are providing outpatient services through hospital-based as well as community-based satellite clinics. In the future, they will organize and deliver multispecialty ambulatory care in clinics far removed from their brick-and-mortar settings (Reece, 2007). To the extent that these clinics offer primary care, they are participating in illness prevention work. There is also some room for health promotion during a health care provider's encounters with the patients in these clinics. "However, patient's medical needs, physician's workloads, reimbursement constraints, and ambulatory practice norms all conspired to make health promotion a low priority in the medical encounter" (Currie & Beasley, 1982, p. 143). This is very likely to change.

To be effective, health promotion programs must be independent entities. At present, some hospitals are entering health promotion programs in the community. Some of these expect their health promotion programs to generate profit, others expect them to break even, and still others offer these programs as a community service.

Although the financial goal of a hospital regarding its health promotion program determines its program-related planning and operation, every hospital that ventures into this area can expect to make some gains. Even the hospital that provides health promotion as a community service stands to improve (a) its image as an agency concerned about the health of the community, (b) the goodwill between itself and the community, (c) the community's familiarity with its services, (d) the cooperation between itself and other health and human service agencies, and (e) its base for referrals for its other services. Perhaps the most important benefit for such a hospital is its enhanced ability to "prepare for future trends in health care that rely on having a solid foundation in areas of ambulatory and health promotion services" (Longe & Wolf, 1983, p. 18).

In the future, more and more hospitals will enter the health promotion business. Their major needs in this regard will be

1. deciding the "what," "where," and "how" of health promotion services;

2. designing and implementing the decided-on programs; and

3. collaborating with the local and state public health departments in disease prevention and health protection work.

Other Organizations

Other organizations engaged in illness prevention and health promotion work are the various voluntary and professional associations, some of which were listed in Chapter 2. Some of these, such as the American Cancer Society, American Heart Association, and American Lung Association, have been among the most ardent health promotion advocates that have contributed significantly to the current levels of awareness about different diseases and measures for their control. These organizations and others that will join this category in the future do not suffer from the constraints and faults of public health departments or hospitals. Public health

departments must satisfy the bureaucratic requirements and whims of politicians, and for hospitals, illness prevention and health promotion represent one of several, often low-priority, missions. Moreover, voluntary organizations can be closer to the people and are generally simpler in their organization, clearer in their mission, and more single-minded in their pursuit of that mission. All these attributes enable them to make their services accessible to people more easily and less expensively.

> The low cost and wide availability of the services offered by these organizations, coupled with their institutional experience and commitment to disease prevention and health promotion, makes them a natural ally of other groups initiating such efforts, and should ensure the growth of their involvement in future health promotion activities. (McGinnis, 1982, p. 413)

The more established of these organizations are quite good at both raising money and providing services. The new ones generally struggle in both of these areas. Their major needs are

1. creating adequate fiscal resources for their programs and activities, and

2. overcoming deficiency in the best knowledge and skills for their programs.

Table 3-B recapitulates the future needs of entities engaged in illness prevention and health promotion work.

Social workers have much to offer illness prevention and health promotion organizations in dealing with their major needs. The concept of "resource" is basic to social work thinking (Siporin, 1975), and social workers understand its various meanings and how to operationalize it. The ability to create, mobilize, and maximize resources is their greatest asset. Similarly, for designing and implementing illness prevention and wellness promotion programs, their *person-in-environment* perspective, grasp of the *systems theory* and concepts of "enabling" and "empowerment," and "community organization" skills will give them an edge over many others.

Table 3-B Future Needs of Illness Prevention and Health Promotion Agencies

Public Health Departments	Generating more funds for personnel and programs
	Reorganizing for greater efficiency and effectiveness
	Intensifying health promotion and wellness activities
Hospitals	Deciding the "what," "where," and "how" of the health promotion services
	Designing and implementing the decided-on programs
	Collaborating with public health departments in disease prevention and health protection work
Other Organizations	Creating adequate fiscal resources for programs and activities
	Overcoming deficiency in the knowledge and skills for programs

FUTURE NEEDS OF LONG-TERM CARE FACILITIES

Although community-based long-term care is viewed as a viable alternative to costly institutional care, both its financing and delivery systems are in need of reform. The cost of nursing home and home-based care is essentially not covered by Medicare or private insurance. Those who need this care must use their own resources, and when those resources are used up, they are forced to turn to Medicaid, a welfare program.

Weissert and Hedrick (1994) reviewed 32 well-designed studies of community-based long-term care programs and concluded that this type of care does not increase survival and does not affect the rate of deterioration in functional status of care recipients. It does reduce unmet needs and increase the life satisfaction of patients and their familial caregivers, but the higher life satisfaction levels diminish with time. Even if the use of institutions (hospitals and nursing homes) is decreased, the decrease is too small to outweigh the costs of additional community-based care. Weiner and Illson (1994) asserted that the long-term care system is broken and needs to be fixed: "Indeed, no other part of the health care system generates as much passionate dissatisfaction as does long-term care" (p. 403). The challenge for long-term care is to become so "good"—appropriate, effective, efficient, and normal—that institution-based care starts being viewed as the alternative care. We look separately at the major needs of the three groups of long-term care settings: nursing homes, community residential care homes, and facilities providing home-based and near home-based care.

Nursing Homes

The essential elements of the nursing home picture and the important needs of nursing homes can be summarized as follows.

The quality of care provided by nursing homes varies greatly—excellent in some and far from acceptable in others. As pointed out in Chapter 2, on the one hand, a few nursing homes not only provide high-quality care but also endeavor to improve the quality of life of their residents by incorporating organizational and architectural changes, pets, plants, community involvement, and self-directed work teams into the nursing home experience (Coleman et al., 2002). On the other hand, there are many nursing homes where not only is the care provided substandard but actual abuse of residents occurs. We previously listed the types of abuse that nursing home residents are known to experience. In nursing homes in the second group, almost any intervention seems to yield measurable benefits for residents, which possibly reflects the general deprivation of the environment (Kane & Kane, 1987). Despite concerted efforts by government and professional agencies to improve the performance of nursing homes (discussed in Chapter 2), the public image of the nursing home as a place that is farthest from "home," dirty, cold, impersonal, and where people go to die persists. The greatest need of nursing homes is to change that image.

Nursing homes have not yet realized the importance of linking with other community services to provide a continuum of care that benefits patients, payers, and providers (Clapp, 1993). We have discussed the health care system of the future being marked by an integrated continuum of comprehensive services. This will be at two levels: one emphasizing continuum and the other integration. Depending on a patient's condition and needs, the principle of continuum of care would ensure his or her smooth movement among hospitals, nursing homes, retirement communities, foster homes, or his or her own residence fortified by appropriate home health and social services. The principle of integration would guide the provision of services by community-based health and human services. This change particularly will affect the care of the elderly. Nursing homes, being an important subacute care setting, will be a significant part of the continuum of care. Nursing homes will need to prepare for this change toward an integrated continuum of comprehensive services.

Nursing homes also will need to extend themselves into the community by making use of their facilities and equipment and by making the services of their personnel available to home-based needy—young and old with disabilities and frail elderly—and other community groups. This can be done directly or through other agencies and programs, some of which even may be willing to pay for those services. Some agencies and programs find purchasing some services less expensive than establishing their own. For improving their residents' quality of life, nursing homes will have to foster the involvement of the community in the lives of those residents.

Thus, the major needs of nursing homes are

1. improving their public image,

2. becoming a part of an integrated continuum of services, and

3. extending themselves into the community.

Community Residential Care Homes

In Chapter 2, we discussed at length assisted living facilities and the difficulty of defining what a typical assisted living facility is. Given the fact that (1) there are many different sponsors of assisted living facilities and many reasons for their entering the business of assisted living, (2) there are many different models of care provided and many variations within those models, and (3) different state governments are creating or modifying assisted living facilities by their payment rules and licensing laws, it is impossible to identify the needs of these organizations across the board. However, according to Wilson (2007), there are three essential components of assisted living: (1) a *residential environment* that provides for a resident's private space as well as public community spaces shared by all residents, (2) an *operating philosophy* that emphasizes a resident's choices and normal lifestyle, and (3) a *service capacity* that delivers routine services as well as specialized health-related services. Given this commonality, we can suggest that the need of assisted living facilities is to improve their commitment and performance in these areas.

We are focusing on smaller entities than assisted living facilities that we have called *community residential care homes*. These are also viable residential alternatives to institutional care. For several reasons, however, they have not received the recognition and support they deserve. While discussing adult foster care, McCoin (1995) said that this type of care suffers from

> the unsocial Darwinistic ethos of being (a) small, (b) qualitatively oriented, and (c) cost-effective. These qualities are antithetical to the "bigness" which seems so necessary to feed that survival of the greediest forces tantamount in today's quantitative/computer/information/politically correct age. (p. 3)

Most public expenditures for long-term care go to institutions, and the nursing home industry sucks up a large proportion of the Medicaid budget. In 2008, 40.6% of the nursing home expenditure of $138.4 billion came from Medicaid (National Center for Health Statistics, 2010b). Whereas nursing homes are paid directly from Medicaid, much of the funding for community residential care comes from the residents' Supplemental Security Income, a much smaller source. These residential care homes lack the organization and voice of the powerful nursing home industry. The advent of the National Association of Residential Care Facilities is an attempt to organize the industry, but this organization is still in its infancy. The major need of these facilities is to organize themselves, improve their visibility, and increase their resources.

Although community residential care homes do provide a family-like atmosphere for their residents, no clear evidence suggests that those residents are integrated into the family of the operator. These settings vary considerably, even in the degree of warmth and family-like atmosphere. Some are like boarding homes, and others are like homes. Ample evidence does suggest, however, that community integration of adults with mental illness and mental retardation residing in the various noninstitutional community living settings has not happened. These settings will need to work for this integration.

Nevertheless, community residential care is proving to be an appropriate and less restrictive option for most children and youths who cannot live with their natural families. Foster care homes serve as the hub of a network of developmental and therapeutic connections for these children (Hess, 1994). This success can be attributed to the training, supervision, and support for the care providers. Similarly, the success of community residential care homes for the elderly sponsored by the Department of Veterans Affairs results from the careful recruitment, training, and ongoing support of "sponsors." Sickman and Dhooper (1991) found that a significantly higher percentage of sponsors who had undergone formal health care training were more competent than those without such training. These settings must improve their performance through systematic training and support. They must ensure that the nurturing environments they provide for those in their care are age appropriate and not infantilizing.

The major future needs of community residential care homes are

1. improving their visibility,
2. increasing their resources, and
3. improving their performance.

Facilities Providing Home-Based and Near Home-Based Care

As is evident from our earlier discussion, there are many variations in the arrangement and provision of home-based services. On the one hand, services provided by hospices are marked by appropriateness, comprehensiveness, coordination, and sensitivity. On the other hand, service goals of many other home care agencies are more often related to the priorities of payers than to the needs of those being served. Even the services approved for payment often lack coordination. In this section, we first discuss the needs of these agencies and then identify the needs of hospices.

Most Facilities Providing Home-Based Care

Several models of home-based care have been proposed, with different rationales, philosophies, and approaches (Malone-Rising, 1994). These models are a definite improvement over the simplistic approach reflected, for example, in Brody's (1977) statement that "the 'well aged' went to homes for the aged, the physically ill to nursing homes, and the mentally impaired to state and private psychiatric hospitals" (p. 262). The narrow perspective of the dominant service model, however, results in the neglect of needs not emphasized by that model. The long-term care needs often are seen as either health or social, as if the two dimensions of life are independent and separate and must compete with each other. Neither the health nor the social service model adequately addresses the functional needs of service recipients.

In Chapter 2, we mentioned studies showing that home- and community-based services are (1) cost-effective and helpful to persons recuperating from a hospital stay; (2) effective in reducing hospital admissions, lengths of stay, and readmission of psychiatric patients; and (3) protective of the physical and mental health of the frail and disabled elderly, reducing their risk for placement in nursing homes. We also discussed the various measures undertaken to improve the quality of in-home care. However, variance in the quality of care is a reality. There is evidence that some home-based care is marked by not only inefficiencies but also shortcomings of a more serious nature, such as unprofessional and criminal behavior of care providers. Although incidents of physical injury, inappropriate care, financial exploitation, intimidation, and disrespect by the care provider may not be frequent, this type of care tends to result in the loss of autonomy and independence of service recipients. Home care agencies must address these quality-of-care issues in view of the following factors.

Home care will continue to be viewed as cost-effective and financially more desirable than institutional care. Almost 6,500 Medicare-certified home health agencies existed in 1993; this number represents a more than 600% increase over the number of such agencies on record at the end of 1966, Medicare's first year (Balinsky, 1994). Since then, the number of Medicare-certified home health agencies has declined and risen because of changes in the Medicare home health coverage and reimbursement. At the end of 2009, there were 10,581 such agencies. When the numbers of Medicare-certified home health agencies, Medicare-certified hospices, and non-Medicare agencies providing care in the home are combined, there now are more than 33,000 providers serving about 12 million individuals (National Association for Home Care & Hospice, 2010). As in the past, proponents of health care reform will continue to advocate for the expansion of home care. The demand for this type of care will rise also because the advances in health care technology will make it increasingly possible to care for more and more sick persons at home who currently must be treated in hospitals and nursing homes. Already, those on dialysis, intravenous chemotherapy, total parenteral nutrition, and ventilators are being cared for at home.

At the individual client level, this care will continue to appeal to people's desire to remain in familiar surroundings, carry on with many activities of daily living, and retain the ability to make small decisions about daily life, such as when to get up, what to wear, what and when to eat, when and what to watch on television, and if or when to turn off the light (Balinsky, 1994; Brickner, 1978). Our forecast about the leaner structure and weaker natural resources of the family in the future also suggests that the basic care provided by family members in the past will not be available in the future. Agencies providing home-based care will be needed for providing more and more of the basic care. They will be seen as helping families stay together.

The need for improvement in the quality of services by in-home and near-home care agencies can be viewed from two angles: one broad and the other narrow. The broad view is represented by the movement away from *quality assurance* and toward *continuous quality improvement* or *total quality management*. The Joint Commission on Accreditation of Health Care Organizations has created new sets of conditions for accreditation that reflect the philosophy of care that continuous quality improvement represents. It is based on the premise that "if it ain't broke, it can still be improved" (O'Leary, 1991a, p. 74). Continuous quality improvement demands that customers come first, which means that the organization must have a formal process that enables it to meet all customer needs and expectations. No longer is the order of priorities structure, process, and outcome; instead, outcome comes first, process second, and structure last (Kirsch & Donovan, 1992). This requirement involves fundamental changes, and all health care organizations will need to prepare for and implement those changes. The narrower view brings to light the major shortcomings of most in-home and many near-home long-term care agencies. Their major needs are

1. improving their assessment of client needs/problems,

2. increasing their ability to provide comprehensive and well-coordinated services, and

3. sharpening their sensitivity to issues of clients' autonomy, independence, and options.

Hospice Care Organizations

These organizations have needs different from those of the home- and community-based agencies discussed above. Of their ongoing needs, the following are the most important.

About 25% of the elderly in the country live in rural areas, and the population of rural America is becoming older (National Advisory Committee on Rural Health and Human Services, 2008). Rural dwellers have less access to and utilize hospice services at much lower rates than do those living in urban areas (Casey, Moscovice, Virnig, & Durham, 2005). Another study (Virnig, Moscovice, Durham, & Casey, 2004) found that rates of hospice care before death were negatively associated with the degree of rurality. The lowest rate of hospice use, 15.2%, was seen in rural areas not adjacent to an urban area, compared with 17% in rural areas adjacent to an urban area and 22.2% in urban areas.

A study by Virnig, Ma, Hartman, Moscovice, and Carlin (2006) used a Bayesian smoothing technique to estimate the ZIP-code-level service area for each Medicare-certified hospice in the United States. They combined these areas to identify ZIP codes not served by any hospice. Their findings are quite revealing. Among the ZIP codes of most urban areas of more than 1,000,000 people, 100% are served by hospice (i.e., 0% are unserved). In comparison, 2.8% of the ZIP codes in urban areas of fewer than 1,000,000 people are unserved by hospice, 9% of ZIP codes in rural areas adjacent to urban areas are unserved, and almost 24% of ZIP codes in rural areas are unserved. About 332,000 elders

live in areas not served by a hospice. More than 15,000 deaths occur in these unserved areas every year. Casey et al. (2005) have estimated that almost one fourth of the 1.7 million elderly Medicare beneficiaries who die every year are rural dwellers.

There are also significant barriers between hospice care services and culturally different minority groups such as African Americans, Latinos, and others, resulting in a lack of access to those services for large numbers of those Americans (Colon, 2005; Reese, Ahern, Nair, O'Faire, & Warren, 1999). For example, Johnson, Kuchibhatla, and Tulsky (2009) surveyed 200 community-dwelling older adults (white, $n = 95$; black, $n = 105$) and found racial differences in their self-reported exposure to information about hospice care. Cohen (2008) did a systematic review of studies that examined rates of hospice use by minority patients compared with white patients. Out of 13 studies, 12 found differences in hospice use between minorities and whites. The major needs of hospice care organizations are

1. improving hospice access to people living in rural areas and

2. reducing barriers to hospice services for minority patients.

Table 3-C shows the differential needs of the three groups of long-term care providers.

Social workers have much to give the long-term care sector as well as hospice care organizations. Because the major recipients of long-term care services are the elderly and persons with disabilities, social workers can contribute their (a) understanding of the needs of these populations, (b) grasp of the major philosophical shifts in the field of disabilities, (c) comprehensive perspective on clients' reality (encompassing both the person and the environment as well as a life span view), and (d) skills in effectively working with these groups. The social work client-worker relationship can become the model for equal partnership between clients and helpers. Social workers also can help long-term care agencies improve their visibility and community

Table 3-C Future Needs of Long-Term Care Facilities

Nursing Homes	Improving their public image
	Becoming a part of an integrated continuum of services
	Extending themselves into the community
Community Residential Care Homes	Improving their visibility
	Increasing their resources
	Improving their performance
Facilities Providing Home-Based Care	Improving their assessment of client needs/problems
	Increasing their ability to provide comprehensive and well-coordinated services
	Sharpening their sensitivity to issues of clients' autonomy, independence, and options
Hospice Care Organizations	Improving hospice access to people living in rural areas
	Reducing barriers to hospice services for minority patients

image, and can make significant contributions to the efforts of hospice organizations in dealing with their problems.

FUTURE NEEDS OF HEALTH CARE PROVIDERS ACROSS SETTINGS

To meet their needs, health care organizations of the future will require the services of personnel who have the necessary knowledge, skills, and commitment. These assets, generally specialized and profession specific, often have to be tailored to the needs of specific client groups for optimal effectiveness. Here, we discuss the major future needs of health care providers on the basis of projections about (a) major consumers of health care services, (b) the state of the art and science of medical and health care, and (c) quality-of-life issues.

Major Consumers of Health Care Services

The major consumers of health care services that most care providers, to varying degrees, will have to know and understand fall broadly into the following groups: (a) the elderly; (b) nonelderly with disabilities; (c) victims of social problems such as homelessness, violence, and alcohol and drug abuse; (d) victims of AIDS and similar new diseases; (e) children; and (f) new immigrants. These groups are likely to be heavy users of all types and levels of health care.

The Elderly

A substantial proportion of the U.S. population in the future will be made up of the elderly, as the 65+ population will double between 2000 and 2050. Those 85 and older are already the most rapidly growing group of the elderly, and it is forecast that their number will double to 8.4 million by 2030 and quadruple by 2050. Although the majority of the elderly will be women, they will not be a homogeneous group; they will reflect the cultural, ethnic, and religious diversity that will characterize the United States in the future. Some facts about the elderly relevant for health care providers are as follows:

- Those 65 and older are substantial users of in-hospital services. In 2007, while accounting for just 13% of the U.S. population, they accounted for 37% of hospital discharges and 43% of the days of care (Hall, DeFrances, Williams, Golosinskiy, & Schwartzman, 2010).
- Despite the centrality of older patients to the economic health of hospitals, most hospitals traditionally have not been good at serving geriatric clients. The following quote from Vladeck (1988) still holds some truth:

  Perhaps most importantly, the increasing body of experience with home- and community-based long-term care services continually reminds us of the capacity of hospitals to mess up even the best-managed long-term care cases. Sooner or later, frail elderly long-term care clients are going to end up in the hospital for treatment of acute problems, and in such instances even care that is minimally adequate by prevailing professional standards may undo months of successful service in terms of functional dependency, self-esteem and self-image, management of depression, or even cognitive orientation and functioning. (p. 42)

- Older adults are highly susceptible to iatrogenic illness.
- Most elderly, when hospitalized, tend to experience confusion and a sense of loss of control. The unfamiliarity of the hospital may precipitate mental confusion, and hospital routines may enforce dependency and disrupt self-care patterns.
- Physical illness necessitating hospitalization may come on the heels of loss of family, friends, and valued roles that the elderly patient was struggling to cope with.
- Any acute episode of illness experienced by older adults may trigger stress-related deterioration and loss of functional ability.

- The primary health problems of older adults are chronic—for example, heart conditions, high blood pressure, hearing loss, glaucoma or cataracts, arthritis, and diabetes. Nearly 90% have at least one chronic condition, and nearly 70% have two or more coexisting conditions (Johns Hopkins University, 2004).
- The acuity of all five senses declines with age, independent of disease.
- Besides multiple chronic illnesses, vulnerabilities of the elderly include large numbers living under conditions of poverty (which adversely affects morbidity and mortality) and being less educated as a group, thereby lacking health literacy (Chen & Landefeld, 2007).
- Depression is common among the elderly. It outweighs physical illness as a risk factor for suicide in late life (Fiske, O'Riley, & Widoe, 2008).
- Maintaining good health consistently is ranked by older adults among their top three priorities, and independent functioning is extremely important to most of them.
- Despite all kinds of reasons against the idea of preventive work with the elderly, it is not only possible but also necessary to consider illness prevention and health promotion work focused on the elderly.
- Elder abuse is being recognized as a serious social problem. With longer-living elderly asserting their claim to societal resources, younger generations becoming resentful of them, the traditional caregivers becoming less available, and caregiving becoming more impersonal, the elder abuse situation will worsen.
- Needs of the elderly are manifold, and no agency's own resources are likely to be adequate to meet all these needs; hence the necessity for knowing about the programs and resources of other organizations, and cooperating and collaborating with them.

Nonelderly With Disabilities

Persons with disabilities are a large, noncohesive group whose members may have only one thing in common. Each has a disability and meets the following criteria: He or she (1) has a physical or mental impairment that substantially limits one or more life activities, (2) has a record of such impairment, and (3) is generally regarded as having impairment. Because of their disability, however, persons with disabilities are vulnerable and share the chronicity of their problems. It is estimated that about 46 million Americans are physically, mentally, or emotionally disabled (Huff, 2010). The following are a few salient facts that should inform health care providers' involvement with persons with disabilities.

- Classifying disabilities into clear-cut, neat groups is difficult. For example, although most physical disabilities fall into three anatomical categories—involving the skeletal system, the muscular system, and the neuromuscular system—some involve more than one anatomical category, and others are independent of these systems.
- The classification of the developmentally disabled includes those with mental retardation, autism, cerebral palsy, epilepsy, and neurological impairment (Velleman, 1990). Public Law 95-502 (Rehabilitation, Comprehensive Services, and Developmental Disabilities Amendments of 1978) defines a developmental disability in terms of functional limitations:

A severe, chronic disability of a person which (a) is attributable to a mental or physical impairment or combination of mental and physical impairments; (b) is manifested before the person attains age 22; (c) is likely to continue indefinitely; (d) results in substantial functional limitations in three or more of the following areas of major life activity: (1) self-care, (2) receptive and expressive language, (3) learning, (4) mobility, (5) self-direction, (6) capacity for independent living, and (7) economic self-sufficiency; and (e) reflects the person's need for combination and sequence of special, interdisciplinary, or generic care, treatment, or other services which are of lifelong or extended duration and are individually planned and coordinated.

- The medical problem necessitating hospitalization for patients with disabilities is superimposed on the existing disability. Its etiology, nature, and consequence must be understood in the context of that disability, and treatment must accommodate the limitations caused by the disability.
- Disability does not make persons with disabilities less human. They should be treated with the same consideration and dignity as others, as persons who *happen to have a disability.* Levitas and Gilson (1987) said people with mental retardation often are treated as if cognitive development is the only dimension of their lives.
- When a person with a disability requests a disability-related service, it may not always be clear if the requested service must be provided under the guidelines of the ADA (Americans with Disabilities Act). In general, if clients without disabilities are eligible for a service, then the person with a disability can expect the same level of service. Most institutions have an ADA compliance officer who can provide answers to case-specific questions. Most accommodations required under the law are made on an individual basis. Therefore, agency personnel, the ADA compliance officer, and the client with a disability should decide jointly on accommodations. If an accommodation is likely to cause undue burden on the agency, then the parties involved should agree to compromise (Huff, 2010).

In the future, advances in medical and health care will save many more from death but not from disabilities; therefore, the number of people with disabilities will grow. They will need services from all types of health care settings for their share of health problems. Care providers must know that people with disabilities may be alike in the social consequences of their disabilities but that each is different in the nature of his or her problem and the range of functional abilities.

Victims of Social Problems

Poverty in all its manifestations, violence in all its forms, and abuse of all kinds of harmful substances will continue to plague the United States in the future. All these problems are interrelated. In a study of 443 impoverished medical patients, Gelberg and Leake (1993) found that 24% were frequent alcohol users and 18% had used illegal drugs recently. Other associated variables included a previous felony conviction and psychiatric hospitalization. We earlier alluded to the health consequences of poverty and homelessness and to the role of alcohol and drug abuse in the incidence of injury, death, and disease. Health care providers—hospital-based providers more than others—will continue to deal with victims of these problems. They will need to know who these patients are.

In Chapter 1, we discussed at length the incidences and consequences of the various types of person abuse—child abuse, partner/spouse abuse, and elder abuse. Here, we look at poverty. Poverty has many faces. As Harrington (1987) put it, "Poverty is an 'integrated' problem: Over two thirds of the poor are white and just under one third are black, Hispanic, Asian, and American Indian. But minority people are significantly overrepresented among people in poverty" (p. 14). The problem of poverty will persist in the future and will continue at higher rates among people of color than among whites. Many of them will continue to "live in a world of self-contained, self-reinforced misery, victims of the hopelessness and the violence which accompanies extreme deprivation" (p. 15). To appreciate the reality of poverty, one can look at homelessness—poverty's most blatant manifestation.

The Homeless

It is estimated that 3.5 million people in the United States are homeless. Even this may be a conservative estimate because many homeless families live in cars, campgrounds, or motels. They avoid contact with social service agencies for fear of losing their children and so are not counted among the homeless (Edelman & Mihaly, 1989). The homeless are not only the skid row alcoholics and happy wanderers they used to be viewed as. Homelessness has the following characteristics:

- The homeless are likely to be younger, more ethnically diverse, and more likely to be members of families than in the past. They include higher proportions of women and minorities and a growing number of people with full-time jobs.

- Among the homeless, 17% are women, who are often victims of domestic violence and sexual abuse. They lack education, affordable housing, child care, and medical care. Many times, they suffer from drug abuse and mental illness. When they are turned away from shelters that are filled to capacity, they often are left with no other option than to attempt to survive on the streets. While the root causes of homelessness, such as poverty, lack of affordable housing, and lack of state support, apply to all homeless populations, domestic violence and sexual abuse impact women disproportionately (Richards, Garland, Bumphus, & Thompson, 2010). An extensive survey of 743 families residing in 14 emergency and transitional family shelters in New York City and northern New Jersey revealed a typical homeless parent to be a young unmarried mother who

1. grew up in poverty;

2. experienced or witnessed domestic violence at some point in her life;

3. never completed high school, often dropping out because of pregnancy;

4. has two or three young children;

5. has at least one child suffering from a chronic health problem;

6. had lived with parents, with a partner, or doubled up prior to becoming homeless;

7. had left her last residence because of overcrowding, a disagreement, or domestic violence;

8. is unemployed because of lack of child care, a lack of work skills, or an inability to find a job; and

9. is entirely dependent on public assistance to support herself and her family (Nunez, 1998, p. 72).

- Women interested in contraception often experience barriers in their effort to prevent pregnancy (Gelberg et al., 2001). Pregnancy can be a challenge for homeless women. Smid, Bourgois, and Auerswald (2010) documented 26 pregnancy outcomes for 13 homeless women (ages 18–26). Of the 26 pregnancies, 8 were voluntarily terminated, 3 were miscarried, and 15 were carried to term. The majority of women who carried to term lost custody of their newborns. Most of those who terminated successfully had sought safe medical care.

- The National Center on Family Homelessness estimates that as many as 1 in 50 U.S. children (1.5 million) are homeless or "precariously housed." Child poverty impacts the development of children negatively, and homelessness further worsens the situation. Both child poverty and family homelessness have been increasing over the past three decades. A study by Schmitz, Wagner, and Menke (2001) found that homelessness leaves children feeling a decreased sense of support and an increased sense of isolation.

- Homeless women are at high risk for physical and sexual assaults. A study by Hudson and her colleagues (2010) assessed the predictors of such assaults. Homeless women with a history of childhood sexual abuse were almost four times more likely to report being sexually assaulted as adults and were two and one third times more likely to report being physically assaulted as adults. Besides childhood sexual abuse, other factors that increase their risk of victimization include substance abuse, lifetime sex trade activity, and previous incarceration.

- *"Homelessness* is a convenient term for those suffering from a range of physical and mental health problems" (Kelly, 2001, p. 229). Health and mental health problems abound in the homeless. A study of the users of four of Detroit's largest homeless shelters found that the homeless had many physical health problems, abused drugs and alcohol, and suffered psychological distress. Dental and vision problems were the most prevalent, followed by neurological, gastrointestinal, and female reproductive problems. Alcohol abusers were significantly more likely to have low blood pressure, symptoms of liver disease, and a history of tuberculosis treatment (Harris, Mowbray, & Solarz, 1994). The history of homelessness—number of homeless episodes, length of time being homeless, and length of time living in unsheltered conditions—has profound effects on the health and use of health services of homeless adults. In general, they are exposed to excessive levels of risk factors for physical illness, such as use of alcohol, illegal drugs, and cigarettes; inadequate nutrition; exposure to contagious diseases such as tuberculosis, hepatitis C and B, and HIV; exposure to the elements; sleeping in an upright position; and walking in poor-fitting shoes (Arangua & Gelberg, 2007). Homeless children experience a higher number of such illness symptoms as fever, ear infections, diarrhea, and asthma. McLean (2004) found that 40% of homeless children in New York City had asthma, which is six times the rate for the general population.

- Physical and mental health problems are much more prevalent among homeless youths. They are also more likely to be exposed to violence and drug use at an early age (Cohen, 2009). Mental health problems they suffer from include poor coping skills, suicidal tendencies, depression, and substance abuse (Arangua & Gelberg, 2007). They have the highest frequency of pregnancy: For girls aged 14 to 17, 48% of those living on the streets and 33% of those living in shelters reported having been pregnant, compared with 10% of those who were housed (Greene & Ringwalt, 1998, as cited in Arangua & Gelberg, 2007).

- A national survey done in 1993 to 1994 and repeated in 2001 found no significant difference in the prevalence of homelessness. Respondents in 2001 had less stereotyped views of homeless people and were more supportive of services for them (Tompsett, Toro, Guzicki, Manrique, & Zatakia, 2006). However, in many cities, policies toward the homeless are hostile and often vicious. The homeless also experience attacks by people, especially young people, and those attacks often result in injuries and even deaths (Kelly, 2001). More than half the homeless reported having been criminally victimized in the past year, compared with 37% of the general population (Burt et al., 1999).

- Homeless shelters are society's response to the problem of homelessness, and the quality of services they provide varies. Relying on field observations and qualitative interviews with shelter residents, DeWald and Moe (2010) analyzed the nuanced ways in which the institutionalization of shelters complicates women's effort to survive homelessness.

- There are ongoing efforts to understand the phenomenon of homelessness and approaches to dealing with this problem. Melamed, Shalit-Kenig, Gelkopf, Lerner, and Kodesh (2004) have developed the concept of *mental home-lessness* to capture the connection between mental illness and housing. They hold that homelessness is a state of mind of which actual physical homelessness may be a manifestation. If a mental patient owns a home, he or she is at high risk of somehow losing it. The HomeBuy5 Program is an approach that has helped many homeless families find an apartment while developing a plan to move them to homeownership (Davey & Ivery, 2009).

- Health care providers in many settings and programs will continue to see the victims of social problems and must learn to relate to them with sensitivity and understanding.

Victims of AIDS and Similar New Diseases

At least for the next few decades, AIDS will continue as a compelling reality. The health and human services professionals will continue to be challenged by the suffering and tragedy at the individual patient/client level and by the social, economic, and political ramifications of this disease for their agencies and programs. Even after a vaccine and a cure for AIDS have been found, the health care system will continue to be challenged by other diseases of the immune system. Service providers in hospitals, outpatient programs, and long-term care facilities will continue being involved in the treatment and care of the victims of those diseases. They will need to look for more effective ways of serving these victims and their families, as well as ways to survive the emotional stress of that work. They must address such complex, persistent, and at times overwhelming themes/concerns as (a) their attitude toward homosexual lifestyles, as well as the fear of being stigmatized because of their work with homosexual patients; (b) their feelings about drug users; (c) their attitude toward women with AIDS; (d) sexuality and intimacy; (e) death and dying; and (f) existential issues such as quality of life, meaning of life, loneliness, isolation, and abandonment (Dworkin & Pincu, 1993).

The following are a few salient facts about AIDS:

- Even more than 25 years into the AIDS epidemics, the prevalence and incidence of HIV/AIDS underscore its power. An estimated 1,039,000 to 1,185,000 people are living with HIV/AIDS in the United States. AIDS is no longer the death sentence it was in the past, but living with it is not easy (Norris, 2010).

- AIDS is no longer the disease of homosexual males concentrated in a few large cities, but a vast majority of its victims (74%) continues to be men. Rural gays and younger gays who do not see themselves as being at risk and men who have sex with other men but do not openly identify themselves as gay are hidden populations that must be given special attention. Of all these male AIDS victims, 45% had sex with other men but did not identify themselves as gay, 27% were infected through high-risk heterosexual contact, 22% were infected through intravenous drug use, and 5% were exposed through sex with other men and intravenous drug use (Norris, 2010).

- Demographic shifts have occurred in the prevalence of HIV infection, with a move from homosexual males to injection drug users—males and females, non-drug-using women, and children. Thus, most injection drug users are at high risk for AIDS. However, victims of AIDS include heterosexuals, both male and female, young and old, white and nonwhite, drug users and drug free, living in urban as well as rural areas. Adolescents are at great risk for the spread of HIV. Other populations of concern are runaways, prostitutes, the homeless, older persons, and those with disabilities.

- Larger proportions of minorities (Hispanic and black), both male and female, are represented among HIV-positive and AIDS patients. For instance, in 2006, the rate of new HIV infection among Latinos was three times that of whites, and in 2005, HIV/AIDS was the fourth leading cause of death for Latino men and women aged 35 to 44 (Norris, 2010). Minorities are likely to continue to be among the major groups of sufferers.

- HIV/AIDS patients are admitted to hospitals for different reasons. Some are admitted because they are too ill to be cared for at home. Others do not know that they have AIDS, but their hospitalization for another illness confirms the diagnosis of AIDS. These reasons create different case dynamics and call for differential interventions.

- Men and women experience differential side effects from AIDS treatment. Women are more prone to lipodystrophy (also called fat redistribution) than are men and experience more dramatic changes in body configuration. Changes in physical appearance can cause them additional stress (Mathews, 2003). They also can have a significant sense of loss—loss of potential love relationships, of family and friends, and of a future with children and grandchildren (Beder, 2006).
- Women also have concerns about their children related to (1) their current or future inability to perform caretaking roles, (2) the fear that they might have inadvertently infected their children while pregnant or through breastfeeding, (3) the difficulty of telling their children of their HIV status, and (4) the effect on the children of the social stigma associated with HIV.
- In many cases, children and adolescents with AIDS feel guilty about having the disease, about their past behavior and lifestyle, and about the possibility of having infected others. They experience sadness, hopelessness, helplessness, isolation, and depression (Lockhart & Wodarski, 1989).

Children

In the future, the proportion of children (those younger than age 18) in the total population (currently 25%) will decline to 23% in 2050, and as a nation, the United States will value children more than it does now. However, in view of the complexity and general lack of stability of the family, ensuring the health and well-being of children will continue to be a societal challenge. Now, almost 44% of children are racial or ethnic minorities, who typically lag behind others in many indicators of well-being. It is forecast that in 15 years, minorities will make up more than half the nation's child population. Despite the progress made during the 20th century, the United States lags behind

many other industrialized countries on major indicators of child health. Among 30 industrialized nations, the United States is

28th in infant mortality rates (the second highest),

21st in low birth-weight rates,

last in relative child poverty,

last in the gap between the rich and the poor,

last in adolescent birth rates (ages 15–19), and

last in protecting children against gun violence.

Other painful facts about U.S. children include the following:

- Every 19 seconds, a baby is born to an unmarried mother (i.e., 4,498 babies are born to unmarried mothers each day).
- Every 32 seconds, a baby is born into poverty (i.e., 2,692 babies are born into poverty each day).
- Every 41 seconds, a child is confirmed as abused or neglected (i.e., 2,175 children are confirmed as abused or neglected each day).
- Every 6 hours, a child is killed by abuse or neglect (i.e., four children are killed by abuse or neglect each day).
- Every 19 seconds, a child is arrested (i.e., 4,435 children are arrested each day).
- Every minute, a baby is born to a teen mother (i.e., 1,210 babies are born to teen mothers each day).
- Every minute, a baby is born at low birth weight (i.e., 964 babies are born at low birth weight each day).
- Every 4 minutes, a child is arrested for a drug offense (i.e., 377 children are arrested for drug offenses each day).
- Every 7 minutes, a child is arrested for a violent crime (i.e., 202 children are arrested for a violent crime each day).
- Every 18 minutes, a baby dies before his or her first birthday (i.e., 78 babies each day die before their first birthday).
- Every 45 minutes, a child or teen dies from an accident (i.e., 32 children or teens die from accidents each day).
- Every 3 hours, a child or teen is killed by a firearm (i.e., nine children or teens are killed by a firearm each day).

- Every 5 hours, a child or teen commits suicide (i.e., five children or teens commit suicide every day; Children's Defense Fund, 2010).

In Chapter 1, we discussed the extent of poverty among children and its adverse physical, psychological, and emotional effects on them. Similarly, we have discussed the ill effects of the problem of child abuse (physical, sexual, and emotional) and neglect. Children who are born poor, at low birth weight, and, thus, without a healthy start in life can fall behind developmentally and have trouble catching up—socially, emotionally, and academically. They fall behind and drop out. Others may be abused or neglected and grow up in foster care. They are more likely to end up in the juvenile justice system. They all face multiple risks that jeopardize their futures. Unmet health and mental health needs greatly increase the likelihood of a child entering the cradle-to-prison pipeline (Children's Defense Fund, 2010). Problems children face are likely to persist in the future. Health care providers will share the responsibility of ensuring the well-being of children.

New Immigrants

In Chapter 1, we discussed reasons why the current rate of immigration is likely to stay steady in the future and why more new people will continue to make this country their home. They will come from all over the world—most from Spanish-speaking lands and islands, and Asian countries, and some from Europe and Africa. Hispanic immigrants will come from North America (Mexico), Central America, the Caribbean islands, South America, and Europe (Spain). Asian and Pacific Islander immigrants will come from 28 different Asian countries and 25 islands in the Pacific. The countries they will come from have different geographical conditions, histories, stages of economic development, customs, languages, religions, and degrees of exposure to Western culture and the English language (Dhooper & Moore, 2001). They will come during periods when immigrants are

welcome and accepted and during times when anti-immigration sentiment prevails and newcomers are resented and rejected. Like others before them, they will experience overt or covert popular and institutional prejudice and discrimination because their looks, speech, customs, and behaviors are different from those of mainstream Americans.

Newcomers bring not only their dreams and hopes for a brighter future and the energy and enthusiasm to make their dreams a reality but also a package full of health-related assets and liabilities. What follows is a list of some of the liabilities. (Most of this material was taken from Dhooper, 2003.)

- Many immigrants bring with them diseases endemic to their native lands, which persist. These can include tuberculosis, hepatitis B, and parasitic infestation.
- Many hold different health beliefs and subscribe to non-Western theories of health and illness.
- Many are unfamiliar with the Western approaches to treatment of illnesses, disease prevention, and wellness. A study of the Southeast Asian population in central Ohio found that 94% of the subjects did not know what blood pressure was, and 85% did not know what could be done to prevent heart disease (Chen, Kuun, Guthrie, Wen, & Zaharlick, 1991).
- Some belong to cultures where certain illnesses are denied and disowned. This is true of both mental and physical illnesses. For instance, some Asian communities believed that HIV was culturally foreign to them or that they were somehow immune to the virus that caused AIDS (Gock, 1994).
- In some cultures, suffering is viewed as inevitable in life and even ennobling for the human soul. Those holding such views tend to ignore their illness and do not seek help.
- New immigrants are unfamiliar with the American health care system and have inadequate exposure and access to it.
- The loss of the extended social support system they had and were used to in their native lands adversely affects their ability to deal with health issues.

- Many acquire new diseases because of the changes in their lifestyle and living conditions.
- They are vulnerable to the physical effects of acculturation-related stress.
- For those who come as refugees, "there is a layer of preimmigration stresses such as the loss of country, home, family, friends, and a way of life and severe forms of physical and emotional trauma" (Dhooper, 2003, p. 65). These add to their problems of survival and acculturation with health consequences.

Their assets, which can be built on when working with them, include the following:

- Most are happy and grateful for their immigration to this country. They want to prove they are worthy of their new status by working hard and doing whatever being "good Americans" entails. They are willing to learn the American way in various dimensions of life.
- In most cultures they belong to, education is highly valued. Therefore, they are willing to invest time, energy, and resources in education—their own and that of their children. In view of this commitment, it is easy to show connections among education, health, and prosperity.
- Religion plays a significant role in the lives of most immigrants. Their faith and religious institutions strongly influence their ability to deal with their problems. These can be viewed as positive forces that health care providers can use to their advantage. A priest or a minister can be an ally who can strengthen their efforts. Similarly, an amulet or talisman worn around the neck or special prayers (said by the patient, the family, or a traditional healer) to ward off disease-causing evil spirits can provide a psychological supplement for the medical treatment.
- Family has a special meaning and place in the lives of most of them. They were socialized to think of the family's needs, prestige, stability, and welfare as more important than the individual's aspirations, comfort, and well-being. Patients' commitment to fulfill their familial obligations can be used to motivate and encourage them to seek help and follow through with treatment plans.
- Despite the tension between the new immigrants' expected treatment modalities based on the system of medicine in their native lands (which in many countries simultaneously addresses illness-related aspects of the patient's body, mind, and spirit) and Western medicine's approach to illness, most are willing to accept Western medicine if it can coexist with the approaches of their native system. Health care providers can determine the extent to which other approaches such as acupuncture, herbal treatment, special diets, fasting, yoga, and meditation can coexist with their treatment methodology.

With a sincere desire to understand, respect for their cultures and worldviews, and accommodation of their needs and situations, health care providers can serve new immigrants effectively.

In general, at all levels and in all health care settings, service providers will need to understand the complexity of the problems these different patient groups face. They will need to change their orientation and responsibilities to serve these groups effectively. That orientation will have to be guided by a new vision of patient care, a vision in which they not only provide their piece but also ensure that the piece fits well in the total picture of patient needs and resources. They will need to recognize, understand, and accommodate patients' situations and problems that impinge on their medical and health needs, and coordinate their services with other community sources of care. Recognizing the need for better integration of the different types of health care and the better use of health and social interventions will involve a conceptual change. It will involve unlearning some ways of thinking about people, their problems, and solutions to those problems. For example, to serve the elderly effectively, hospital-based service providers will need to (a) improve their knowledge about the elderly and their sociomedical needs; (b) sharpen their skills to meet those needs; (c) realize that their "traditional motivation to cure must be complemented by the idea that caring rather than curing is the reality of later life, and that maximization of function is the most appropriate goal to achieve" (Eisdorfer & Maddox, 1988, p. 9); (d) appreciate that a comprehensive assessment

of the elderly requires the skills of many professionals working as a team; (e) recognize the
importance of better integration of hospital-based
and community-based care; and (f) accommodate
elderly patients' expectation for sympathy and
understanding, clarity and completeness of communication, sensitivity about their functional
difficulties, comprehensive assessment and intervention, support and guidance in decision making, and ability to balance the use of high-tech
measures with quality-of-life considerations
(American Hospital Association, 1989). What
Eisdorfer and Maddox (1988) said almost 25 years
ago is still valid:

> The practice of adequate medical care for older
> persons must involve the recognition that a differ-
> ent style of practice is needed. This style of prac-
> tice would appreciate the range of variables that
> affect functional capacity and incorporate into
> patient management a similar range of nonmedical
> adaptive approaches—from prostheses to social-
> ization, day care, homemaker services, and
> "friendly visitors." (p. 17)

Similarly, service providers will need to
change their attitudes toward other patient populations, such as the poor, the homeless, the
abused, substance abusers, and new immigrants.
These patients often are viewed as responsible
for their problems. For example, it is not uncommon for health care providers to hold on to such
myths about the poor as (a) only welfare mothers and their children are poor, (b) most welfare
recipients are too lazy to work, and (c) families
on welfare spend their money on luxuries. Nor
is it uncommon for health care professionals to
believe that victims of abuse, rape, and other
forms of violence somehow brought their painful experience on themselves. Health care professionals will need to (a) learn not to be blinded
to the plight of victims by their belief in the
myths, simplistic explanations, and half-truths
about these problems; (b) realize that blaming
the victim does not help in generating patient
trust in the professional and the patient's faith in
him- or herself necessary for the success of the

intervention; (c) understand that, given the deficits of their internal and external resources,
these patients require the use of more intensive,
coordinated, and multidisciplinary skills for
even minimal impact of the intervention; and
(d) consider the coming of these patients for
medical assistance as an opportunity to help them
go beyond the immediate problem.

State of the Art and Science of Medical and Health Care

In the future, advances in biomedical knowledge and health care technology will make the
medical miracles of today commonplace occur-
rences. The ability of physicians to diagnose and
treat most diseases will have improved manifold.
They will be able to detect diseases long before
symptoms of those diseases appear and, thereby,
prevent the degree of damage caused. They also
will be able to monitor the organ functioning of
patients at high risk for failure of those organs.
The therapeutic tools at their disposal will be
many and more sophisticated. They will treat illnesses with more powerful drugs administered in
newer, more reliable, and better-controlled ways.
They will use more sophisticated surgical instruments and techniques, as well as human and
artificial organs and tissues for repair, correction,
and replacement of damaged and diseased body
parts. If the required replacement part is not
available, physicians will have found newer
approaches to keeping a patient alive while he or
she waits for the needed part. For illnesses that
do not respond to chemotherapy and do not lend
themselves to surgical treatment, physicians will
use more powerful radiation and laser treatments
with more effective devices and techniques.
What is high-tech now will be considered old-
fashioned in the future.

To deliver the much more sophisticated high-
tech medicine, physicians of the future will be the
masters of these life-saving machines and techniques, each specializing in the use of a particular
set of machines and methodology for correcting a

particular part of the body. The science of medicine will have reached its pinnacle and, in the process, reduced its practitioners to super-technicians. The tendency to treat the damaged and diseased body parts rather than the whole person will continue to pull physicians away from a holistic view of people and their problems. This pull will persist as a threat to the art of medicine. Physicians will need to discover and rediscover the importance of caring as a vital part of the curing business. High-powered physicians also will experience ambivalence about treating the patient as a partner. This ambivalence and the struggle in the task of combining the caring and the curing—the art and the science of medicine—will be reflected in the behaviors of many other health care providers as well. Studies of hospital-based professionals have found that all professionals are strongly influenced by the attitudes, stances, and behaviors of physicians. Looked at from another perspective, the practice of high-tech medicine also may be a source of frustration for the practitioner. Mishel and Murdaugh (1987) called modern medicine a halfway technology, because, no matter how wonderful, it does not completely cure illness. Patients do live longer, but medical illness often is replaced by psychosocial problems.

In the future, the institution of the family will have undergone so much change that it will be hard to agree on what a "normal" family is. The image of the family as a symbol of cohesion, stability, and everything positive in life will be a thing of the past. People will search for warmth of concern and understanding from all kinds of formal and informal groups and health and human service organizations. Health care organizations, directed by the needs of the consumers of their services, will demand that service providers shift their focus from the problem to the person with the problem. Service providers will need to make that shift and deal with whatever such a shift entails. A more holistic view of the patient and the patient's problems will force physicians and other health care providers to realize that the expertise of any one professional

is inadequate for the job of treating the whole patient and that meaningful sharing and collaboration among many professionals are necessary for effective service. Similarly, determining how medical care will enhance a patient's quality of life will require the input of many disciplines. Hospital-based service providers will need to change many of their attitudes and behaviors accordingly.

Quality-of-Life Issues

Quality of life will become a touchstone for quality of medical and health care services in the future. Health care organizations and professionals will be judged not by the adequacy, correctness, and efficiency of their equipment and procedures but by the outcome of their service as it affects the quality of the patient's life. Emphasis on quality of life in the context of care is growing rapidly. There is a significant change in the definition of success of health care measures.

> Historically, evaluation of the success of medical therapies has focused on specific clinical parameters and survival. However, the recent surge of interest in patient-centered endpoints has generated great support for the medical outcomes movement. Not only clinicians but also payers and managers are interested in assessing outcomes to begin measuring quality of care. (Ganz, Litwin, Hays, & Kaplan, 2007, p. 187)

Outcomes of care are increasingly including health-related quality-of-life variables, and measures of patients' evaluation of the results of health care continue to be developed. According to Ganz et al. (2007), whereas there was not a single publication on the topic of quality of life identified in PubMed in 1972, the database identified 5,399 articles using the "quality of life" key word in 2004.

What is quality of life? There is no consensus about what it is and what it entails. Andrews and Withey (1976) identified more than 800 overlapping dimensions of quality of life. The general concept encompasses a range of human experience: access to daily necessities of life such as food and shelter, intrapersonal and interpersonal response to life events, and activities associated with professional fulfillment and personal happiness (Patrick & Erickson, 1993). A group of researchers at the University of Minnesota have proposed 11 domains of quality of life in long-term care: (1) a sense of safety, security, and order; (2) physical comfort; (3) enjoyment; (4) meaningful activity; (5) reciprocal relationships; (6) functional competence; (7) dignity; (8) privacy; (9) individuality and the ability to express one's identity; (10) autonomy and choice; and (11) spiritual well-being (Kane, 2001).

Today, transplantation of vital organs such as hearts, kidneys, livers, and lungs is considered the miracle of medical care that saves and prolongs life, but does it improve the quality of life of the organ recipient? Divergent views abound. For example, on the one hand, Simmons and Abress (1990) compared 766 patients on one of the three treatment modalities—center dialysis, continuous peritoneal dialysis, and kidney transplantation—and found that transplant patients scored significantly higher on almost all measures of quality of life than both dialysis groups. On the other hand, Baumann, Young, and Egan (1992) studied the recipients of heart transplants and concluded that the experience of living with a heart transplant should be understood as a chronic condition. They found that although life improved for the majority of their sample, transplant recipients continued to experience work problems, financial burdens, family role changes, lifestyle changes, and side effects of the long-term drug treatment. According to Johnson (1990), transplantation does not cure disease: "It extends life by trading one chronic disease (of the organ) for another (a chronically compromised immune system). Under these circumstances, the quality of life for those who survive surgery and their families will vary dramatically" (p. 177).

The necessity for operationalizing the concept of "quality of life" will continue to provide a challenge and an opportunity to health care providers.

> For other caring health professions, such as nursing, social work, and occupational and physical therapy, it [quality of life] provided a firm set of criteria to demonstrate more convincingly their contribution to patient health and well-being. And for medicine, it represents a reaffirmation of one of its most important missions. (Levine, 1987, p. 5)

The objective and the subjective are the two dimensions of quality of life that everyone agrees on. Objective indicators of quality of life include a return to work, functional ability, and health status, whereas subjective indicators of quality of life include well-being, life satisfaction, psychological affect, and happiness (Evans, 1991). Both dimensions, the subjective more than the objective, are influenced by a person's culture—values, worldview, and meaning of life. In the future, the challenge for determining the quality of life of recipients of health care will be monumental. The populations to be served will be much more culturally diverse, and many more people will have chronic problems. The situations demanding the (a) incorporation of the individual's subjective dimension of the quality of life into the decisions for medical care when it is at variance with the ideas and values of professionals, (b) appropriate use of high-cost health care technology, and (c) equitable distribution of technological and other resources will create a host of ethical conflicts and dilemmas for health care providers. Providers will need to seek solutions to such problems from joint deliberations. That will involve sharing with, depending on, and benefiting from everyone's knowledge and skills. Table 3-D below recapitulates the future needs of all health care providers.

In all the problem areas discussed above, social workers can help other health care providers improve their understanding, skills, and performance. A deeper knowledge of the lives and needs of victims of social problems and a unique perspective on ethically challenging situations and quality-of-life issues, as well as a willingness to cooperate, skills for collaboration, and

Table 3-D Future Needs of Health Care Providers Across Settings

- Regarding major consumers of health care services

  The elderly

  Nonelderly with disabilities

  Victims of violence and abuse (child, spouse, and elder abuse)

  The homeless

  Alcohol and drug abusers

  Patients with AIDS and new diseases

  Children

  New immigrants

- Regarding the changing state of the art and science of medical and health care
- Regarding quality-of-life issues

strategies for conflict management, qualify social workers for that helping role. Also, "their grounding in systems theory, expertise in working with diverse systems, knowledge of small group theory, and skills in communication and tension reduction are significant assets" (Dhooper, 1994b, p. 106).

Critical Thinking Questions

1. Given the major philosophical shifts in the fields of gerontology and disabilities, what and how can social work assets (practice principles and methodologies) give social workers an edge over other health care professionals?

2. In some cultures, suffering is not only seen as inevitable but even considered ennobling for the human soul. How can social work philosophy and approaches guide your intervention with individuals holding such beliefs?

4

SOCIAL WORK IN ACUTE CARE

Chapter 3 identified the future needs of health care settings and health care providers. The major needs of acute care hospitals include (a) reorganizing to gain or retain a position of leadership in the community, (b) delivering ambulatory care to the sufferers of chronic medical ailments and victims of social health problems, (c) providing effective and comprehensive patient-as-a-partner as well as family-centered inpatient care, and (d) maintaining a quality of both inpatient and outpatient services that meet the highest professional standards and that are technologically sophisticated, ethically correct, and financially cost-effective. The future needs of hospital-based service providers include (a) understanding their patients, patients' problems, and patients' situations, and relating to their patients as partners; (b) coexisting and teaming up with other professionals to provide comprehensive patient care; (c) knowing how best to deal with ethically problematic patient care situations; and (d) contributing to the hospital's community-oriented activities.

HISTORY OF SOCIAL
WORK IN ACUTE CARE SETTINGS

Acute care generally is provided through emergency rooms, trauma centers, intensive care units, newborn nurseries, general medical and surgical departments, and other specialty care units of hospitals. Emergency rooms, urgent care centers, and outpatient surgery clinics are included among ambulatory care settings. (The past and future of social work roles in those settings are discussed in Chapter 5.) In this chapter, our focus is on hospitals, which are the center of most acute care activity. The presence of social workers in hospitals can be traced back to 1905, when Dr. Richard Cabot hired the first social worker for his clinic at Massachusetts General Hospital in Boston. Dr. Cabot, the chief of medicine at the hospital, believed that the effectiveness of medical treatment depended on a complete diagnosis, for which it was necessary to have information on the patient's home, family, work, and problems. He had been associated with the Boston Children's Aid Society and observed social workers in action. He had listened to their case discussions and studied their case records. "Later, when he saw some of the same children in his clinic, he realized how much better he was able to understand them and their home backgrounds and other environmental factors" (Morris, 1971, p. 90). His venture was considered an experiment. The social work program was referred to as an "unofficial department" in the hospital's 1896 annual report, and funds for it came from Dr. Cabot, his personal friends, and other contributors (Cannon, 1952). The experiment was highly successful, and the social work unit at his hospital became a model for the establishment of similar units in other hospitals across the United States. Within a decade, more than 100 hospitals employed social workers (Barker, 1991). Initially, social workers were not allowed on the hospital wards and were not involved with inpatients. The realization that they could make positive contributions to the care of inpatients came slowly. Massachusetts General Hospital officially recognized social work activities on the wards in 1914.

World War I also created a need for social workers. They were needed in army hospitals overseas to work with injured soldiers and in U.S. Public Health Service hospitals at home to work with returning veterans and their families (Kerson, 1979). In 1920, the American Hospital Association sponsored a formal survey of hospital social services that led to the formation of a committee on training for hospital social workers. The American Association of Hospital Social Workers, formed in 1918, set standards for the curriculum components designed to prepare medical social workers at the schools of social work, several of which had been established by then. The Association also pioneered the working relationship between schools and hospital social service departments regarding students' fieldwork (Bernard, 1977; Shevlin, 1983). In 1928, minimum standards for social service departments were included in the hospital standards published by the American College of Surgeons (Nacman, 1977). The standards of social work practice in hospitals have changed over the years to reflect the evolution of that practice in response to the changing needs of patient populations and hospitals.

From the 1930s on, medicine became increasingly more specialized and resulted in the fragmentation of health care. No one was responsible for coordinating the care a patient could be receiving from many different specialists and facilities simultaneously.

> Patients may as a result receive incompatible medications and conflicting instructions: Families may be treated in an atomized fashion, as though the baby's illness or the father's unemployment had nothing to do with the mother's ulcer, headaches, or mental illness. (Furstenberg, 1984, pp. 28–29)

Although their activities were a part of the solution to the problems of specializations in medicine, social workers were not unaffected by the idea of specialization. Social workers also became more specialized, and "serious fractures between medical and psychiatric social work were well established by the 1940s" (Bracht, 1978, p. 13). During the 1940s and 1950s, social workers became involved in health care teams and comprehensive health care projects to address the lack of coordination of care (Bracht, 1978). By the 1950s, newer illnesses such as heart disease, stroke, and cancers had replaced tuberculosis, polio, and other infectious diseases, and medical care of acute and chronic problems was fusing with the concept of "rehabilitation" (Nacman, 1977). In the 1960s, the civil rights and welfare movements led to changes, including the passage of Medicare and Medicaid, which in turn created more demand for social workers in hospitals. In the 1970s, the establishment of a patient's bill of rights sanctioned the advocacy role of social workers (Nacman, 1977). In the 1980s, societal concern about rising health care costs led to the institution of prospective payment systems (using diagnosis-related groups, or DRGs), social workers became involved in hospitals' utilization review work, and their discharge planning function acquired an unprecedented importance. The problem of providing increasingly technologically sophisticated care and of cutting costs for that care persists.

Throughout its history, while responding to the demands of its environment, hospital social work has created a professional repertoire consisting of theoretical explanations (and a conceptual grasp of the various realities of patients, health care providers, and their institutions), practice principles, models of intervention, strategies, and techniques. The needs of patients and organizations have guided the development of the various models of practice.

Some of these provide general approaches and tools for psychosocial assessment and interventions. Others are site, problem, and population specific. Still others focus on the major social work functions such as case management, interdisciplinary collaboration, discharge planning, documentation, and community liaison. (Dhooper, 1994a, p. 50)

Still others are aimed at improving social workers' effectiveness and efficiency, professional accountability, and autonomy.

The early "friendly visitors" have been succeeded by well-trained, qualified social work practitioners who provide services to patients and their families through a multiplicity of professional techniques. The role of social worker as assistant to the physician has evolved into the social worker as a dynamic contributing member of the interdisciplinary team. (Shevlin, 1983, p. 13)

Despite this impressive history of growth and development, social work has not become a core profession in hospitals and other health care institutions. In view of projections about the demands of the future on hospitals and hospital-based health care providers, where should social work fit into the world of the hospital of tomorrow, what roles should social workers take, and what functions should they perform?

While discussing the domain of social work in the health care field, Meyer (1984) said that the social worker's unit of attention (the individual, family, group, population at risk), social work method (casework, group work, community organization), and social work processes (direct practice, policy analysis, program planning, administration) are not sufficient as explanations of domain because "other disciplines share our interests in all of them, often even in the arena of values . . . that which we have held so dearly and have thought to be uniquely held by social workers" (p. 7). The blurring of professional boundaries, mentioned earlier, will continue in the future. Hence, the search for a social work domain in health care must continue. We as social workers must constantly remind ourselves that we do

have a perspective on the reality of individuals, families, organizations, and communities that is particular to social work.

The bio-psycho-social framework that characterizes our work governs the way we perceive the phenomena, the goals we construct, and the interventions we employ. That is how we recognize the social work domain in whatever field of practice we work in. But domain is not the only territory to be staked out . . . it is not social work because we have planted a flag on it. It is only social work if social workers apply themselves to defining it, to understanding it, to working with it effectively, and to assuming responsibility for it. (p. 11)

Changes in society and health care institutions in the future will offer new opportunities for social workers to define their domain and take responsibility for it. Social workers are qualified to make significant contributions to the efforts of hospitals and hospital-based health care providers to serve their constituents and clients effectively. As Huntington (1986) put it,

Well-trained social workers can work with intrapersonal issues raised by a particular illness or condition, those of body image, stigma, and self-esteem; the interpersonal issues involved in the patient's relationships with his most significant others; the person-institution issues of his relationship to work, education, recreation, and other social institutions; and the person-environment issues of relationship to neighborhood, community, and society. Social work's focus and targets of intervention include institutions and environments outside the patient, which can facilitate or inhibit his well-being. (p. 1155)

FUTURE SOCIAL WORK ROLES IN ACUTE CARE SETTINGS

Social workers will play several roles regarding the needs of acute care settings. The scope of those roles will depend on such factors as the intensity of specific needs; size, purpose, and location of the hospital; and the resources of its social work component. Whether a hospital is a part of a large multihealth corporation or an independent entity will also determine the role of a social work administrator, the scope of social work activities, and the resources for the social work unit.

Multihealth corporations are characterized by horizontal and vertical integration made possible by mergers or takeovers of several health care organizations:

> An example of a health care system that is integrated horizontally and vertically would be a corporation that includes a number of acute care hospitals of varying sizes and with various specialties (horizontal), as well as urgent care centers, a home health care agency, a hospice, a nursing home, and a rehabilitation facility (vertical). (Kenny, 1990, p. 23)

The job of social work administrators in hospitals that are parts of multihealth corporations is likely to be more difficult because of the complexity of the organizational structure and a different set of demands made by the nature, goals, and priorities of the corporation. Kenny (1990) included in those demands the need to balance three, often conflicting, identities: corporate, institutional, and professional. Social work administrators will have to sharpen their skills appropriate for operating within a political arena of multihealth systems. (In Chapter 8, we discuss approaches to gaining and retaining power that social workers, in both administrative and non-administrative positions, will find helpful.) Social work administrators in all hospitals should function as patient advocates at the corporate level and seek to influence the direction of the organization with their expertise and information on psychosocial aspects of patient care, gaps in service, unmet needs, and issues of access (Rosenberg & Clarke, 1987). By doing so, they will be advocates for social work and social workers. They also should diversify their departmental activities and services.

> Strategically, diversification balances the vulnerabilities of our departments. Providing only one

product or service is a risk few can afford. The specialties of today may become extinct tomorrow. Departments that demonstrate sensitivity in meeting the needs of their institution as well as the needs of their clients are most likely to endure. (Butcher, 1995, p. 5)

Although for different reasons, both independent community hospitals and those owned and operated by multihealth corporations will go beyond the traditional boundaries and extend themselves into the community. This expansion will provide social workers excellent opportunities for improving their value for those institutions. Thus, they will widen the definition and scope of their work and take on newer roles while retaining the traditional ones.

Cost consciousness will continue to pervade all hospital operations, and efforts to find ways of maximizing efficiency will be ongoing. Already, many hospitals are experimenting with unit-based management, and physician assistants and nurse practitioners are performing more and more of the functions traditionally seen as a physician's responsibility. Besides being a part of the hospital's newer cost-effective ventures, social workers will critically examine social work functions to determine which of those can be delegated to others who do not have formal social work training. These others may be volunteers and/or less highly paid personnel with or without people-oriented skills. Training and supervision of these assistants or extenders of the social worker will become a part of social work responsibilities.

Social workers will continue their involvement with individual patients and their families (in both inpatient and outpatient programs), and through this case activity, they will act as non-threatening role models for other service providers regarding family-centered comprehensive patient-as-a-partner care. Besides the role of caseworker, they will play many other professional roles, including that of coordinator of services, discharge planner, coordinator of multi- and interdisciplinary teams, advocate, community organizer, consultant, and researcher. These roles will involve the performance of several functions.

Regarding social work roles in relation to the future needs of hospitals and hospital-based health care providers, hospitals will need to (a) venture into the community; (b) provide patient-centered, high-quality care; and (c) meet the special needs of major patient groups. The major need of care providers will be understanding and relating to patients as partners, coexisting with other professionals, and dealing effectively with ethically challenging situations. Table 4-A lists the major future social work roles in hospitals.

Table 4-A   Future Social Work Roles in Hospitals

- Community liaison and community organizer
- Collaborator and consultant
- Discharge planner and resource mobilizer
- Caseworker and counselor
- Demonstrator of patient-as-a-partner and family-centered care
- Contributor to the care of special patient groups

Social Work Role in the Hospital's Expansion Into the Community

The role of social work in hospital expansion into the community will involve such functions as assessment of the community's social health needs, participation in community coalitions for change, participation in planning for community activities, and involvement in joint programs with other agencies demonstrating the hospital's commitment to an integrated network of care, and/or laying the groundwork for its solo efforts. There are many examples of such ventures [1], including an early intervention program for infants with chronic health impairments and developmental disabilities, a pain management clinic, a rehabilitation program for substance abusers, a rape crisis center, a program for abused women, a day hospital for the elderly, and a home health program for the elderly and chronically ill. It is unlikely that all hospitals will offer hospital-based ambulatory programs or venture into joint projects with other community agencies. A hospital's commitment to the provision of comprehensive health care services, however, will give social workers many opportunities to play many more roles than are available today. Social workers will be not only the bridge between the hospital and the community but also the vehicle for taking the hospital into the community. Their major roles will be the hospital's *community liaison* and *community organizer.*

Social Work Role in the Hospital's Patient-Centered High-Quality Care

Examples of efforts by hospitals to create collaborative models of patient care have started appearing in the literature (DiMatteo, Giordani, Lepper, & Croghan, 2002; Gance-Cleveland, 2005; Institute for Family-Centered Care, 2004; Kitchen, 2005; Ponte, Connor, DeMarco, & Price, 2004; Zimmerman & Dabelko, 2007). These models establish mutually beneficial partnerships among patients, family members, and health care providers. The social work role in the hospital's patient-centered high-quality care will require the social worker to act as a collaborator and a consultant. The collaboration will be aimed at bringing about a unity in the diversity of health care professionals and approaches through teamwork. The relevant functions will include (a) coordinating teamwork, (b) exploring the patient-as-a-partner practice, (c) showing and sharing culturally sensitive approaches to patients and their problems, (d) demonstrating family-centered care, (e) planning and monitoring comprehensive services, and (f) dealing with quality-of-life questions and resolving ethical conflicts and dilemmas. Besides work with the patient care team, there will be room for the social worker's contribution to the hospital at the organizational level. He or she will function as a member of its continuous-quality maintenance and ethics committees. The continuous-quality maintenance work will include implementing collaborative models of patient care that emphasize sharing of responsibility in the planning, delivery, and evaluation of health services among patients, families, and care providers.

Consultation will be a case-level as well as an issue-related organizational-level activity. It may be related to the hospital's (a) ambulatory care work—both the ongoing programs (e.g., emergency medical services) and new programs of nonemergency health services, illness prevention, and primary care; (b) quality-assurance and cost-effectiveness activities that would require participation in the utilization and review work and involvement in the work of the ethics committee; and (c) research (disciplinary and interdisciplinary) on patients, their care, and outcomes. The social worker's major roles will be *collaborator* and *consultant.*

Social Work Role in the Hospital's Response to the Needs of Special Patient Groups

The special patient groups that will tax the creativity and resources of hospitals in the future are the elderly, patients with disabilities, those with AIDS, and victims of violence and abuse. These groups have been considered special because they are medically more vulnerable than others. The term *vulnerable* derives from the Latin word for wounded. "In a sense, medically vulnerable populations are those that are wounded by social forces placing them at a disadvantage for their health" (Grumbach, Braveman, Adler, & Bindman, 2007, p. 3). Vulnerable patients experience a triple jeopardy. They are more likely to be ill, more likely to have difficulty accessing care, and more likely to receive suboptimal care (Schillinger, Villela, & Saba, 2007).

The Elderly

Vulnerabilities of the elderly include multiple chronic illnesses, large numbers living under conditions of poverty (which adversely affects morbidity and mortality), and being less educated as a group and thereby lacking health literacy (Chen & Landefeld, 2007). The elderly will continue to be major consumers of hospital services and will demand comprehensive services in terms of both inpatient treatment and after-discharge care. In the future, the elderly will be healthier, better informed, more diverse, more politically active, and generally more assertive than they are today. At the same time, their kinship support networks will be much thinner and weaker because there will be fewer younger people and more of the traditional caregivers will become a part of the workforce.

Social work is the only profession whose primary responsibility is to attend to the psychosocial needs of patients and their families. Every other profession has as its central task the delivery of physical interventions (Brown & Furstenberg, 1992), and "practitioners of psychiatry and geriatric psychotherapy have not yet fully overcome Freud's skepticism about the treatability of those who are aging, despite the vigorous and at times overoptimistic reactions against this skepticism" (Monk, 1981, p. 62). Hence, minimally, hospital-based social workers will (a) enrich the understanding of other professionals about the patient and his or her total situation encompassing medical and psychosocial needs, (b) attend to the psychosocial aspects of the patient's medical condition and hospitalization, and (c) plan for the patient's postdischarge care. As society's recognition of the elder abuse phenomenon increases, they will play an important role in the hospital's organizational response to it. That response may be in creating protocols for dealing with cases of elder abuse or in establishing a multidisciplinary center that ensures specialized assessment and intervention and close collaboration with relevant outside social, legal, and penal agencies.

Patients With Disabilities

Patients with disabilities are not a single group. Disabilities are diverse in their causes, nature, and personal and social implications. *Disability* is an umbrella term for impairments, activity limitations, and participation restrictions. Disability has the potential to affect patient-clinician communication and the treatment plan if the disability is not appropriately incorporated into the plan (Kushel & Iezzoni, 2007). As with the elderly, the medical problem necessitating hospitalization for patients with disabilities is superimposed on the existing disability. Its etiology, nature, and consequence must be understood in the context of that disability, and treatment must accommodate the limitations caused by the disability. Social work in these cases would involve (a) a thorough psychosocial assessment, (b) offering assistance to other professionals in understanding and dealing with the patient, (c) acting as liaison between the hospital and the community service system active with the patient on an ongoing basis, and (d) discharge planning.

Patients With AIDS

Social workers have been pioneers not only in establishing HIV/AIDS services but also "in creating the very definition of AIDS as a biopsychosocial phenomenon that goes beyond an entrenched, narrow biomedical perspective" (Getzel, 1992, p. 2). AIDS is no longer a death sentence, but living with it is not easy.

> Many practical and financial problems have developed for many who spent their life savings, sold their life insurance, resigned from the world of work, and foreclosed relationships, all because they assumed that death was imminent and they did not dare to hope that they may have a future. (Beder, 2006, p. 100)

HIV/AIDS patients are admitted to hospitals because they are too ill to be cared for at home. In the case of hospitalization for another illness that confirms the diagnosis of AIDS, the social worker's activity becomes much more intense. In general, the major areas of hospital-based social work involvement in AIDS cases will continue to be (a) the patient's need to accept and adapt to the reality of his or her illness; (b) the needs of the patient's family; (c) facilitation of access to appropriate financial, housing, home health, transportation, supportive counseling, and other needed services; and (d) discharge planning and case management.

Victims of Violence and Abuse

Admittance of victims of violence and abuse to the hospital depends on the medical seriousness of their injuries. Abused children may be admitted to the hospital until protective services can ensure the safety of their homes or find alternative arrangements for their discharge; most adult victims of violence—abused spouses (victims of intimate partner violence) [2], abused elderly [3], and casualties of street violence—are treated in emergency departments and discharged or transferred to intensive care units for necessary medical and surgical intervention.

Hospitals have clear protocols for dealing with cases of child abuse, and the social work role and functions are specified. The future will see a similar uniform approach to cases of elder abuse and intimate partner violence. The Joint Commission on the Accreditation of Health Care Organizations already requires that, to qualify for accreditation, hospitals have a program in place for identifying and treating patients who are victims of domestic violence. This requirement has not yet created universal compliance. Some hospitals may even have hospital-based special units for serving adult victims of abuse. Minimally, the social work functions will be (a) attending to the psychosocial needs of the victims, (b) mobilizing their social support system, and (c) hooking them up with the appropriate community resources. Social workers can also help in the formulation of institutional protocols for dealing with such cases and for creating special units to serve these patients. The major social work roles regarding these special patient groups will be *clinician, discharge planner,* and *resource mobilizer.*

Social Work Role in Demonstrating Viable Approaches to Patient-as-a-Partner and Family-Centered Care

Social workers will be involved in case activity in both inpatient and outpatient care. Their major case-related functions in inpatient care will include (a) preadmission screening/planning, (b) psychosocial assessment, (c) short-term social work treatment, (d) advocacy for patient and family, (e) discharge planning, and (f) post-discharge follow-up. The case-level activity in outpatient care will minimally include (a) psychosocial assessment, (b) crisis intervention, (c) ongoing counseling, and (d) coordination and monitoring of social, psychological, and medical services. The counseling of patients and families (in both inpatient and outpatient care) will include helping them (a) adjust to ever-changing health care technology and advances in the science of genetics, (b) make difficult personal decisions, and (c) act as partners of service providers and organizations.

The difficulty of decision making can be understood by imagining the options of a young woman at genetic risk for conceiving an unhealthy child: She may choose not to have children, to adopt, or to have children anyway. "Other options include artificial insemination by donor, egg donation, in vitro fertilization and implantation, surrogate motherhood, and selection and/or freezing of only healthy embryos" (Weiss, 1995, p. 16). The social work activities will demonstrate how to treat clients (patients and their families) as equals and how to encourage them to participate in their treatment and care as active partners. The major social work roles will be *caseworker* and *counselor.*

SOCIAL WORK KNOWLEDGE AND SKILLS FOR ROLE-RELATED INTERVENTIONS

In this section, we discuss the knowledge and skills needed for hospital-based social work in relation to the major roles identified in previous sections.

Social Worker as Community Liaison and Community Organizer

In the future, most hospitals—particularly primary and secondary care hospitals—will be actively involved in the community. This involvement may take several forms, such as (a) the creation and implementation of new hospital-based, as well as community-based, services that are needed in the community; (b) the coordination of community health and human services; and (c) collaboration with other health and human service agencies. Several examples of such activities are already available (see Note 1). Some of these examples of hospitals' successful community-oriented programs are the result of the creativity of social workers. In the future, the hospital's community-service orientation and social work's increased emphasis on the integration of micro and macro modes of practice will converge. No specific delineation exists between micro and macro social work. Macro issues are just micro issues that have been repeated many times (Butcher, 1995). The potential for social work contributions is endless.

Given the hospital's resources and commitment to community service, a critical look at the community's social health needs will reveal many avenues to explore. Spitzer and Neely (1992) described the role of hospital-based social work in developing a statewide intervention system for first responders delivering emergency services. The realization that fire, rescue, medical, and law-enforcement personnel serving as first responders to often dangerous situations are highly vulnerable to acute and cumulative stress led to the creation of a statewide program. "The social work contribution, which received state and national recognition, united local fire, ambulance, clergy, mental health, and medical professionals into one of the largest critical stress debriefing teams in the United States" (p. 56). Sulman, Kanee, Stewart, and Savage (2007) described the approach of an urban Canadian teaching hospital to promotion of an equitable and inclusive diverse environment. It established an office of diversity and human rights responsible for education, training, policy development, and complaint management. That office is staffed by a social worker. Most social workers will not be expected to be this ambitious. They should, however, realize the importance of thorough community needs assessment, because each community is different. The uniqueness of the community must guide the development of the hospital's community programs.

An extensive literature describes approaches to community needs assessment. These approaches have been classified variously. For example, Rubin and Babbie (1993) categorized them as (a) the key informant approach, (b) the community forum approach, (c) the rates under treatment approach, (d) the social indicator approach, and (e) the community survey approach. Siegel, Attkisson, and Carlson (1995) divided them into (a) indicator approaches, involving analyses of social and health indicators as revealed in the available secondary data; (b) social survey approaches, involving analyses of service providers and resources and citizen surveys; and (c) community group approaches, using community forums, nominal groups techniques, the delphi technique, and community impressions. Social workers should keep abreast of the know-how of these approaches and other community needs assessment methodologies.

It will be helpful to remember that the existing data in the form of demographic and other vital statistics are generally in the public domain and easily available. The Centers for Disease Control and Prevention conduct surveys in each state using the "Behavioral Risk Factor Surveillance System" questionnaire and gather information on behaviors ranging from calories consumed to cancer screening. That information is also available. The approaches involving contact with key informants and the general public in community forums and focus groups require the use of social casework and group work skills. For the community survey approach, social workers will have to use their knowledge of the research methodology. Bosworth (1999) recommends that a community health needs assessment have the following five elements: (1) *an assessment plan*—lays out the reasons for the needs assessment, its goals and objectives, and the methodology and time frame for achieving those goals; (2) *a community profile*—assembles all the information (from various sources) about

the community; (3) *key health needs of the community*—specifies the key health problems of the community and identifies underserved groups; (4) *an estimate of the health status of the community*—provides an analysis of the community's health needs and problems (based on a survey of health-related behaviors); and (5) *recommendations for action.*

Once the needs have been determined and the hospital's new role agreed on, the organizational response to those needs may take several forms. Jones (1979) suggested a number of new hospital roles classified by different levels, such as local system, organization, medical model, programs, capacity management, and resource management. For example, programmatically, hospitals can start a hospice, a rehabilitation center, an innovative emergency medical service, a day-care program, and a home care program. From a capacity management perspective, they can create swing beds, convert to ambulatory care, and change into a long-term care facility. The role options from the medical model of care perspective can include preacute/acute/postacute, wellness, and holistic care. From an organizational perspective, multi-institutional systems, mergers, innovative medical staff alternatives, and corporate reorganization are some possible options.

Social workers serve every health and human service agency, and hospital-based social workers, in their role as caseworkers, deal with social workers and other professionals in other agencies. These client- and program-related dealings, as well as other formal and informal contacts within the local professional community, create a network of relationships. Most social workers are also members of various coalitions and special-interest groups. Hospital-based social workers should build on these existing contacts and relationships to perform functions pertaining to their community liaison and community organizer roles.

They should also recognize and address the barriers to interagency collaboration. The first step in addressing the problem is to initiate or renew communication. "Once two or more agencies agree to talk, the next step is to assess the problem and to identify both obstacles to coordination as well as favorable factors" (Bond & Duffle, 1995, p. 48). Various tools can aid in accomplishing this. Focus groups are quite common. Another tool is the "organizational mirror." Agencies prepare lists for one another covering strengths and weaknesses, as well as an empathy list that states the perceived difficulties of the other's role (Iles & Auluck, 1990). The next steps are to formulate mutual goals and to plan strategies for working toward those goals.

> For progress to occur, a "level playing field" is necessary. This may not happen easily; it may be necessary to address negative attitudes toward each other. Conflict may occur. Working through the conflict is necessary to developing trust. The change agents need patience and the ability to focus on the goal despite frustration. Frustration with the process may cause people to drift away. The change agents need to keep bringing people to back the effort if this occurs. (Bond & Duffle, 1995, p. 49)

Social workers should realize that their group work skills and their basic problem-solving expertise not only are good for micro situations but also are invaluable for their community liaison and community organizational work. Social work differs from other health professions primarily in its acceptance of responsibility for vulnerable people (Caroff, 1988). That responsibility has meant sensitivity and empathy for and an ability to relate to and work with vulnerable populations. These assets of social workers, plus their networking and community organizational skills, will enable them to identify leaders of the poor and minorities who can enrich public representation in the hospital's policymaking bodies.

Social Worker as Collaborator and Consultant

Collaboration

In the future, teamwork will be the hallmark of health care. A more holistic view of the patient and patient problems, the need to relate health care to the patient's quality of life, ethical issues raised by complex medical technology, and the necessity for coexistence among many diverse professionals will highlight the importance of collaboration. Despite its need and importance, however, collaboration will not happen easily. Everything encourages competition, which "in Western society has become so ingrained in the fabric of our culture that it has become a primary value" (Kraus, 1980, p. 25). Collaboration—a cooperative venture based on shared power and authority—is the opposite of competition.

Over the past several decades, the term *teamwork* has become commonplace in health care organizations. Teams are viewed as important functioning units, and the current and potential benefits of teamwork are recognized and applauded. At the same time, the nature and quality of teamwork vary tremendously, and there is still much truth in the conclusions that "interprofessional health care teams may never have been fully and consciously planned, tried, or studied" (Brown, 1982, p. 17) and that, at times, "the team is only an illusion held by more powerless providers who are dependent upon an integrated practice" (Nason, 1983, p. 26). Nevertheless, the need for collaboration expressed as teamwork will continue to create opportunities for social workers in the role of collaborator. No other professionals have the assets for this role that social workers possess. Social work values mediation, cooperation, mutual respect, participation, and coordination (Abramson, 1984). Social workers are grounded in systems theory, understand small-group theory, have experience working with many different systems, and have skills in communication. They are superbly qualified to be the coordinators of and consultants for various efforts and activities. We discuss the social worker's collaborator role at two levels: with other professionals around case activity and in organizational committees on policy and procedural issues.

Collaboration is the best type of teamwork—working together in a joint venture. Collaborative teamwork requires communication, cooperation, and coordination. Collaboration can also be conceptualized as one end of a continuum; at the other end is competition, with communication, cooperation, and coordination falling between the two extremes and each representing an increasingly higher level of working together (Dhooper, 1994b). Thus, there are degrees of teamwork. Collaboration involves a level of integration of the various team members' knowledge and skills that results in synergy—the total being more than the sum of the separate knowledge and skills of the individuals involved. Depending on the level of integration, teamwork is distinguished by such terms as *multidisciplinary, interdisciplinary*, and *transdisciplinary.* In *multidisciplinary teamwork*, individuals from different disciplines are involved, but each is responsible for only his or her disciplinary activities, relationships between disciplines are not explicated, and each member is affected very little by the efforts of others (Clark & Connelly, 1979; Halper, 1993). *Interdisciplinary teamwork* presupposes interaction among various disciplines. The members perform their disciplinary activity but are also responsible for the group effort and common group goals. It has a fluidity of disciplinary boundaries and flexibility of roles. *Transdisciplinary teamwork* has these characteristics to a greater extent. "Representatives of various disciplines work together in the initial evaluation and care plan, but only one or two team members actually provide the services" (Halper, 1993, p. 34).

Social workers as team builders must determine whether interdisciplinary or transdisciplinary teamwork is the desired goal for the collaborative effort. Teams go through a sort of "evolutionary" process in their development, major elements of which are leadership, communication pattern, approach to conflict resolution, and decision-making strategy. They should also monitor that process. Two sets of variables—people related and place related—influence teamwork and determine the unique characteristics of particular teams. People-related variables include the individual characteristics of team members, such as personality, attitude, knowledge, and skills. Place-related variables include the setting,

resources, stability, goals, organizational culture, and reward system. Both sets of variables can be manipulated. Similarly, communication, cooperation, and coordination, the major components of teamwork, can be improved and enhanced. These are facilitated by (a) clear common purpose, goals, and approach; (b) an understanding of the roles, functions, and responsibilities of all members; and (c) continuous team-building efforts directed at both monitoring team development and seeking organizational support.

Social workers as coordinators of patient care teams can benefit from the following suggestions:

1. *Apply the problem-solving approach to teamwork.* The generic components of the collaborative problem-solving approach are (a) problem specification—specifying the patient's condition or problem that requires interdisciplinary cooperation; (b) statement of the collaborative purpose—identifying the interdisciplinary services and the form of collaboration needed; (c) goal specification—specifying the objectives necessary for realizing the collaborative purpose; (d) task identification—identifying the specific activities essential for providing and/or coordinating services; (e) role designation and intervention—designating specific roles and responsibilities for each member; and (f) evaluation and revision—continuously assessing each component of the process and revising if required (Carlton, 1984). This process effectively deals with the major challenges of teamwork, which Drinka and Clark (2000) identified as goal conflict, role conflict, decision-making difficulties, and ineffective communication.

2. *Be aware of the barriers to teamwork and consciously work on removing or reducing them.* These barriers can be organizational and structural, philosophical and professional—or what Stewart (1990) called "bureaucracy of the mind"—and practical. Many hospitals are experimenting with unit-based management, and in the future, decentralized organizational structures will likely become more popular. Despite other faults, such structures can create an environment

in which teamwork as a concept is understood, studied, and practiced (Lowe & Herranen, 1981) and interprofessional collaboration becomes possible in substance and not merely in form.

The influence of organizational and structural factors can be minimized by twofold efforts directed *within* at the team members and *outside* at the organizational bosses. Given our definition of collaboration as a cooperative venture based on shared power and authority, within-the-team efforts should be directed at encouraging participative decision making. This can be done by (a) de-emphasizing roles and focusing on the functions of the various members in relation to the problem at hand; (b) recognizing the importance of the process as well as the product—both the teamwork and the task work (teamwork emphasizes the interactions among team members essential for coordinated action; task work focuses on behaviors related to the tasks to be performed by individual members); (c) fostering mechanisms for building, recognizing, and supporting interdependence; (d) operating as an open system with many channels of formal and informal communication; and (e) continual ongoing feedback, evaluation, and modification of both the group and the individual. Outside-directed efforts should be aimed at securing recognition, autonomy, resources, and support for teamwork from the top officials and a shift in the reward system from "hierarchical components to explicit positive recognition of the team delivery model" (Lowe & Herranen, 1981, p. 6). This can be done by (a) keeping top officials informed of the accomplishments and successes of the team; (b) highlighting the tangible and intangible benefits of the team approach; (c) negotiating for resources, change in the institutional award system, and greater consonance between institutional and team goals; and (d) using appropriate institutional change strategies.

3. *Work on changing the "bureaucracy of the mind" by becoming nonthreatening teachers of other professionals.* This task can be facilitated by (a) reminding other professionals of the purpose, the common goal of the team; (b) focusing on the needs of the patient/client and the problem at hand; (c) highlighting the different dimensions of the problem and how they are beyond the expertise of any one professional; (d) emphasizing the appropriateness of different skills for effective problem solving; (e) respecting the knowledge and skills of other team members; (f) providing much-needed emotional support and understanding; and (g) demonstrating how decisions are better implemented when implementers are decision makers as well.

4. *Attend to the practical barriers that may be the cause or effect of a lack of congenial environment for team meetings and deliberations.* Finding a comfortable place at a time convenient for team members is an example of overcoming a practical barrier. The social work skills of resource creation and mobilization and of manipulating the environment can deal easily with these barriers.

5. *Remember that team building is a continuous process and that the relationships among team members must be constantly nurtured.* The most important skills are "communication skills (listening, reflective questioning, restatement), conflict resolution skills, information gathering skills (brainstorming, networking), and decision-shaping skills (negotiating, consensus-building)" (Carlett, 1993, p. 30). Teams progress through identifiable stages variously labeled as orientation, accommodation, negotiation, operation, and dissolution (Brill, 1976), and forming, storming, norming, and performing. The social worker should monitor these stages and ensure that the movement is from "I" to "we" to "it" (the task). Conflict in the team should not be denied or ignored and should not be defined as any one member's problem. It should be viewed as belonging to the whole group and dealt with in a way that avoids win-or-lose solutions. Chapter 8 provides more strategies for thriving in interprofessional settings.

This section ends with a list of major attributes of teamwork on which the STEAMWORK model proposed by Maple (1992) is built: *sensitivity—* being sensitive to the problem-solving process and to one another; *tolerance*—listening for similarities among differences; *empathy*—putting oneself in the place of others; *acceptance*—making efforts to accept others; *maturity*—sitting back and observing one's own behavior and being willing to change; *wisdom*—recognizing that one does not have all the answers, being willing to learn, and knowing when to speak and when to be quiet; *ownership*—owning a piece of the picture to complete the process; *responsibility*—accepting that where we are is not always someone else's fault; and *kindness*—being kind even when familiarity tends to breed contempt (p. 146). Social workers should realize that they already possess in abundance many of these attributes. Kitchen and Brook (2005) described and evaluated a project in a teaching hospital that placed the social worker in a facilitative role within the medical team.

Social workers can also assist the team in dealing with ethical issues at the case level. Exploring the psychosocial dimensions of the illness experience of patients and their families gives social workers a special understanding of those patients and their situations. The value system of social workers has generated such moral imperatives as the client's right to self-determination, respect and acceptance, caring, confidentiality, and regard for individual differences (Goldstein, 1987), and throughout their history, social workers have had to struggle with and resolve value conflicts (Reamer, 1998). Their understanding of patient situations, their sensitivity to human problems, and their value system can enrich the deliberations and decision making of the team in ethically challenging cases. Social workers can draw on the growing social work literature on approaches to resolving ethical conflicts and dilemmas. For example, Bennett (1988) listed the following guidelines, from which all helping professionals can benefit:

- Accept the idea of the adequate—not perfect—condition.
- Choose the least restrictive intervention when the need for protective measures is obvious.
- Accept the idea of limited or partial decision-making capacity in clients.

- Provide desirable decision-making environments.
- Search out what the individual's "best interests" are when he or she is unable to participate in planning.

At the organizational level, as members of hospital committees, social workers can use some of the same skills of collaboration that are valid for creating and functioning in patient care teams. The purpose of each committee, however, will determine the type of knowledge appropriate for meaningful contribution to the process and product of committee work. We discuss the potential social work role on a hospital ethics committee as an example. Following the recommendation of the President's Commission for the Study of Ethical Problems in Medicine and Biomedical and Behavioral Research (1983) that hospitals try committees to improve decision making regarding clinical care, many hospitals have established these committees, often called ethics committees. In a few states (e.g., Maryland), social work representation on these committees is mandated by law. In others states, social workers are sometimes included among the committee members. In the future, the need for such committees will grow, and the social work perspective will have significant relevance for their work. To be effective as members of ethics committees, social workers should do the following:

1. *Improve their understanding of the "what" and "why" of these committees.* Whereas Furlong (1986) identified education, policy development, and case consultation and review as the major functions of these committees, Levine (1984) listed many more functions these committees can perform. He divided these into prospective consultation on individual cases and retrospective review of decision-making functions. The *prospective consultation* functions include determining that all relevant information has been obtained and communicated to decision makers; suggesting additional sources of information where appropriate; identifying ethical issues, as opposed to emotional, legal, religious, or professional issues; spelling out conflicting values, interests,

and duties at stake; facilitating communication and helping resolve disagreements resulting from lack of information or misunderstanding of facts or principles; providing support to staff and families; and recommending, wherever appropriate, that the hospital seek recourse to courts. In *retrospective review,* these committees may determine that appropriate decisions were made, identify cases involving inappropriate decisions, formulate guidelines for difficult types of cases or procedures, and educate hospital professionals about the moral issues in clinical care. Some committees are also concerned with issues of social justice—questions of equitable allocation of expensive medical technology.

2. *Use their knowledge and understanding of the realities of patients and their situations, including quality-of-life concerns based on comprehensive psychosocial assessments.* Social workers should always remember that they represent the only profession with a history of, mission to, and qualifications for advocating and intervening on behalf of vulnerable populations.

3. *Familiarize themselves with the major approaches to ethical reasoning and resolving ethical issues to better appreciate the perspectives of others.* At the same time, they should develop personal ethical guidelines based on social work values and standards.

4. *Deepen their understanding of group dynamics and sharpen their group work skills.* As Baker (quoted in Furlong, 1986) put it,

> Here [in the Institutional Ethics Committee], the social worker uses knowledge of group dynamics and functioning and the skills of purposeful exploration and nonjudgmental listening to help balance the group and to enable each member to express his/her opinion despite possible intimidation from stronger, more powerful groups or staff members. (p. 98)

5. *Develop or refine the skills for building value consensus.* Helpful techniques include reviewing the codes of ethics of other professions and having informal discussions with other committee members; encouraging fellow members to learn a common moral language (shared meanings of such concepts as "autonomy," "confidentiality," and "quality of life"); encouraging them to spend time clarifying and prioritizing their own and the group's values and ethical principles; helping the group develop a procedure for analyzing complex ethical dilemmas; and creating an atmosphere that allows for the expression of thoughts and feelings, reduces ambiguity, and tolerates disagreement (Abramson, 1984).

Consultation

In many situations, at both the case and organizational levels, social work collaboration will take the form of consultation. *Consultation* is the activity in which expert knowledge, experience, skills, and professional attitude and values are transmitted in a relationship between consultant and consultee (National Association of Social Workers, 1981). Its purpose is to enhance the consultee's skills to do his or her job, which requires the consultant to be a *content expert* as well as a *process helper.* Each mode of consultation—content and process—involves a different set of activities. A distinction is made between internal and external consultants, and there are differences between working as an internal or external consultant. Most principles and processes used, however, are the same. Consultation is work related, issue focused, voluntary, and nonjudgmental.

Most of the literature, theory, and models relating to consultation focus on the relationship of the consultant to the consultee (Kurpius & Fuqua, 1993). Kurpius (1978) identified the following four generic modes of consultation: (a) *provision*—the consultant provides direct service or product; (b) *prescription*—the consultant diagnoses the problem and gives direction for its treatment; (c) *collaboration*—the consultant works with the consultee in defining, designing, and implementing a planned change process; and (d) *mediation*—the consultant identifies a need, gathers data, and shares relevant data and observations as a means of focusing the consulting effort. The mediation mode is more applicable to internal consultants.

Gallessich (1982) discussed six models of consultation: (1) organizational, (2) program, (3) education and training, (4) mental health, (5) behavioral, and (6) clinical consultation. Social workers should learn about the various models, theories, and principles of consultation (e.g., Brack, Jones, Smith, White, & Brack, 1993; Caplan & Caplan, 1993; Fuqua & Kurpius, 1993; Jacobsen, 2005; Kurpius, Fuqua, & Rozecki, 1993; Lippitt & Lippitt, 1978; Rockwood, 1993; Sears, Rudisill, & Mason-Sears, 2006; and Stroh & Johnson, 2006). Sabatino (2009) provided an excellent example of how the various models are used in school social work consultation.

The following practice principles are suggested for effective consultation:

- The consultant should discuss with the consultee their expectations of the process, objectives, and respective roles so that there is clarity about these areas.
- The consultant should be sure that he or she has the needed competence to provide the requested consultation.
- "Occasionally, it becomes clear that the consultee is really seeking supervision, therapy, or even a substitute to take over a troubling situation; it is important that the consultant not assume these roles" (Germain, 1984, p. 206). Instead, he or she should convey the willingness to help through a mutual process of problem solving.
- Consultation is a problem-solving process. Social workers' skills in problem solving can be used in consultation. Problem-solving approaches to consultation have been of great value to people in organizations (Kurpius & Fuqua, 1993).
- The consultant should ask the consultee for specific data about the problem, what has been done about it previously, and how it is similar to or different from his or her usual array of problem situations (Germain, 1984).
- The consultant should remember that problem formulation guides the selection of an appropriate model of consultation (Sabatino, 2009).
- The consultant should avoid rushing in with a solution to the problem, as the questions asked may help the consultee understand the situation better, think about it differently, and come up

with his or her own solution (Collins, Pancoast, & Dunn, 1977).
- The consultant should present his or her ideas as possibilities rather than as the right solution to the problem. "Presenting the consultee with several ideas increases his own cognitive and decision-making powers and hence his competence in his own profession" (Germain, 1984, p. 207).
- The consultant should realize that an understanding of systems theory can be a definite plus in consultation, because, "whether implicitly or explicitly, current models of organizational consultation are based upon systems theory" (Brown, Pryzwansky, & Schultz, 1987, p. 99).

Social Worker as Discharge Planner and Resource Mobilizer

Discharge Planning

Weak social support systems, as well as the large numbers of elderly and chronically ill people living in the community, will force hospitals to expand the definition of discharge planning in the future. Discharge planning will begin even before a patient comes into the hospital and will continue after he or she has gone back into the community. It will include preadmission planning, discharge planning, and postdischarge follow-up, and that expanded definition will also fit into the hospital's efforts to go beyond the provision of illness care to provide wellness and health maintenance services. Social workers' current discharge planner role will grow into the role of social health care manager, the provider of psychosocial services aimed at helping patients and families with the transition to and from the hospital.

The expanded discharge planning role of social work is conceived as having three major parts. The first provides social health care services to complement medical treatment beginning prior to admission where possible and in at least the emergency room. The second encompasses the social health care services normally provided during hospitalization. In the third part, posthospital social health care and treatment services are included for those chronically ill patients and their families who are connected to hospital physicians or to hospital services. (Blumenfield & Rosenberg, 1988, pp. 38–39)

Our discussion of the knowledge and skills needed for the expanded discharge planner role is woven into an account of the social work efforts to conceptualize and operationalize discharge planning in the past. Social workers have a rich past on which to build the future. The "what" and "how" of preadmission planning and discharge planning are addressed in this chapter; postdischarge follow-up is discussed in the next chapter as part of case management.

Preadmission planning is a method of increasing the efficiency and effectiveness of social work with hospitalized patients. Theoretically, this is possible in all nonemergency admissions. A social work contact with a patient prior to his or her admission can result in an initial psychosocial assessment of the patient, the beginning of the patient-worker relationship, the determination of the type and extent of social work involvement needed, and the setting of the stage for social work activity, including discharge planning. It would allow social workers to alert physicians and others to psychosocial problems that may be important to consider before performing medical procedures. It can accomplish the psychosocial preparation of the patient for (a) the upcoming hospital experience (by providing the planned procedure-related education, reducing preoperative anxiety, and increasing pain tolerance) and (b) the posthospital experience (Berkman, Bedell, Parker, McCarthy, & Rosenbaum, 1988). For the hospital, social work preadmission screening can shorten the length of hospital stays and reduce unnecessary readmissions and/or emergency department visits.

Despite its importance, preadmission screening has not been a part of regular social work activity in hospitals. A national study of hospital discharge planning found that very few hospitals (17%) screen patients prior to admission (Feather, 1993). Not much has been written about preadmission screening and planning in the social

work literature. Studies by Reardon and his colleagues (Reardon, Blumenfield, Weissman, & Rosenberg, 1988) and Berkman and her associates (1988) and the ideas of Blumenfield and Rosenberg (1988) are indicative of future possibilities but are not reflective of the current reality. Reardon et al. (1988) found that patients viewed preadmission screening as an indication of genuine concern for them and as a commitment to help ease the transition in admission to and discharge from the hospital. A study of preadmission assessment for elective surgery done in Australia (Velecky, 1995) found support for preadmission screening and provision of social work intervention prior to admission. Another study done in Israel (Epstein et al., 1998) also evaluated the impact of preadmission social work intervention on patient satisfaction and length of hospital stay. That study used a modified posttest control group design. The study group patients were screened before hospitalization and offered services on admission, whereas control group patients received standard care. Study group patients were significantly more satisfied with services, but impact on the length of stay was not demonstrated. However, postoperative complications were related to longer lengths of stay, and unlike control group patients, study group patients did not have significantly longer lengths of stay.

In the future, preadmission screening and planning should become an important element of hospital-based social work. It will give patients a greater sense of control, and making them a part of the planning, even before admission, will be an important part of the process of treating the patient as a partner.

Combining the tools used for postadmission high-risk screening done by hospital social workers today with appropriate psychosocial assessment tools can accomplish the purpose of preadmission screening and planning. With the availability of advanced telecommunication technology in the future, it can be done by social workers themselves or by social worker extenders. This service can be marketed to prospective patients via the media, by word of mouth, and by referral from outpatient clinics and physicians' offices. As Blumenfield and Rosenberg (1988) suggested, hospital support can be sought because "it fits well with strategies to (1) attract patients, (2) prepare them for the hospitalization experience, and (3) begin planning for posthospital care prior to admission" (p. 41).

The institution of preadmission screening and planning will make a significant difference in the process of *discharge planning* but is not likely to change its nature. Discharge planning is part of the history of the hospital. Even in the middle ages, the person leaving the "hospital" was given "bread for the road" (Mullaney & Andrews, 1983). Discharge planning has been one basic function of hospital-based social work all along, although its importance has waxed and waned among social workers. Back in 1913, Ida Cannon recognized that a patient who left the hospital too early or without convalescent plans risked "grievous results of an incomplete recovery" (Cannon, 1913). In the 1920s, social workers embraced Freud's theoretical framework that directed attention to intrapsychic causes of suffering, and in order to establish themselves as experts on psychosocial aspects of health care, they began regarding discharge planning as an unprofessional chore (Blumenfield, 1986). Nevertheless, they retained the discharge function because of its relevance for patient care but accorded it a low professional status (Davidson, 1978). Also, until the introduction of the prospective payment system (using DRGs), the discharge planning activity did not receive organizational appreciation and encouragement. In those days, the integration of acute services and long-term care did not benefit hospitals directly. On the contrary, hospitals had financial incentive to keep patients hospitalized longer (Hall, 1985). In the 1970s, social workers rediscovered the importance of discharge planning as reflected in the following words of Fields (1978):

> Discharge planning is where medical care interfaces with quality-of-life concerns. It is where human care needs clash or mesh with our technical cure capability. It is where institutions must validate

their mission and raison d'etre. It is where the action is, and we belong there. Let us hold that territory with courage, compassion, resourcefulness, and pride. (p. 5)

Now, discharge planning is required by both the Joint Commission on Accreditation of Health Care Organizations and the Professional Standards Review Organizations, and the institution of DRGs has made it a key element of hospital survival. The Omnibus Budget Reconciliation Act of 1986 made discharge planning a separate condition of hospital participation in the Medicare program rather than a part of quality assurance. In the future, the law will provide for uniform needs assessment aimed at evaluating (a) the functional capacity of each individual, (b) his or her nursing and other care needs, and (c) his or her social and familial resources to meet those needs (Feather, 1993). The importance of discharge planning will increase in the future because people will live longer and medical technologies will enhance the ability of hospitals to ameliorate and cure diseases.

> Indeed, stays in hospitals will become part of the expected life experience rather than an exception. Institutional care for some part of life may become the norm rather than a failure of the medical system to cure, and discharge planning will become an increasingly significant role for social workers in health care settings. (Ciotti & Watt, 1992, p. 502)

Discharge planning helps ensure not only the optimum use of hospital beds but also the continuity of care by providing for the posthospital needs of patients. Research studies have demonstrated its importance for reducing the hospital length of stay, as well as readmission rates (Andrews, 1986; Cable & Mayers, 1983; Morrow-Howell, Proctor, & Mui, 1991; Proctor & Morrow-Howell, 1990). More recently, a study (Lechman & Duder, 2009) compared predictors of length of stay for a sample of patients referred to social services in three large urban hospitals and examined changes in patient characteristics and the nature of social work practice. A significant relationship between severity of patients' psychosocial problems and length of stay was found, confirming the important role that social workers can play in controlling hospital costs. Auerbach, Mason, and Laporte (2007) reported the value of social work through a tracking system that monitored social work discharge services and compared the outcome with non-social-work discharges. The sample consisted of 64,722 patients admitted to the med-surg unit of a hospital over a period of 2 1/2 years. Of the total, 15.7% (10,156 patients) had social work involvement. The mean length of stay of social-work–served patients was significantly longer than non-social-work patients. However, the social-work–served group included older and hard-to-place patients. The majority had to be placed in institutions, which involves such matters as availability of beds, insurance/Medicare/Medicaid eligibility, and agreement of the family with the discharge plan.

What does discharge planning involve as a social work activity? The position statement of the Society for Hospital Directors, issued in 1985, includes the following components:

- Development of systems that ensure timely and efficient identification of patients who require discharge planning
- Assessment of the psychological, social, environmental, and financial impact of illness on patients and families
- Provision of psychosocial services to patients and families
- Coordination of the contributions of the health care team
- Development and maintenance of liaison with local, state, and federal resources
- Establishment of systems to monitor and evaluate the effectiveness of the discharge planning process
- Identification of services that are not available to meet the posthospital needs of patients and families with a view to effecting the development of needed resources ("Role of the Social Worker," 1986)

The specific case situations determine the degree of emphasis on any of the above components, and the complexity of discharge plans varies from case to case. The above-named document describes four outcome levels of discharge planning: (a) patient and family understanding of the diagnosis, anticipated level of functioning, prescribed treatment, and plan for follow-up; (b) specialized instruction so that the patient and the family can provide posthospital care; (c) coordination of the essential community support system; and (d) relocation of the patient and coordination of support systems or transfer to another health care facility.

The above lists highlight only some of the things that social workers do. Social work activity with the patient and the family is based on a grasp of the psychosocial context within which illness or injury, hospitalization, and discharge occur. Viewing this phenomenon from the role theory perspective, Blazyk and Canavan (1985) said,

> Hospitalization validates the definition of the patient as "ill." The need for discharge, therefore, is often seen as incongruent with this identity. Discharge planning demands a sudden reversal of the patient role, in that the individual, family, or society must quickly resume responsibility for activities and burdens suspended during hospitalization. (p. 491)

Discharge often involves substantial life reorganization and is not simply a return to the life before hospitalization. It may represent a crisis, and the worker must treat it as such.

Discharge planning may also involve ethical conflicts and dilemmas for the worker. The very idea of DRG raises the issue of "averageness versus individualization" (Blumenfield, 1986)— all patients having the same diagnosis are assumed to have similar needs, strengths, and resources, and patients are not given the right to refuse a discharge. In some situations, the obligation to the institution and the needs of the patient conflict. Blumenfield and Lowe (1987) listed several ethical conflicts involved in discharge planning. Similarly, the social worker may have to deal with legal issues (e.g., see Mullaney & Andrews, 1983). In working with patients and their families, social workers should use all the necessary therapeutic skills. Discharge in the case of victims of catastrophic illnesses, "where recovery is minimal or moderate and significant deficits remain, is often viewed by the patient and/or family as symbolizing failure, loss of hope, and abandonment on the part of the medical staff" (Blazyk & Canavan, 1986, p. 23). The social worker should help them reframe the meaning of discharge and shift from a loss orientation to one of problem solving and planning for the future.

Resource Mobilization

Resource mobilization for effective discharge planning can be conceived of as a two-pronged activity directed at human and material resources within the hospital and at the sources of support in the patient's social world and the larger community outside. Work on behalf of the patient takes special significance in discharge planning. It calls for collaboration with other professionals within the hospital and health and human services outside. In his study of hospital discharge planning effectiveness, Feather (1993) tested the importance of four sets of variables: role and procedural clarity, power, discharge planning model, and hospital characteristics. He found that the power and role clarity variables were the most important. These explained almost 50% of the variance in effectiveness. The power variables included discharge planner influence, physician support, and hospital administration support. Of these, support and cooperation from physicians was the most important factor. As Feather recommended,

> Instead of concentrating solely on improving the process within the discharge planning program, they [discharge planners] must devote substantial effort to enhancing their visibility in the hospital at large. . . . In the long run, effectiveness will be enhanced through activities that increase power and clarity, such as participation in hospital-wide committees, providing seminars on discharge planning for physicians and other hospital personnel, or developing a brochure that clearly explains the function of discharge planning. (p. 12)

Chapter 8 presents strategies for attaining and retaining power that social workers in all health care settings can practice. Here, it will suffice to point out that the sensitivity and skills that social workers bring to bear on their work with clients are equally effective in educating and influencing other professionals.

> To the extent that we help patients leave the hospital because "the doctor wants the bed" or "UR is pushing us," we act as demeaned instruments of a system we neither understand nor can hope to impact. To the extent we look behind those presenting requests and identify the sources of pressures, assessing their nature, strength, and legitimacy, we will be able and trustworthy helpers to patients and families, and responsible colleagues to physicians and administrators. (Fields, 1978, p. 5)

In teaching physicians and others, social workers may emphasize the patients' rights related to discharge planning:

> A right to receive certain basic services that will facilitate and optimize transfer from the hospital, a right to receive information about his or her illness and what he or she needs to do about it, a right to understand the support he or she needs and the resources available to provide that support, and a right to secure those resources. (Rehr, 1986, p. 47)

Social workers should sensitize physicians and others to the complexity of discharge planning by helping them realize that (a) all patients who are bright and alert may not be financially and/or mentally competent; (b) all family members who profess to want their relative home with them may not be guided by the best interests of the patient and may have other motives, such as guilt or greed; (c) families that do not want the responsibility of care for their relative do not say so clearly—their indirect signals often fail to change the conviction of discharge planners that home is the best place for the patient to go; (d) patients who are dependent on frail elderly spouses for care are putting themselves and their spouses at risk; (e) the information given by patients or families with memory impairments cannot be taken at face value; and (f) the weak and the infirm may be abused, neglected, or taken advantage of at home, and if this possibility is unheeded, the patient is being returned to a dangerous environment (Ciotti & Watt, 1992).

Discharge planning work on behalf of the patient and family outside the hospital requires knowledge of community resources and the skills of identifying or creating and mobilizing resources, advocacy, linking and matching patients and resources, and monitoring. Formal and informal contacts with community agencies, updated resource manuals and continually refined information systems, and streamlined procedural matters will help improve these skills. Quality discharge planning will be a mark of the quality of hospital-based care in the future, and social work has much to contribute to that.

Social Worker as Caseworker and Counselor

In the *caseworker and counselor role,* the social worker not only serves the patient and the family but also demonstrates a service that is patient and family centered, comprehensive, and well coordinated. Differences will exist in the intensity of social work involvement, depending on the level of care provided by the hospital. In general, however, (a) advances in medical technology, (b) the use of diverse health care approaches and personnel within the hospital, and (c) the need to be more closely bound with the health, mental health, and social service systems in the community will make hospitals more complex. The following observations and suggestions will be helpful for this role:

1. In the future, patients—the consumers of health care—will be better informed and more active and will demand to be treated as partners in their treatment and care, and health care organizations will accommodate those demands. Patients, thus, will have more choices and consequently greater difficulty in making decisions. The counseling aspect of social work activity

will involve not only helping patients understand and cope with their illness and its treatment—the hospitalization, medical procedures, and their consequences—but also teaching them and their families how to make decisions. Ways of helping them gain greater control and decision-making power can include (a) consulting and involving the patient and the family in the establishment and implementation of daily care routines; (b) providing accurate and clear information about the illness, the "what," "why," and "how" of the treatment plan, and alternatives, if any; (c) manipulating the environmental arrangements so that the patient has both greater privacy and less isolation; (d) pointing out the validity of their decisions and highlighting their efforts and progress; and (e) encouraging their meaningful participation in discharge planning.

2. Advanced technology will add to the importance of the within-the-institution advocacy part of social casework. Social workers should use their knowledge, values, and skills to demystify sophisticated medical technology. While noting that the principle of respect of human dignity is particularly vulnerable to the press of technology, Abramson (1990) said,

> By nature of the fact that social workers are not responsible for applying the technology as are doctors, nurses, physical and occupational therapists, and other health care personnel, social workers can hold onto the thread of autonomy and dignity by questioning the purpose of the technology, and encouraging dialogue and negotiation amongst all the participants, and by advocating for the patient when s/he is not able to do so for him/herself. (pp. 12–13)

3. The personal social support systems of patients will be much thinner and weaker in the future. Social work practice has always recognized the role of the family in the illness, coping, recovery, and wellness of the individual, and the reciprocal impact of illness on the family. The changed family forms and weaker social supports, however, will make it necessary to put extra efforts into identifying, involving, and mobilizing patients' families and making the care family

centered. The family will have to be defined more broadly, such as "a social system comprised of individuals related to each other by virtue of strong reciprocal affect who share a permanent household or group of households that endure over time" (Caroff & Mailick, 1985, p. 20). Such a definition covers all kinds of familial structures and memberships that may emerge in the future.

4. The social work literature is rich with ideas for effective assessment of and intervention with families of hospitalized patients (e.g., Caroff & Mailick, 1985; Cowles, 2003; Dillon, 1985; Germain, 1984; Kemler, 1985). On the basis of an extensive review of the relevant literature, Bergman and her associates (1993) identified four key family characteristics that may significantly impact the course of recovery and ongoing functioning of patients: family cohesion, adaptability, social integration, and degree of family stress. Family *cohesion* is the degree of emotional bonding between family members and of individual autonomy experienced by each member. Cohesive families are marked by mutual appreciation, commitment and support, open communication, individual differentiation, and group consolidation. They avoid the extremes of enmeshment and unconcern. Family *adaptability* is the degree of flexibility in terms of the family's structure, roles, and relationship rules that allows it to respond to situational and developmental stress. A family's *social integration* is its degree of involvement with its social network, which is a significant source of support. The *degree of family stress* existing at any given time affects the family's response to stressful events. Exploring these characteristics can easily be made a part of the psychosocial assessment, and a variety of assessment tools are available for the purpose. Such an assessment will help the worker target the particular dimensions of the patient's social reality for intervention.

5. Advances in medical technology will continue to result in more patients surviving serious injuries and diseases, substituting chronic illnesses for life-threatening conditions, introducing a strong element of uncertainty and

unpredictability in many situations, and adding another layer of stress for the patient and the family. The social worker should use a systems perspective for a comprehensive view of the total impact of illness on the patient and his or her family and for planning to intervene at different points and levels of the familial system. "Working within a family systems perspective can be especially useful in terms of opening lines of communication, helping family members support each other in the tension of the uncertainty, and dealing with dyssynchrony when it occurs" (Kemler, 1985, p. 49). In the desire to protect their members from anxiety, many families do not allow open talk or discussion of a member's illness, its prognosis, and consequences. This reluctance often results in the family's failure to deal with its situation realistically, to use its internal and external resources optimally, and to protect its members from avoidable anxiety, suffering, and disease.

6. For helping the hospital and fellow professionals from other disciplines provide family-centered care, social workers should build into their casework, teamwork, advocacy work, and other activities the principles presented in Table 4-B. These have been adapted from the critical components of family-centered care defined by the Association for the Care of Children's Health (Shelton, Jeppson, & Johnson, 1987).

Below, we discuss the knowledge and skills required for the social worker's caseworker and counselor role in relation to the special needs of major patient groups. These groups include the elderly, patients with disabilities, patients with AIDS, and victims of violence and abuse.

The Elderly

To serve elderly clients more effectively, social workers will find the following suggestions helpful:

1. Social workers should know that the general principles of aging are that (a) functions decline and (b) variability increases. Although

---

Table 4-B   Principles of Family-Centered Care

- Recognize that the family is the constant in a patient's life, whereas service systems and their personnel fluctuate.
- Facilitate family/professional collaboration at all levels of hospital, home, and community care.*
- Provide families complete and unbiased information in a supportive manner at all times.
- Incorporate into policy and practice the recognition and honoring of cultural diversity,** strengths, and individuality within and across all families.
- Recognize and respect different methods of coping and implementing comprehensive policies and programs for meeting diverse needs of families.
- Encourage and facilitate family-to-family support and networking.
- Ensure that hospital, home, and community service and support systems are flexible, accessible, and comprehensive in responding to family-identified needs.
- Appreciate families as families and patients as patients, and recognize that they possess a wide range of strengths, concerns, emotions, and aspirations beyond their need for health services.

---

*Family/professional collaboration should be at all levels: (a) care of the individual; (b) program development, implementation, and evaluation; and (c) policy formation.

**Cultural diversity should be defined widely to include ethnic, racial, spiritual, social, economic, educational, and geographic variations.

---

decline in the body's functioning is inevitable in old age, the degree and form of decline varies immensely among the aged. A person's chronological age does not tell much about him or her.

2. Social workers should know that most elderly, when hospitalized, tend to experience confusion and a sense of loss of control. The unfamiliarity of the hospital may precipitate mental confusion, and hospital routines may enforce dependency and disrupt self-care patterns. Patients may feel overwhelmed emotionally by their situation, and surgical anesthesia may exacerbate confusion (Furstenberg & Mezey, 1987). A study of adverse events in the hospitalized elderly by Foreman, Theis, and Anderson (1993) found that 54% of their sample had experienced some degree of acute confusion during hospitalization.

3. Social workers should know that physical illness necessitating hospitalization may come on the heels of losses of family, friends, and valued roles with which the elderly patient was struggling to cope.

4. Social workers should realize that depression is common among the elderly and that the prevalence rates of major depression and depressive symptoms in hospitalized, medically ill elderly are high. Depressive symptoms, when combined with medical illness, have additive effects on the patient's function and well-being (Kurlowicz, 1994). Depression outweighs physical illness as a risk factor for suicide in late life (Fiske, O'Riley, & Widoe, 2008).

5. Social workers should sharpen their assessment skills and use them so that a comprehensive picture of the patient's life situation emerges. With a view to ensuring effective discharge planning, social workers should enrich their assessment skills with elements of functional assessment. The gerontological literature contains several models of and tools for functional assessment. Functional assessment is evaluative in its thrust. "There is an implied asset-versus-liability, positive-versus-negative judgment made about every attribute being assessed" (Lawton, 1986, p. 39). Lawton proposed a framework for functional assessment

that he called "the good life." The good life is indicated by positively assessed qualities in four sectors: (a) behavioral competence, (b) psychological well-being, (c) perceived quality of life, and (d) objective environment. Weissensee, Kjervik, and Anderson (1995) devised a tool to assess the cognitively impaired elderly whose legal competency is in question.

6. In their dealings with elderly patients, social workers should guard against ageism creeping into their approach to working with them. Behaviors that indicate ageism include pigeonholing the elderly and not allowing them to be individuals, avoiding them, and discriminating against them in terms of access to services. Social workers should always remember that the rationale for a distinctive social work purpose with regard to the aged is the premise that "the individual has the right to complete his or her natural life cycle, with its expectable flow and sense of continuity, without culturally imposed inhibiting restraints" (Monk, 1981, p. 63).

7. Social workers should be conscious of the possibility of countertransference and other attitudes affecting their professional behavior. The following reasons for negative staff attitudes toward treating older persons that the Committee on Aging of the Group for the Advancement of Psychiatry (1971) report listed are still valid: (a) The aged stimulate the therapist's fear about his or her own old age; (b) they arouse the therapist's conflicts about his or her relationship with parental figures; (c) the therapist believes he or she has nothing useful to offer older people because he or she believes they cannot change their behavior or that their problems are a result of untreatable organic brain disease; (d) the therapist believes that his or her skills will be wasted because the aged are near death and not really deserving of attention; (e) the patient may die while in treatment, which could challenge the therapist's sense of importance; and (f) the therapist's colleagues may be contemptuous of his or her efforts on behalf of aged patients. In the future, geriatric medicine and geriatric psychiatry will have gained

unprecedented respectability, and no one will consider the work of these disciplines to be a morbid preoccupation with death. Some of the above attitudes will persist, however, and the scope of geriatric medicine and psychiatry's activities will continue to be narrower than social work's.

8. In view of the sensory losses and other physical impairments of elderly patients, social workers should pay attention to these patients' need to communicate adequately and be involved in their care by "making sure that eyeglasses are available and clean, hearing aids are available and have working batteries, and patients are well oriented to their surroundings with the use of orientation boards" (Maus, 2010, p. 226). Social workers should also learn to use nonverbal communication along with various "leads" that encourage the elaboration of feelings, thoughts, and concerns. These leads include restatement, clarification, interpretation, general leads, and summary leads (Kermis, 1986). The use of computers and other communication devices in the future will make communication with such elderly easier. Social workers will have to acquire the skills to use those devices.

9. Social workers should make their intervention with the elderly empowerment oriented, one that enhances the patient's sense of control and capability to exert influence over the hospital and its service providers. Empowerment can be understood in terms of both the content—the specific activities—and the process of empowerment. We discuss both of these aspects of empowerment at length in the next chapter. Tactics of empowerment suggested by Brown and Furstenberg (1992) include contracting, setting small goals, encouraging client self-monitoring, creating room for decision making, reinforcing the perception of control, and organizing for self-advocacy.

10. Social workers will continue to be responsible for discharge planning (earlier we discussed the knowledge and skills appropriate for discharge planning). In planning the discharge of elderly patients, social workers should take into consideration the unique needs of the individual

patient and try to find the best possible match between those needs and the available resources. They should also familiarize themselves with the various approaches to resolving ethical conflicts and dilemmas, because several ethical issues can be involved in discharge planning. Blumenfield and Lowe (1987) and others (e.g., Abramson, 1983; Reamer, 1986) have discussed these issues and suggested ways of resolving them.

11. Social workers should constantly enrich their professional repertoire with ideas for therapeutic interventions from the gerontological literature.

Patients With Disabilities

Work with patients with disabilities demands extra sensitivity and commitment to the principles of individualization and to comprehensive assessment. In discussing persons with mental retardation who are also old, Howell (1987) wrote,

> Some health problems in clients with mental retardation arise as a consequence of institutional care. Obesity, for instance, may be in part the result of a diet scant in fresh fruits and vegetables and whole grain foods, and overburdened with simple carbohydrates; sugary foods may have been given as rewards. Similarly, addiction to tobacco or to caffeine may reflect the use of these substances as positive reinforcers. Dental problems may be a consequence of the unavailability of dental care. Cardiovascular and musculoskeletal fitness may be less than optimal if the client has had little access to exercise facilities, and little encouragement. A history of use of psychotropic medications may result in impaired function of liver, kidneys, or thyroid, cataracts, or tardive dyskinesia. Other health problems related to institutionalization include exposure to hepatitis B and the possibility of a residual carrier state; a history of sexual and/or physical abuse; and habits of public masturbation or self-inflicted injury, sometimes (but not always) associated with boredom and lack of opportunities for social, physical, sexual, and mental engagement. (p. 101)

In assessing and working with inpatients with disabilities, social workers should seek and build on the information, assistance, and involvement of community-based service providers active with the patient. Social workers should be aware of their attitudes toward those with disabilities and consciously guard against their negative attitudes influencing their professional behaviors.

Social workers should ensure that people with disabilities are treated with respect and dignity like everyone else. Disability does not make these patients less human. Levitas and Gilson (1987) said people with mental retardation are often treated as if cognitive development were the only dimension of their lives.

Social workers should practice (and urge others to practice) the principles of individualization and avoidance of overprotection in treating patients with disabilities, because "normalization" and "mainstreaming" are the goals as well as the major principles of work with these patients in the community. They should realize that allowing the hospitalized person with a disability to do as much as he or she can with respect to personal hygiene, individual activities, planning for treatment, and care may require much patience and time.

We present some helpful suggestions for effective interaction with patients with disabilities in Table 4-C below. These are taken from Baladerian, as cited in Brandle et al. (2007), and from Huff (2010).

The need for comprehensive services in response to the unique problem and situation of each patient highlights the importance of (a) the principle of individualization, (b) the necessity of a comprehensive assessment, and (c) concerted efforts to coordinate services. In the future, hospitals will be committed to providing comprehensive patient- and family-centered care, and patients will insist on being treated as partners. With client autonomy and self-determination as the essential philosophical bases of their practice, social workers will also have opportunities to help the organization and other professionals in the creation of an atmosphere appropriate for that type of care.

Table 4-C Suggestions for Effective Interaction With Patients With Disabilities

- Do not assume that a person with a disability has a cognitive limitation.
- Treat adults as adults regardless of any disability they may have.
- Look and speak directly to the person being interviewed, rather than at the interpreter or others in the room.
- Use simple language when communicating with a person with a cognitive disability. Avoid abstractions and "confusing" questions about time, sequences, or reasons for behavior.
- Take time and do not rush the interview.
- Use open-ended and nonleading questions whenever possible.
- Do not hesitate to ask the patient to repeat the sentence if his/her speech is difficult to understand.
- Do not avoid such words as *walking*, *running*, *standing*, and *seeing* in talking with patients with disabilities. Persons with disabilities use these terms just the same as persons without disabilities.
- When it appears that the patient may need assistance, ask if you can help.
- Use extra care while interacting with patients with low or no vision* and those with hearing problems.**

*While interacting with patients with low or no vision,

1. identify yourself by name—do not assume that you will be recognized by the sound of your voice;
2. maintain eye contact even if the patient does not look back at you; and
3. be sure that there is no change in the tone of your voice.

**While interacting with patients with hearing problems,

1. speak clearly and directly—do not exaggerate or shout;
2. do not cover your mouth, as the patient may depend on reading your lips to understand the conversation;
3. be visual—use your hands and body to make gestures and expressions that help communicate your verbal message;
4. use a sign language interpreter if the patient is familiar with sign language; and
5. communicate the message in writing if you are not communicating as effectively as you would like.

Patients With AIDS

The need for self-awareness on the part of the social worker is, perhaps, nowhere as real as when working with patients with AIDS. Social workers should, therefore, practice the principle of self-awareness, which involves consciously examining their own attitudes, beliefs, and feelings and the ways these affect their actions and responses (Furstenberg & Olson, 1984).

The principle of individualization is of immense significance in working with AIDS patients. Social workers should know that patients' adaptive tasks include maintaining a meaningful quality of life, retaining intimacy, coping with the loss of function, confronting existential and spiritual issues, and planning for the survival of family and friends (Moynihan, Christ, & Gallo-Silver, 1988; Siegel & Krauss, 1991). Patients who are gay men, injection drug users, women, and children, as well as the families of these patients, have differing needs and adaptive tasks. For example, individuals with transfusion-related HIV infection have the additional adaptive tasks of "coping with feelings of victimization, sadness, anger, and isolation; decision making concerning their medical treatment in the context of preexisting medical condition; and rebuilding trust in relationships with health care professionals" (Gallo-Silver, Raveis, & Moynihan, 1993, p. 66).

Over the years, more and more women are being diagnosed with HIV. This is attributed to their "having been victims of sexual assault, having had sexual partners who were infected, using intravenous drugs, or having unprotected sex with drug users" (Beder, 2006, p. 111). Mathews (2003) discussed differential side effects of treatment on women. They are more prone to lipodystrophy (or fat redistribution) than are men and experience more dramatic changes in body configuration. Changes in physical appearance can cause them additional stress. They can feel a significant sense of loss, "loss of their future, of potential love relationships, of family and friends, and of a future with children and grandchildren" (Beder, 2006, p. 111). Furthermore, they have concerns about their children related to their current or future inability to perform caretaking roles, the fear that they might have inadvertently infected their children while pregnant or through breastfeeding, the difficulty of telling their children of their HIV status, and the effect on the children of the social stigma associated with HIV. Thus, their needs are different from those of other patient groups.

In many cases, children and adolescents with AIDS feel guilty about having the disease, about their past behavior and lifestyle, and about the possibility of having infected others. They experience sadness, hopelessness, helplessness, isolation, and depression (Lockhart & Wodarski, 1989). Haney (1988), an AIDS patient himself, said, "AIDS has become closely associated with horrifying negative pictures of incapacitation, abandonment, rejection, hatred, physical and mental deterioration, and deformity. When one is faced with these bleak and barren prospects associated with AIDS, suicide becomes a viable alternative" (p. 251).

While working with AIDS cases, social workers must define families as more than families of origin and families of procreation and include what Bonuck (1993) called a "functional family," a group marked by committed relationships among individuals that fulfill the functions of family (Anderson, 1988). The emotional and tangible effect of AIDS on the family varies by the type of family and such factors as social stigma and isolation, fear of contagion on the part of family members, fear of infecting one's loved ones, fear of abandonment, guilt, and psychological and physical fatigue (Bonuck, 1993). Social workers should know that the family's ability to be involved in the care of the patient also depends on such factors as coping characteristics and resources, perceptions of self-efficacy, perceived adequacy of social support, familial obligation and affection, fears of being infected, the degree to which the patient is held responsible for the illness, and acceptance of homosexuality (McDonnell, Abell, & Miller, 1991).

Social workers should use their casework and counseling skills in meeting the differential needs of patients and patients' families. To counteract the pervasive helplessness, hopelessness, and isolation, empowerment techniques should be built into the work done with these clients. Some of these techniques can focus on the positive and less fatalistic aspects of AIDS, connect patients with sources of support, and help them regain and retain power and control over their lives and illness. Borden (1989) recommended life review and reminiscence as a helpful technique for working with young adults with AIDS, because reminiscence processes work to preserve a sense of ego integrity, order, coherence, and cohesiveness.

Discharge planning for AIDS patients requires extra work and care. Social workers should supplement their skills with measures to deal with the following obstacles to effective case management that Roberts, Severinsen, Kuehn, Straker, and Fritz (1992) identified: (a) stigma of AIDS and homosexuality; (b) lack of family support; (c) impact of AIDS dementia, which has been observed in 60% to 80% of AIDS patients; (d) ethical dilemmas in discharge planning, such as the patient's wish for confidentiality about his or her disease and the need to involve his or her family; (e) conflicts in advocacy process within the hospital (if the patient insists that his or her familial visitors not know of his or her AIDS and if dementia makes his or her behavior unpredictable); (f) lack of adequate resources; and (g) issues of countertransference, which may include fear of the unknown, fear of contagion, fear of death, denial of helplessness, homophobia, overidentification, anger, and the need for professional omnipotence (Dunkel & Hatfield, 1986).

Many gay patients who have not fully accepted a personal identity of being gay may put geographic distance between themselves and their kinship networks and thereby deprive themselves of their natural supports, as well as local gay support. That deprivation makes discharge planning more difficult. Social workers' advocacy skills become much more important in such cases.

Victims of Violence and Abuse

We suggest a threefold social work contribution to the hospital's service to victims of violence and abuse: (1) direct work with the victims, (2) creating a culture of understanding and help for victims of violence, and (3) creating a special program or unit to address their needs. We discuss the social work crisis intervention skills appropriate for dealing with victims of violence and their families in Chapter 5.

For creating an organizational culture of understanding and help, social workers can help in (a) establishing a screening, treatment, and safety protocol; (b) providing ongoing training for all staff; (c) incorporating written and electronic chart prompts; (d) assessing adherence to the protocol through routine studies; and (e) making resources available to patients, regardless of whether victims of abuse, for example, have disclosed intimate partner violence. This can be done through (1) placing posters prominently in different parts of the institution, (2) placing small safety cards in private places such as bathrooms and examination rooms, (3) advertising and educating all patients about intimate partner violence services, and (4) posting the crisis phone number for the national hot line, 1-800-799-SAFE (Kimberg, 2007).

In creating a center or program for the service of abused women, social workers can benefit from a few impressive examples. Edlis (1993) described a hospital-based rape crisis center in Haifa, Israel. That center has been in existence since 1980, and its success has encouraged the development of similar centers in other hospitals in that country. Such a center has several advantages: (a) It is open and accessible to rape victims 24 hours a day, 7 days a week; (b) skilled professionals are on duty at all times; (c) it provides access to a full range of needed medical examinations and tests; and (d) it has the ability to centralize services and act as a liaison to agencies outside the hospital. The hospital's social work department developed procedures, guidelines, and protocols for the center, conducted training seminars for the hospital staff and community organizations, and created a plan for crisis intervention (Edlis, 1993). To establish and run such programs, social workers should increase their understanding of the different approaches to serving battered women and models of women's shelters (e.g., N. J. Davis, 1988).

Brandle and her colleagues (2007) provided the following helpful suggestions for interviewing victims of elder abuse.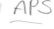

1. Take time to build rapport with the patient.

2. Interview in a private place out of the earshot of others, who may include the abuser.

3. Start with general questions leading to more specific ones.

4. Questions to elicit information about the abuse can include the following:
   - How is your social life? When was the last time you went out with friends or family?
   - Who makes decisions in your house? Who decides how your money is spent?
   - How are things going with your spouse/partner, caregiver, or adult child?
   - Is there someone in your family who has an emotional or drinking or drug problem?
   - Are there strangers coming in or out of your house without your permission?

- Are you afraid? Has anyone made you feel uncomfortable?
- Have you ever been hit, kicked, or hurt in any way?
- Does anyone threaten you or force you to do things that you do not want to do?
- Have you ever been forced to do sexual acts you did not wish to do?
- Is any of this going on now?

They also listed signs and symptoms of physical abuse, sexual abuse, emotional abuse, neglect, and self-neglect.

Wolf and Pillemaer (1994) presented four "best practice models" in elder abuse programming: (a) a multidisciplinary team approach of the San Francisco Consortium for the Prevention of Elder Abuse; (b) the Senior Advocacy Volunteer Program in Madison, Wisconsin; (c) the Victim Support Group of the Elder Abuse Project of the Mount Sinai Medical Center, New York; and (d) a social work master's level training unit within Adult Protective Services in Hawaii. Two of these—(a) and (c)—can easily be hospital based. A few medical centers across the country have created interdisciplinary centers or teams responsible for providing consultation and support to hospital staff in cases of elder abuse and assisting in the multidisciplinary evaluation of and planning for those cases. These also serve as the link between the hospital and outside agencies/personnel concerned about elder abuse, such as adult protective services, police departments, civil/criminal lawyers, and victim advocates (Brandle et al., 2007). Social workers play an important part in those organizational responses to this problem. Where such a center or team does not exist, social workers can help create one. They can benefit from the example and experience of the existing programs.

We have chosen to postpone the discussion of social work with culturally diverse patients. Cultural diversity will pervade all dimensions of life and will need to be accommodated at the case as well as the organizational levels in all sectors of health care. Ideas about effective social work approaches to working with culturally diverse populations are presented in Chapter 8.

RELEVANT ETHICAL CONSIDERATIONS

In every health care setting, social workers are likely to experience ethically challenging situations. However, the complexity and fast pace of health care activities in acute care settings make those challenges more difficult. Discharge planning is the major function of social workers in acute care settings and is often performed in ethically challenging situations. We discuss ethical questions and concerns pertaining to discharge planning in this section.

As we pointed out earlier, the importance of the discharge planning role of social workers in acute care settings has been growing over the past 30 years. It has now taken center stage. However, in some settings, social workers are sharing this role with others—paraprofessionals and nurses—in response to the hospital's cost-cutting measures. In such settings, they are generally responsible for dealing with more difficult cases. The difficulty of those cases is reflected in the following conditions, listed by Cowles (2003).

- The patient is insufficiently recovered from the acute health condition to take care of him/herself.
- The patient is mentally confused, emotionally depressed, or otherwise mentally impaired—permanently or temporarily.
- The patient needs oxygen, an indwelling catheter that requires irrigating and changing, assistance with eating, dressing, walking, bathing, toileting, and so forth.
- The patient has a new baby with special problems but has never cared for an infant before.
- The patient now has a seizure disorder, and his or her family has never seen a grand mal seizure before.
- The patient has been advised not to climb stairs but lives in a second-floor apartment with no elevator access.

- The patient has AIDS, and the family has not yet been informed.
- The patient is a young man, now permanently paralyzed from the waist down, and his family lives in a rural mountain area several hundred miles away.
- The patient is a young mother with several children to care for, but she will be unable to do any lifting for several weeks, and the father is undependable.
- The patient will need to return to the hospital twice a week for an indefinite period of time for kidney dialysis treatments, and he or she has no personal transportation (p. 167).

We earlier discussed the complexity of discharge planning by quoting Ciotti and Watt (1992). Some of the possible causes of complexity are worth reiterating here: (1) Patients who look bright may not be competent to follow postdischarge instructions; (2) families that do not want to or cannot provide care for their relative may not say so clearly; (3) families wanting their relative home may have reasons other than the best interest of the patient; (4) sending a patient home in the care of a frail elderly spouse may put both spouses at risk; (6) postdischarge instructions given to a patient or a family member with memory impairment may result in a disaster for the patient; and (7) the weak and the infirm may be abused, neglected, or taken advantage of if discharged to a potentially dangerous environment.

Despite the complexity and difficulty of discharge planning, social workers play the role of discharge planner admirably and feel satisfied with their performance. Resnick and Dziegielewski (1996) studied social workers and others involved in discharge planning and found that a vast majority (86%) of them reported satisfaction with their jobs. Satisfaction was linked to (a) finding purpose in what they do, (b) being able to see the outcome of their work, (c) having contributed positively to a patient's life, and (d) believing that what was done benefited the patient served.

Discharge planning and all it involves have an important ethical dimension. At the organizational level, there is the possibility of a conflict between patients' rights regarding discharge planning and the institution's need for efficiency and cost savings. Discharge planning may also involve ethical conflicts and dilemmas for the social worker. As Blumenfield (1986) pointed out, the very idea of DRGs raises the issue of "averageness versus individualization." All patients having the same diagnosis are assumed to have similar needs, strengths, and resources, and patients are not given the right to refuse a discharge. In some situations, the obligation to the institution and the needs of the patient conflict. Discharge planning becomes an ethically challenging activity because social workers are the main performers on the stage and are expected by the institution to ensure the success of the show. They are working in complex bureaucratic settings where the fiscal health of the institution is more important than the health of individual patients. They are also functioning in multidisciplinary settings where other professionals are guided by their own ethical values and guidelines, and the degree of congruence on what is in the best interest of the patient may be low. Blumenfield and Lowe (1987) identified several ethical conflicts that may be involved in discharge planning, and those conflicts are as valid today as they were 25 years ago. We list those conflicts below.

1. A conflict between two ethical principles held by the worker

2. A conflict between two possible actions in which some reasons favor one course of action and the others militate against this course

3. A conflict that exists between two unsatisfactory alternatives

4. A conflict between one's principles and one's perceived role

5. A conflict between the need to act and the need to reflect

Conflicts 4 and 5 are setting/context related. A conflict between one's principles and one's role manifests itself as a conflict between the desire to do what is right for the patient and the role of a "team player" or "discharge planner." A conflict between the need to act and the need to reflect arises in difficult discharge planning situations. The worker is urged to come up with and implement a discharge plan quickly, while a worthwhile plan would require reflection, exploration, and collaborative interchange about its ramifications.

In resolving these and other such conflicts, social workers will find the following suggestions helpful.

- Understand social work values as codified in the National Association of Social Workers (2000) Code of Ethics.
- Let your professional values supersede your personal values if there is a conflict between personal and professional values.
- Adhere to professional values that stress maximum participation, self-determination, autonomy, and informed choice of the patient.
- Do not look for ethical certainty, because ethical issues and conflicts arise in situations that defy a simple, universally correct response. Ambiguity can prevent rash actions or easy solutions that cannot be reversed.
- Gather all the facts relevant to the situation and do a thorough assessment. The lack of all the factual information reduces the possible choices and leads to poor decisions (Gelman, 1986).
- In dealing with others on the health care team, enrich their understanding with our holistic perspective, grasp of the dynamics of the patient's situation, and quality-of-life issues involved in the case.
- Make sincere efforts to understand the perspectives of others. Ethical reasoning can be guided by various ethical principles, each of which has equal moral force when viewed in the abstract.
- Use a decision-making model. The following model, one of many available in the literature, is from Joseph (cited in Garrett, 1994). It requires the following steps:

1. Definition of the dilemma
2. Looking at all the relevant facts and developing valid arguments for various courses of action
3. Consideration of practice wisdom, personal beliefs, and values, and how these may influence the final decision
4. Developing options, exploring compromises, and evaluating alternatives in an attempt to find a course of action with the least negative effect
5. Choosing a position that you can defend

Critical Thinking Questions

1. How does the interplay of personal (lifestyle, knowledge, preference, etc.), institutional, and social factors generate and perpetuate health problems?
2. How do personal beliefs, values, and assumptions about vulnerable patients affect a professional's ability to create a context for effective interventions?

NOTES

1. Some hospitals have established hospital-based hospice programs; others have gone into the nursing home business by creating both swing beds within the hospital and separate entities in the community. Some hospitals provide home care services; others are trying ambulatory care options such as hospital-based primary care centers, health management organizations, specialized clinics for chronic pain, sleep disturbance, and so forth, as well as community-based satellite clinics and health promotion programs (Bayles, 1979; DeSpiegler, 1979; Drew, 1979; Justins, 1994; McInerney, 1979; Smith, 1979; Wilson, 1979; Yanni, 1979). Rock, Haymes, Auerbach, and Beckerman (1992) described a hospital-sponsored community residence program for the chronically mentally ill.

The possibilities for a hospital's becoming the coordinator of community health and human services or for collaborating with other agencies and programs are immense. Long, Artis, and Dobbins (1993) described a hospital-based program for family-centered early intervention for infants with chronic health impairments and developmental disabilities. Patterson (1995) described the University of Maryland Hospital's comprehensive family-centered pediatric AIDS program. Rubin and Black (1992) described a joint program of two hospitals in Pittsburgh designed to provide community-based health education to seniors. Those hospitals conduct a semiannual town meeting, one or the other taking the lead in its organization; costs are divided equally and topics and format developed jointly. This program has benefited both hospitals by enabling them to improve their services for the elderly. All such ventures have a social work component and call for either initiative or input from social workers. The Pittsburgh Town Meeting program used the skills of a social worker as its part-time executive director.

2. *Intimate partner violence* is the term recommended by the Centers for Disease Control and Prevention, which defines it as violence committed by a spouse, ex-spouse, current or former partner (of the same or opposite sex) in any of the following four forms: physical, sexual, threats of physical or sexual violence, or psychological/emotional abuse. There are other, more elaborate definitions of this term, such as the following:

> Intimate partner violence is a pattern of assaultive and coercive behaviors that may include inflicted physical injury, psychological abuse, sexual assault, progressive social isolation, stalking, deprivation, intimidation, and threats. These behaviors are perpetrated by someone who is, was, or wishes to be involved in an intimate or dating relationship with an adult or adolescent, and are aimed at establishing control by one partner over the other. (Family Violence Prevention Fund, 2002, p. 2)

3. Elder abuse includes several different types: (1) physical abuse, (2) sexual abuse, (3) emotional abuse, (4) financial exploitation, (5) neglect, (6) self-neglect, and (7) abandonment. Wolf (2000) captured the reality of elder abuse in the following words:

> Unlike some child abuse, which focuses solely on the child and parent (or surrogate parent), and relationship or spouse abuse, which deals with intimate partner relationships, elder abuse covers a wide range involving adult children, intimate partners, more distant relatives, friends, neighbors, caregivers, and other people in whom the older person has placed his or her trust. In addition to multiple relationships, each with its specific set of interpersonal dynamics, elder abuse has a financial component too not associated with either child or battered women. Pensions, Social Security, and home ownership have made elders easy prey for unscrupulous caregivers, business service personnel, and even family members. (pp. x–xi)

5

Social Work in Ambulatory Care

Ambulatory care is perhaps the most important element of the health care system. This is where the patient first comes into contact with the system and continues to stay in it. Ambulatory care services are also a major source of intake of patients for other health care sectors. Chapter 2 described the various definitions of and the different services encompassed by ambulatory care, the long history of this type of care, and the numerous settings through which it is provided. In the future, the demand for ambulatory care will increase, leading to growth not only in the number and popularity of services but also in the variety of care providers and organizations. Even though the provision of primary care will be the minimal expectation from ambulatory care settings, the increased demand for services will put greater strain on the system's resources, accompanied by questions of equity and quality of services. Provision of patient-centered, comprehensive, and coordinated services and attention to the special health care concerns of major population groups will be the main needs of all ambulatory care settings in the future.

History of Social Work in Ambulatory Care Settings

Social work has been a part of many ambulatory care settings for a long time. In 1893, Jane Addams established a free medical dispensary at Chicago's Hull-House. Other social workers were involved in the opening of similar dispensaries in many other cities (Bracht, 1978). From the late 1800s onward, social work, "medicine's first professional ally from the social field" (Simmons & Wolff, 1954, p. 12), contributed impressively to the development of social medicine and public health. Physicians and medical establishments began seeing the utility of social work methodology and social workers for improving their understanding and treatment of poor patients. Since the middle of the 19th century, physicians such as Dr. Elizabeth Blackwell of the New York Infirmary, Dr. Dwight Chapin of the New York Postgraduate Hospital, and Dr. William Osier of Johns Hopkins Hospital and University in Baltimore had used hired help, volunteers, or medical students as "friendly visitors" for reporting home conditions of patients to the physician and for interpreting the physician's instructions to patients and their families (Cannon, 1952).

In 1903, Dr. Richard Cabot, chief of medicine at Massachusetts General Hospital in Boston, introduced a social worker into his medical clinic. He was convinced that a person's personal difficulties may be the cause and not the result of his or her illness (Nacman, 1977). He considered medical and social work to be "branches split off a common trunk: the care of people in trouble" (Cabot, 1915, p. 91). Serving the poor—essentially, the entire clientele of health centers and clinics—was a frustrating experience for both service providers and recipients because of the social and cultural gap between the two. The caregiver was frustrated because of the lack of appreciation and absence of expected results. The recipient was frustrated because of the lack of opportunity for self-expression and unwillingness to accept the stipulations required for receiving service (Ginker et al., cited in Nacman, 1977).

Case management

The social work role in outpatient clinics involved four major functions: (a) educating the physician about the patient's domestic and social conditions, (b) helping the patient comply with the physician's orders, (c) alleviating the patient's social problems that interfered with medical care, and (d) providing a link between the health care setting and community agencies. Although the earliest health social workers, mostly nurses, had little or no formal training in social work, they were expected to be "all-around human beings who can supplement the necessary and valuable narrowness of the physician" (Cabot, 1915, p. 176). Ever since, social workers have been adding a unique dimension to health care.

> The contribution that social work makes to health care is in its holistic approach to problems of both body and mind. . . . Social work's uniqueness comes from its persistent focus on the physical, sociopsychological, and environmental health needs of clients. (Bracht, 1978, p. 13)

That was the beginning of social work's involvement with ambulatory care settings. With the growth of these settings in their numbers, auspices, foci, and purposes came increased presence

of social workers. The creation in 1912 of the U.S. Children's Bureau (the first five chiefs of which were social workers) led to the discovery that infant and maternal mortality rates were significantly related to social and economic factors. That finding resulted in the birth of the first grant-in-aid programs in the health field under the Maternal and Infancy Act of 1921 (Kerson, DuChainey, & Schmid, 1989). Social workers were employed in public health clinics as a part of the maternal and child health programs. Similarly, after World War I, the National Venereal Disease Control Act provided financial assistance to state and local health departments for clinics for surveillance, early diagnosis, and treatment of venereal disease. Social workers were a part of those clinics as well. Their interventions were focused on educating victims and families about the causes and dissemination of syphilis, tracing the syphilitic's sexual contacts, and encouraging the patient to comply with the treatment (Kerson, 1979). Earlier, social workers had been heavily involved in tuberculosis control programs, working with both patients and their families. In 1935, the Social Security Act created the maternal and child health program and the crippled children's program. In the 1950s, programs to coordinate medical and social services for unwed mothers were developed. Now, such comprehensive programs are mandated by Title V of the Social Security Act (Kerson et al., 1989). In the 1960s, new health care organizations and programs appeared. These included Office of Economic Opportunity neighborhood health centers, expanded programs for the prevention of maternal and infant problems, special outreach programs for the rural poor, and community mental health centers. Social workers made substantial contributions to all of these (Bracht, 1978).

Thus, social workers have been important elements of many ambulatory care programs. They have worked not only in generic such settings as public health departments, health centers, and health maintenance organizations but also in such specialized settings as clinics for genetic counseling, family planning, prenatal and postnatal care, care of the newborn, diagnosis and treatment/management of persons with disabilities, and service to those with AIDS, and they work with victims of child abuse, rape, and spousal abuse. They have also been involved in such acute ambulatory care settings as emergency rooms and ambulatory surgery centers.

Both nonacute care and acute care settings are likely to continue as the sites for ambulatory care in the future, providing varied opportunities for social workers to make significant contributions to those settings. Social workers will be able to take on important roles in helping these settings meet their needs. Their knowledge and skills will be appropriate for (a) comprehensiveness of care—they will assess the total situation of patients and attend to the psychosocial dimensions of patients' health needs; (b) coordination of care—they will be responsible for ensuring that all the pieces of care for and on behalf of the patient are coordinated; (c) integration of care—they will be the major link between the ambulatory care setting and other health and social service resources; and (d) patient-centered patient-as-a-partner care—they will demonstrate how to relate to patients as partners in their care through their involvement with those patients. They will also help in meeting the special needs of major patient groups. Social work contributions will be equally valuable for acute and nonacute ambulatory settings.

The needs of patients using acute care settings such as emergency rooms for emergency as well as nonemergency problems are different in their nature, intensity, and urgency from those of patients seen in other ambulatory settings. Social work's contribution to the care of the two groups would be different in the degree of involvement, as well as in the use of knowledge and skills. Ambulatory care, therefore, can be divided into (a) acute ambulatory and (b) nonacute ambulatory care. We discuss social work roles and functions in each of these separately.

FUTURE SOCIAL WORK ROLES IN ACUTE AMBULATORY CARE SETTINGS

In the future, with expanded access to health care, all kinds of nonacute ambulatory care settings will try to attract and retain patients. For example, many pharmacies are already offering flu shots and welcome walk-ins. Also, coordination of services between those settings and other community health and human services will be better. Those changes will reduce somewhat the inappropriate use of acute care settings. Acute ambulatory care settings such as emergency rooms, however, will continue as a part of the infrastructure of primary care in the United States. Their greatest attraction will continue to be convenience of access to care. "No physician will be available 24 hours a day, 7 days a week for his/her patients" (Young & Sklar, 1995, p. 669). Moreover, advances in information technology will ensure continuity of information for patients with chronic problems who come to acute care settings. Thus, these settings will add *continuity of care* to *convenience of access to care* as their attributes. Then there will always be patients whose problems do not fit into a neat service category, who misjudge the nature of their need or exaggerate the seriousness of their problem, and who end up in acute care facilities. They will need someone to listen to their story, help them put the situation in the correct perspective, and steer them in the right direction. In all the situations described above, the social worker will continue to play professional roles distinct from those of others—roles for which other professionals do not have the appropriate and necessary attitudes, knowledge, and skills. In dealing with people with nonemergent health and nonhealth needs, the social worker's attitude is often in complete contrast to that of others. These patients are generally viewed as abusing the facility, inappropriately taxing its resources, and threatening its routine order. This attitude tends to translate into impatience, intolerance, and callousness on the part of the staff. Sometimes, even the legitimate health-related complaints of these patients would be ignored if the social worker did not intervene.

In acute ambulatory care settings, four distinct situations are/can be encountered: (a) true medical emergencies, (b) social emergencies, (c) nonemergency health and social needs, and (d) a medical emergency created by an act of terrorism. We have separated the terrorism-related emergency situation from other medical emergency situations because it has a character of its own. Social work intervention will be different in each of these.

Social Work Role in True Medical Emergencies

Burns, cardiac problems, poisonings, and traumas are among the true medical emergencies. All these have some common characteristics: They are generally unexpected, happen suddenly, and endanger the patient's life, and the patient and/or the family are not prepared for their occurrence. Discussing trauma patients, Moonilal (1982) said that these patients may experience shock, excessive blood loss, severe respiratory distress, or cardiac arrest.

> Victims of multiple trauma are usually products of motor vehicle accidents, shootings, stabbings, or suicide attempts and are generally in shock, unconscious, or near death. Most arrive at the hospital with paramedics—a few are brought in by family or friends. (p. 16)

Immediately on their arrival, these patients become the object of intense life-saving medical activities on the part of physicians, nurses, and paramedical staff. The situation, at the same time, also generates important nonmedical needs. These include notifying the family if they are not aware of the sudden illness or injury of the patient and dealing with their reaction to what is generally experienced as an acute emotional crisis. In all emergency care settings, although physicians and nurses are specially trained and skilled for the medical treatment and care of severely ill and injured patients, a person is seldom clearly designated and trained for contacting the family of the critically ill, dying, or dead patients. That job is performed by different persons in an ad hoc, generally inconsistent, and sometimes haphazard manner. Part of the reason for inconsistency is the differing access to information and different perspectives on the situation.

> For example, the physician focuses on diagnoses and prognoses; the nurse is familiar with the

patient's vital signs and observable behavior; and the registration staff members are most informed about the location of the incident and have first-hand reports relayed by ambulance personnel. (Robinson, 1982, p. 616)

Clark and LaBeff (1982) studied how different professionals—physicians, nurses, law enforcement personnel, and members of the clergy—delivered news of death, and they discovered five strategies of delivery. The strategy chosen seemed to depend on such factors as the personality of the person and the circumstances of the situation. The inconsistency in the manner of notification of families of acutely ill and dying or dead patients, whether because of different information, perspective, or personality of the notifier, can have adverse effects on the family. In the future, with computers taking over many functions performed by people today, the likelihood that this need of such families will be handled impersonally and insensitively will be even greater.

Depending on the nature of the emergency, a family's immediate reaction may be disbelief, confusion, anxiety, fear, anger, guilt, or grief. "Unanticipated medical emergencies can overwhelm the unsuspecting family, making coping impossible" (Silverman, 1986, p. 312). Thus, the need for intervention is urgent. A family faced with the possible loss of a loved one needs help.

The emergency may end in the patient's (a) dying; (b) being transferred to a hospital's intensive care unit with an uncertainty about survival, the prospect for survival with long-term disability, or the hope for complete recovery; (c) being transferred to a medical facility for less intensive further treatment; (d) being sent to a penal institution in the case of crime-related injuries; or (e) being discharged home. All these possibilities involve uncertainty, numerous questions, a flood of emotions, and the need for the family to plan a response to the situation. Families need help in reducing the degree of uncertainty, in understanding and gaining control of the situation, in expressing and getting validation of their emotions, in obtaining honest answers and consistent information, and in preparing for whatever may be happening and being planned for the patient. They must be prepared for even looking at the loved one, who may have been badly disfigured by the trauma and is sure to be hooked up to several machines. Acute care units "generate fear, provoke anxiety, and heighten the family's awareness that the patient is seriously ill and may not live" (Dhooper, 1994b, p. 42). Regarding the powerful impact of these units, the following observation of Hay and Oken (1972) is essentially as true today as it was 40 years ago.

> Initially, the greatest impact comes from the intricate machinery, with its flashing lights, buzzing and beeping monitor, gurgling suction pumps, and wheezing respirators. . . . Desperately ill, sick, and injured human beings are hooked up to that machinery. And, in addition to mechanical stimuli, one can discern moaning, crying, screaming, and the last gasps of life. Sights of blood, vomitus and excreta, exposed genitalia, mutilated wasted bodies, and unconscious and helpless people assault the sensibilities. (p. 110)

A social worker's services should be made available to the families of seriously ill patients.

> If a social worker is not available, the family will find another, perhaps less professionally trained, supportive liaison. At some point, the barrage of outside stimuli will begin to overwhelm the system. Once saturated, the family system will close, making intervention difficult. (Silverman, 1986, p. 311)

Social workers in all acute care settings, including acute ambulatory care centers/units, should consider attending to the needs of families as their major function and take on this responsibility. Their understanding of crisis theory, sensitivity for individuals in crisis, and skills in crisis intervention make them the best qualified for the job. Moreover, their contacting the family can set the stage for their subsequent activity with the family. Their focus should be on alleviating the impact of the crisis-created stress and helping the family grasp the situation and mobilize its internal and external resources to deal with it. This function would involve activity

with the family and on behalf of the family both within the center and outside. Social work activity with the family would include assessment, consultation, crisis management, grief counseling, and termination (Moonilal, 1982).

Although the focus of social work intervention is on the family, depending on the nature and severity of the patient's medical condition, there may at times be room for some social work activity with the patient himself or herself. That usually would involve a psychosocial assessment (to enrich the medical personnel's understanding of the patient) and discharge planning. The activities in cases of acutely ill, dying, or dead patients (for which the anxiety level of the patient's family, friends, and relatives is high), as suggested above, would represent the social work role of *family crisis counselor, provider of concrete services,* and *liaison* between the family and others inside and outside the health care setting.

Social Work Role in Social Emergencies

Ours is a culture of violence that is "reflected in the history, attitude, belief systems, and coping styles of the population in dealing with conflicts, frustration, and the quest for wealth and power" (Shachter & Seinfeld, 1994, p. 347). Our society is not likely to disown or reform this culture. Violence will continue to be legitimated and rationalized. When violence is directed toward those who are weak and defenseless, however, it results in social emergencies that, of course, have significant medical dimensions.

We include in social emergencies cases of child abuse, spousal abuse, elder abuse, and rape. These are invariably encountered in ambulatory acute care settings, particularly emergency departments and centers. Sometimes, the reality of these emergencies is obvious, but many times, it has to be looked for. Physicians and nurses are generally quite good at looking for the signs of physical abuse in children, easily detecting the incidence of physical neglect in children, and often suspecting child sexual abuse. The same may not be true of their ability to look for or sensitivity to the possibility of spousal and elder abuse in the cases they treat.

Similarly, every state has legal requirements with clear institutional protocols for reporting cases of child abuse. Several states have parallel reporting requirements regarding elder abuse, but hardly any have the same regarding spouse abuse. Most acute care settings lack clear procedures and protocols for intervention in cases of these types of abuse, despite the Joint Commission on the Accreditation of Health Care Organizations requirement regarding the treatment of victims of domestic violence. This situation will improve in the future. However, social workers will continue to add to the health care setting's ability to identify cases of abuse, manage the emergency situation, improve the quality of its responsiveness to the victim's need, and set in motion the process of correction.

Child Abuse

Child abuse in all its forms—physical abuse, physical neglect, sexual abuse, and emotional abuse—is a problem that continues to defy efforts to prevent and correct it, and it is likely to persist in the future. Children are seen in acute care settings for all types of urgent and nonurgent health problems, including abuse. Sometimes a child is brought in for the confirmation and validation of abuse because it is suspected and child protection officials are already involved. The social worker's role in ambulatory acute care settings in such cases is to (a) attend to the emotional (and informational) needs of the child and his or her parent if accompanying the child; (b) interview the child and/or others and supplement the findings of the medical examination and tests with a psychosocial assessment; and (c) coordinate the setting's case activity with that of the child protection agency.

Very often, a child is brought in for a health complaint that may or may not be the result of abuse. The discovery of abuse may depend on the suspicion of the health personnel. The suspicion may be substantiated by medical examination and

tests or may remain only a suspicion. A study by Lane and Dubowitz (2009) assessed the self-reported experience, comfort, and competence of primary care pediatricians in evaluating and managing cases of child maltreatment, in rendering opinions regarding the likelihood of child maltreatment, and in providing court testimony. The majority had little experience evaluating and reporting suspected child maltreatment. While they felt competent in conducting medical exams for suspected maltreatment, they felt less competent in rendering a definitive opinion and did not generally feel competent to testify in court. Their sense of competence was particularly low for sexual abuse.

The major social work functions in cases of child abuse are as follows:

- Raising medical personnel's index of suspicion
- Reducing the likelihood of an abuse situation going undetected and unconfirmed by a thorough psychosocial assessment that adds to the diagnostic work of the physician
- Attending to the emotional needs of the child and the parent
- Preparing the child and the parent for the sequence of events that follow the suspicion of abuse
- Informing and cooperating with child protection agency personnel

The performance of these functions is aided if the hospital's emergency department has a protocol for crisis intervention. The Boes and McDermott (2000) protocol suggests the following for assessment and intervention in child abuse cases:

1. Visual assessment of the patient's suspicious injuries, such as (1) bruises of several colors (indicating different times of abuse); (2) bruises that have odd shapes, are clustered, or are located in places where they could not be the result of an accident; (3) retinal damage (from being shaken); (4) orbital or facial fracture (if the child was not in a car accident); (5) rope burns or marks from restraints; (6) signs of hair pulling (bald spots, loose hair, or swollen scalp); and (7) "fearful behavior" reflected in

the patient speaking very softly, looking around when answering questions, and questioning the confidentiality of the interview.

2. Verbal inquiry that includes (1) an interview with the patient without family present, seeking to know (a) what events led to the patient's coming to the ER, (b) who composes the patient's household and what the family members' ages and health statuses are, (c) whether any family members were ever treated for mental health problems, (d) what the patient's past medical history is—whether he or she has had similar injuries in the past, and (e) how the patient's caretaker expresses anger, and (2) an interview with the person who brought or accompanied the child to the ER to see if there is any conflict of information between the two sources.

3. Patient being stabilized and transferred to the hospital's children's ward or children's hospital for further treatment, if needed.

4. If abuse is suspected, reporting the case to the local child protective service agency as well as the state's child abuse hot line.

5. Interviewing the mother (if she brought the child) privately to ascertain whether she is also a victim of abuse.

Spouse Abuse/Intimate Partner Violence

As pointed out above, cases of intimate partner violence (IPV), which are mostly battered women, are not looked for and treated with the same degree of concern as shown to victims of child abuse. Battering accounts for more than 25% of ER visits by women, yet even in hospitals with protocols for dealing with such cases, fewer than 1 in 25 are accurately diagnosed (Stark et al., 1981). Pagelow (1992) conducted an extensive review of the literature on women battering, which included several studies that found non-identification of victims of spousal abuse by medical personnel. Randall (1990) quoted one physician as saying, "The only physicians who ask about violence are psychiatrists, and they're only interested if it occurs in a dream. They rarely ask about the violent events that occur in real life" (p. 939). Pagelow (1981) found a pattern of disdain for battered women and considerable victim blaming on the part of physicians and nurses, who often attributed victims' returning home to abusive men to psychological defects in them. Pagelow (1992) concluded, however, that the situation is slowly changing, with nurses in emergency settings voluntarily reporting cases of wife abuse to police departments. This situation is likely to continue to change in the future, with more women in positions of authority—as physicians and managers—in health care settings. More and more physicians (particularly those in internal medicine, family practice, and ob-gyn) will include screening for IPV in their work with female patients. Trabold (2007) reviewed studies on intervention for IPV and found that screening (verbal and written) yields increased disclosure of IPV and provides an opportunity to make the needed resources available to victims. The perspective of medical personnel, however, is not expected to equal that of social workers in its comprehensiveness. Social workers will also continue to be the best liaisons between their health care setting and mental health and social services in the community. The social work functions in cases of IPV will include the following:

- Sensitizing other staff to the plight of IPV victims
- Advocating IPV screening and training for members of the health care team
- Advocating the development of an adult abuse protocol [1]
- Doing psychosocial assessment in cases of abuse
- Attending to the emotional needs of victims
- Enlarging the scope of intervention beyond the treatment of the medical problem
- Empowering victims with encouragement, information, and options
- Connecting victims with the appropriate abuse-related sources of support in the community, including spouse abuse shelters
- Linking victims with regular health care resources

Violence against women has both short-term and long-term effects on their physical and psychological well-being. Victims of abuse are much more likely than nonvictims to have poor health, chronic pain problems, addictions, problem pregnancies, depression, and suicide attempts (Plichta, 1992).

Screening for IPV should include the following questions (Kimberg, 2007):

> "Has your partner ever hit you or hurt you?"
>
> "Has your partner ever threatened you or frightened you?"
>
> "Has your partner ever forced you to have sex when you did not want to?"
>
> "Does your partner yell at you or frequently criticize you?"

The Committee on Violence (2004) has suggested the mnemonic RADAR for clinicians: **R,** *routinely screen*; **A,** *always ask*; **D,** *document response*; **A,** *assess safety and lethality*; and **R,** *respond.*

Assessment should include the following:

1. Current IPV: (1) victim's safety—threats of homicide, weapons involved, history of strangulation or stalking; (2) suicidality and homicidality; and (3) safety of children

2. Past IPV: (1) pattern of abuse and (2) history of effects of abuse, such as (a) injuries/ hospitalizations, (b) physical and psychological health effects, and (c) economic, social, and other effects

3. Support and coping strategies and readiness for change (Kimberg, 2007)

Intervention in cases of IPV should include the following:

1. Encouraging the victim to file a police report.

2. Explaining to the victim her options for ensuring her safety. She can take out a Protection from Abuse Order on a 24-hour basis or have the abuser arrested and held in custody. Also, electronic devices are available that aid in the protection of victims, such as alarm/security systems; electronic bracelets and pendants (worn around the neck) that, when activated, send a silent alarm to the police; cell phones preprogrammed to 911 for an emergency police response; and instant cameras that provide photographic evidence of abuse.

3. Encouraging the victim to call a hot line for counseling, information about shelters for women and children, and legal advice.

4. Assisting the victim in making such a call from the ER.

5. Being alert to the possibility of abuse and neglect of the victim's children (Boes & McDermott, 2000; Roberts & Roberts, 2000).

Elder Abuse

Elder abuse encompasses physical abuse and neglect, psychological and social abuse, and financial exploitation. Except in cases where the signs of physical abuse are obvious, the detection of even physical abuse in the elderly is difficult. Cognitively impaired and often confused elderly cannot tell about the abuse, and even those not so impaired often do not share their unpleasant secret because of denial, shame, or fear of a consequence worse than abuse. It is not uncommon that the abuser is the elderly person's caregiver. Other forms of abuse generally go unrecognized. Denial and improper assessment by health care professionals are also factors in the nonidentification of elder abuse (Benton & Marshall, 1991). All 50 states have legislation to protect elderly victims of domestic abuse and neglect, and 42 states have mandatory reporting laws, but there is significant inactivity in response to the legal mandate. Ehrlich and Anetzberger (1991) surveyed state public health departments on procedures for reporting elder abuse. All 50 states responded. Although 94% of respondents were aware of the state law, only 20% to 28% reported the use of written procedures or training materials specifically designed for health care personnel.

It is forecast that, in the future, the social scene will be dominated by more and more longer-living elderly who will assert their claim to societal resources, younger generations will become resentful of the elderly, traditional caregivers will become increasingly less available, and caregiving will become more impersonal. This forecast gives little hope for the elder abuse situation improving in the future. However, there will be a comprehensive approach to the detection of elder abuse through the use of standard assessment instruments such as the one proposed by Fulmer (1984). This instrument has eight sections that together cover assessment of all dimensions of an elderly person's life, such as mental status; hygiene and nutrition; usual lifestyle; interactions with significant others; the presence of bruises, contractures, pressure sores, and lacerations; and other medical signs and symptoms of possible abuse or neglect. Despite the use of such instruments, the difficulty of determining the reality of abuse will persist. When an alert and oriented elder chooses to deny or deliberately hide the existence of abuse, its detection requires extra sensitivity for, strong ability to relate to, and sharp skill in assessing that patient's situation. Social workers in acute ambulatory care settings can make a significant difference in the need for early detection of and appropriate intervention in cases of elder abuse. Because of their training and the major purpose of their activity, social workers possess these professional attributes more than do other health care providers. Their functions in these cases would be similar to those in the case of IPV:

- Supplementing the medical diagnosis with psychosocial assessment
- Attending to the immediate nonmedical needs of the patient
- Reporting abuse to the appropriate authorities
- Coordinating the acute care setting's case activity with the work of the adult protection agency
- Planning for discharge of the patient

Rape

As a traumatic experience, rape is unique because it is the quintessential violation of a person and leaves the victim feeling used, damaged, and defiled (Soskis, 1985). Norris (1992) examined the frequency and impact of 10 potentially traumatic events among 1,000 adults and found

1 in 3 female

that, whereas tragic death occurred most often and motor vehicle crashes presented the most adverse combination of frequency and impact, sexual assault yielded the highest rate of post-traumatic stress disorder. Although men are raped with equally devastating effects, the majority of victims seen in health care settings are women. Frazier and Cohen (1992) reviewed research on prevalence and effects of three types of sexual victimization of women—child sexual abuse, sexual assault, and sexual harassment—and concluded that these experiences are quite common among women and have serious detrimental effects on their mental health.

The societal picture of rape as a major problem is not likely to change substantially in the future. Two parallel but opposing forces will continue to operate. On the one hand, historically, the trend has been toward a gradual decrease in the prosecution of and penalty for rape. During the 17th, 18th, and 19th centuries, rape was not as prevalent as it became in 20th-century America, but it was viewed with horror and was severely punished (Crossman, 1992). *Rape myths,* defined as prejudicial, stereotypical, and false beliefs about rape, rape victims, and rapists, continue to be accepted by people from varied walks of life, including women (Tabone et al., 1992). The convicted sexual offenders are extremely heterogeneous, which makes focused preventive work impossible. On the other hand, social workers will continue to improve their understanding of the phenomenon of rape (Ellis, 1991; Haggard, 1991; Lakey, 1992; Malamuth, 1991; Prentky & Knight, 1991), leading to better preventive and therapeutic programs. Steinberg (1991) suggested that Title IX be amended to define rape as sex discrimination. Such efforts will be made to increase rape prosecution rates.

Rape victims being seen in the ambulatory acute care setting often have no physical injury and are there for the physical examination and specimen collection necessary for evidentiary reasons. They are invariably in a state of acute emotional crisis, which must be handled with utmost care and understanding. Responding to such crises is in the appropriate domain of social work expertise. Social work functions in these cases are as follows:

- Ensuring that the rape patient is not kept sitting in the waiting room like most patients with nonurgent medical problems
- Listening to the patient with empathy and acceptance of her emotions
- Helping her deal constructively with feelings of guilt and shame
- Restoring her sense of control in whatever ways the situation will permit
- Contacting the local rape crisis center and putting the resources of that agency at her disposal
- Helping her identify and mobilize her own social supports
- Being available for follow-up and linking her with the appropriate mental health, legal, and social services

Social work functions in the social emergencies discussed above will require the social worker to assume the role of *helper with the crisis* the patient is in, *advocate,* and *coordinator of services* of the health care setting and other appropriate agencies.

Social Work Role in a Terrorism-Related Medical Emergency

The medical response to such an emergency will vary according to the type of weapon used in the terrorist attack and the nature of injuries resulting from that weapon.

> Thus, if a terrorist's weapons are conventional explosives, trauma surgeons and anesthesiologists are likely to be called to service. If chemical or radiological agents are dispersed, toxicologists, radiologists, and pulmonologists might be engaged. If biological agents are released, specialists in infectious disease and dermatology could be essential. (Shapira, Hammond, & Cole, 2009, p. 4)

As per these authors, this type of emergency also requires advanced knowledge and preparation on the part of medical care providers, their ability to treat a large number of casualties, protocols for incident management, stockpiling of supplies in accessible locations, and a communication system that connects the hospital with other hospitals, law enforcement authorities, and families of victims. Victims are likely to be not only many but also with multiple impairments. They are invariably innocent people. They are likely to be overwhelmed by a sense of rage, grief, despair, and abject powerlessness (Larkin & Woody, 2005; Miller, 2004).

Patients arriving at an ER show a variety of psychological reactions. Some may be calm, while others may be extremely distressed. This distress often includes

> anxiety symptoms: crying, shaking, and agitation. It can also manifest as dissociation: Patients feel as if they are not "there," but are watching themselves, or have such vivid intrusive images of the attack that they are not aware of their immediate surroundings. (Freedman, 2009, p. 417)

The symptoms of PTSD (posttraumatic stress disorder) are common in these victims but should not necessarily be considered pathological. The main aim of nonmedical intervention is to "stop" the traumatic event for the patient. Patients may be confused about what really happened to them, have difficulty locating their family and friends, and be unsure about the medical procedure they will be undergoing. Providing the needed information and help while assuring them that they are now in a safe place will help stop the traumatic event (Freedman, 2009). Larkin and Woody (2005) advise against detailed questioning about the traumatic experience because patients "are often in a state of heightened arousal, and verbalization and elaboration of a traumatic experience at this point can exacerbate distress" (p. 391). Social workers are superbly qualified to perform the vital tasks mentioned above. They will also be helping the patients' loved ones as they pour in. Other tasks they are likely to perform have been discussed in regard to their roles in true medical emergencies.

Social Work Role in Nonemergency Health and Social Needs

Earlier, we talked about a large proportion of the patient population of acute care settings consisting of those who do not have an emergency situation. Most of these people come to the acute care settings because they have nowhere else to go. They all have a need that they believe deserves immediate attention and assistance. Some have medical problems that could be treated in a nonacute ambulatory setting if one were accessible to them financially and logistically. Others have nonmedical problems that they are able to couch in medical terms. Still others have problems that are simply nonmedical but cannot be taken to social service agencies because these agencies are not open in the evenings, at night, and on the weekends. The greatest attraction that acute ambulatory care settings, particularly emergency rooms, have is that they are open 24 hours a day, 7 days a week. As Soskis (1985) put it,

> A sizable proportion of people visiting emergency rooms have no major medical complaint or sometimes no medical complaint at all, and often few or no resources—social, economic, or otherwise—to help them cope with the problems that brought them in. This group comes to the emergency room because the emergency room is always open, because they can usually get there (by police, fire rescue, or similar transport), and because they know that they will be seen. (p. 3)

In the group of people who come to these settings without legitimate health problems, Soskis (1985) included alcoholics, the homeless, runaways, persons with psychiatric conditions, and "space cases." The space cases are the chronic former mental patients living on the streets but shunned by other homeless. All these are unwelcome because they are seen as inappropriately using and abusing the resources of an acute care setting. Talking of the homeless as ER patients, Beder (2006) says that the mind-set of administrators in many inner city hospitals is to "Treat 'em and street 'em." Some are more unwelcome than others, however. They include (a) those who

have chronic and complex problems, come frequently, and are demanding and hostile; (b) those who are emotionally disturbed or have drug and alcohol problems and who come in after fights or accidents, have attempted suicides and homicides, and are disruptive; and (c) the elderly whose presenting problems are related to aging, such as sleeplessness, loss of mobility and memory, aches and pains, malnutrition, and feelings of being unable to cope (Soskis, 1980).

Social work activity in regard to these patients is fourfold: (1) assessing their needs; (2) ensuring that they are medically screened and treated, if need be; (3) providing the necessary concrete social services; and (4) referring them to an appropriate community social service, mental health service, or other health care resource (discharge planning). Sometimes, social workers are able to go beyond these actions. One of the ER social workers whom Beder (2006) interviewed talked about a satisfying case of a *repeater* (a patient who came to the ER frequently). Over time, the worker got to know this homeless woman, who was in her mid-50s with a history of extensive alcoholism. On each visit, she was put into a cubicle, fed, and allowed to sleep off her intoxication. The worker, who spent some time listening to her story, concerns, and fears, was able to persuade her to try to stop drinking and seek admission to a homeless shelter. A protocol for crisis intervention in the hospital emergency room, developed by Boes and McDermott (2000), includes assessment and intervention strategies for homeless, substance abuse, and psychiatric patients. The following suggestions taken from that protocol can be incorporated into the fourfold activity mentioned above.

Homeless Patients: Assessment and Intervention

Assessment: Explore all possible places where the patient could stay. Helpful questions include, (1) How long have you been without shelter? (2) Where did you stay last night? (3) Do you have friends or family in the area who can provide shelter? (4) Have you ever been in a shelter before? If yes, which one? (5) Are you willing to go to a shelter now?

Intervention: If the patient is willing to go to a shelter, contact various shelters in the area to see if a bed is available. If there is evidence of a mental health problem, contact the appropriate mental health unit/agency and arrange for an evaluation. If no beds are available in the local homeless shelters, call the Office of Service to Homeless Adults for assistance. When a bed is found, arrange transportation for the patient to go there.

Psychiatric Patients: Assessment and Intervention

Assessment: Important suggestions for assessment are as follows: (1) Observe the patient's behavior to determine if it poses a danger to him or her or others. If so, talk to the medical staff to determine if restraints are necessary. (2) Review the patient's chart and consult with the person who accompanied the patient to the ER and the physician regarding the patient's present condition and past mental health history. (3) Observe and interview the patient for signs of mental illness such as agitation, depression, disorientation, and suicide attempts. (4) Obtain the usual information on (a) the presenting problem, its symptoms and duration, and precipitating events leading to the patient coming to the ER; (b) any history of drugs or alcohol abuse, arrests, other medical problems and their treatments; and (c) the patient's living situation and its stability, social support system and its resources, etc.

Intervention: Intervention will depend on such factors as whether (1) the patient is medically cleared for discharge but is a threat to himself or herself or others, (2) the patient is not medically cleared and is admitted to the hospital voluntarily, and (3) the patient is not medically cleared and has to be admitted to the hospital involuntarily. 6404

1. *The patient is medically cleared for discharge but is a threat to himself or herself or others.*

   a. Call for a psychiatric consult for evaluation.

   b. If the consulting psychiatrist thinks that the patient requires inpatient treatment and the patient is willing to enter treatment voluntarily and has the health insurance coverage for that treatment, the psychiatrist will arrange for his or her admission to the appropriate facility. If the patient is willing to go for inpatient treatment but has no insurance, arrange for placement in a public mental hospital and have him or her sign the necessary voluntary commitment form.

   c. If the psychiatrist has recommended inpatient treatment and patient is resistant, involuntary placement is required. The ER physician and the psychiatrist have to complete the involuntary commitment form, petition for the patient's placement, and contact the appropriate mental health facility.

   d. Arrange for the patient's transportation to the mental health facility, as he or she must be transported by ambulance.

2. *The patient is not medically cleared and is admitted to the hospital voluntarily.* The hospital physicians will deal with the case and consult a psychiatrist if considered necessary.

3. *The patient is not medically cleared and has to be admitted to the hospital involuntarily.* In such cases, only a judge can issue an emergency medical commitment order. Contact an administrator of the hospital who will contact the appropriate authorities and find a judge to issue such an order.

Alcoholics/Substance Abuse Patients: Assessment and Intervention

Assessment: The questions that should be woven into the assessment interview are, (1) When did you last use the substance? (2) What is it and how much was used? (3) What was the method of use (e.g., drinking, smoking, snorting, injecting)? (4) How often do you use the substance? (5) How long have you been using it? (6) Have you ever been in detoxification or rehabilitation? (7) If yes, when and where was it and what was the result? (8) Are you willing to enter such a program now? (9) If yes, would you prefer an inpatient or outpatient program? (10) What kind of health insurance coverage do you have, if any? (11) If you have health insurance, can you show me your insurance card? Look for the physical symptoms of substance abuse such as shakes, blackouts, and seizures.

Intervention:

If the patient is interested in entering a detoxification or rehabilitation program, make sure that the patient is medically cleared for transfer to a detox or rehab facility. Make sure that he or she is willing to go immediately. Contact the patient's health insurance company for precertification. The insurance company will determine where the patient will be referred, will find a bed, and will confirm admission. When that happens, arrange for his or her transportation to the facility.

If the patient is not interested in entering a detoxification or rehabilitation program or would like outpatient help, make a referral to an appropriate outpatient program and encourage the patient to follow through on that referral. If it is after hours, give the patient the pertinent information (the name, address, phone number, and contact person at the agency) and explain the procedure so that he or she can follow up the next day or when ready.

As we will see later in this chapter, the advocacy skills of the social worker become most important in dealing with patients who come to acute care settings for nonacute and nonmedical needs. The social worker has to be an advocate for these patients while contacting resources outside as well as inside the unit, because these patients do overtax the emotional resources of the staff. Therefore, in cases of these "abusers" of the facility, the social work role is that of *advocate* within and outside the setting, *broker,* and *provider of concrete services.*

Other Social Work Roles in Acute Ambulatory Care

Besides the patient-oriented roles, the social worker will continue to play two other roles: one focused on other professionals/service providers and the other related to the environment of the setting. The social worker plays the role of an *educator* when he or she

a. provides information on the patient's social, emotional, and demographic situation;

b. interprets the patient's needs and/or helps the patient articulate those needs beyond vague complaints;

c. enables medical professionals to discover the not-so-obvious cases of physical, sexual, and other forms of abuse; and

d. helps those professionals not be blinded to the real health problems by stereotypical views of the homeless, substance abusers, those with chronic mental illness, and difficult patients.

The social worker helps his or her fellow care providers keep their morale high and stress low by managing the social dimension of the ever-occurring crises. He or she can also play the role of a *therapeutic helper* by enabling these emergency health care workers to deal with the *critical incident stress,* particularly after their involvement in terrorism-related emergencies. Larkin and Woody (2005) defined critical incident stress as "an unusually strong emotional, behavioral, psychological, physiological reaction of an emergency worker who is confronted with an acute traumatic event outside the usual human experience" (p. 393). Critical incident stress management is done through debriefing, and social workers have the skills for this. Larkin and Woody (2005) presented the process and techniques for debriefing [2].

The social worker also plays the role of *stabilizer* of the health care setting. By attending to the patients and/or their families—who must wait, at times, for hours—the social worker contributes to making the setting's atmosphere less aversive and more supportive (Soskis, 1985).

We end this section with a recap of future social worker roles in acute ambulatory care settings in Table 5-A.

Table 5-A   Future Social Work Roles in Acute Ambulatory Care Settings

- Social work role in true medical emergencies
- Social work role in social emergencies
- Social work role in a terrorism-related medical emergency
- Social work role in nonemergency health and social needs
- Other social work roles in acute ambulatory care

FUTURE SOCIAL WORK ROLES IN NONACUTE AMBULATORY CARE SETTINGS

In the future, health care will have changed so that most care will be (a) provided by groups or teams of professionals, (b) geared to accommodate the specific needs of special groups, and (c) marked by such attributes as accessibility, comprehensiveness, coordination, and accountability. The limelight will be on ambulatory care settings, and they will be expected to demonstrate and reflect these changes and attributes. Social workers will significantly contribute to that reality. This chapter elaborates on the above attributes of care to highlight social work roles and functions.

"Accessibility refers to the responsibility of the health provider team to assist the patient or the potential patient to overcome temporal, spatial, economic, and psychologic barriers to health care" (Wallace, Goldberg, & Slaby, 1984, p. 29). With the implementation of the new law, financial barriers to care will be removed in the future, but other barriers will persist. Social work skills will be valued in helping patients overcome those barriers.

An Institute of Medicine (1978) report defined comprehensiveness as the ability and willingness of the primary care team to handle most of the health problems in the population it serves. It is estimated that between 20% and 70% of all visits to general medical clinics involve such problems as substance abuse, domestic violence, sexual dysfunction, stress reactions, grief, anxiety, and depression (Rosen, Locke, Goldberg, & Babigian, 1972), which are more psychosocial than medical. Comprehensiveness demands that these problems be handled and monitored in the health care setting.

> Since such patients appear with problems at medical settings, and since such problems are intertwined in a complex fashion with bodily symptoms and feelings, the responsible course is to develop a strategy for patient management at the point at which help is sought. (Mechanic, 1980, p. 18)

Moreover, many patients do not want to go to mental health or social service agencies because of the stigma attached to seeking help there. Social workers are skilled at handling these problems. They can enhance the setting's ability to provide comprehensive services.

Coordination of services is the next attribute of primary care and involves the responsibility of ensuring that all the pieces of care provided to the patient (within the setting and outside by medical specialists and others) fit together and yield the maximum benefit. Even if the care coordinator is a medical person,

> the role of patient care coordinator at times calls for the contribution of the team social worker, particularly when environmental/network/systems issues both within and without the health care establishment appear to threaten, disrupt, or preclude the process of diagnosis and treatment. (Wallace et al., 1984, p. 31)

Netting and Williams (2001) reported the results of their examination of nine projects, funded by the John A. Hartford Foundation, to develop care coordination models based in physician offices. These projects employed different personnel as care coordinators, called intervention agents. These included nurses, physician assistants, and paraprofessionals. Two projects used social workers in case-management–type roles and one as a consultant with nurse practitioners. The project physicians referred to older patients' life problems as "cans of worms," "Pandora's boxes," and "seas of trouble." Dealing with those problems required skills in advocacy, mediation, negotiation, and community relations—skills that social workers have acquired as part of their education and socialization.

Continuity of services is dependent on their accessibility, comprehensiveness, and coordination, as well as the setting's ability to accommodate other subjective and objective patient-related variables affecting the patient's willingness to continue. It may require individualizing, reaching out to, and understanding the unique reality of patients and their families. Social workers have an edge over other professionals in accomplishing these tasks. Again in the words of Wallace et al. (1984),

> The contribution of social work to primary care is essential when it comes to ensuring continuity of care with poor, uneducated, perpetually crisis-prone, or barely functioning patients. Intervention with these cases often requires experience with a particular set of values and with a lifestyle, which is distant from middle-class proprieties and preoccupations. (p. 32)

Accountability is an attribute not unique to primary care. An Institute of Medicine (1978) report recommended that, to ensure accountability, the primary care practice should regularly review the process and outcomes of its care; establish a policy of providing information to the patient about the risks, undesirable effects, and unexpected outcomes of treatment; and follow sound fiscal management policies and procedures. Social workers will have as much to offer to the realization of accountability as other members of the group.

In the future, ambulatory care settings will make concerted efforts to acquire, incorporate, and practice these attributes and, in the process, will experience a shift in the perspective on care from biomedical to biopsychosocial. As it is acknowledged that the social element can be as life threatening as the physical and psychological illness, the "social" dimension of care will become as important as the "biological" and the "psychological," and with that will come a deeper appreciation of the contributions of nonmedical health care providers such as social workers.

> The true foundation of primary care lies in the realization that operationalizing comprehensive models of health care requires collaborative effort beyond the expertise of medicine no matter how less specialized it becomes. The foremost responsibility of medicine and its unique area of expertise will be the biological dimension of health care. In essence, the primary care physician is the biomedical specialist as part of the primary care team, appreciative of the psychosocial and social

dimensions but not inexpertly attempting to provide them. (Wallace et al., 1984, p. 65)

Social workers will have made tremendous contributions to that biopsychosocial model in the future. The major social work roles in nonacute ambulatory settings will include both patient-focused and other roles.

Patient-Focused Social Work Roles

Patient-focused social work roles will include the following:

1. *Clinical work with patients and their families.* This work may be necessitated by (a) concerns of the well and the worried well, (b) difficulties in coping with the stresses of life that find expression as somatic and psychosomatic complaints in some patients, (c) primary psychosocial problems of others threatening to jeopardize their physical health, and (d) psychosocial problems accompanying disease—problems in understanding and accepting diagnosis, coping and following through with treatment, living with its physical and emotional effects, and dealing with the social consequences of illness. Work with families has been a neglected area of primary care. Even physicians trained as family practitioners have, in actual practice, focused on the individual rather than the family. Social workers will be able to fill that gap. Their clinical work may involve such diverse modalities as providing information, crisis intervention, short-term therapy, and long-term casework. The strength orientation of social work will pervade these interventions and will be viewed as a distinguishing and valued mark of the contribution of social workers.

2. *Coordination of services for patients and families provided by several agencies and programs.* Other agencies may be hospitals and medical centers providing more intensive secondary and tertiary health care or mental health centers and social work programs providing nonmedical services. There will always be patients

whose problems are so complex as to make the resources of an ambulatory health care setting inadequate.

3. *Education as part of disease prevention and health promotion activities.* Most nonacute ambulatory care facilities will provide disease prevention and health promotion programs as part of their comprehensive services. These programs will offer health education and social support groups for those struggling with different types of problems.

> Health-related problems, such as obesity, substance abuse (including smoking), prolonged stress, child abuse, child sexual abuse, terminal illness, and behaviors leading to high-risk pregnancy, could be the focus of such group activities. (Greene, Kruse, & Arthurs, 1985, p. 63)

Social workers will be involved as organizers, facilitators, and educators of these groups.

Other Social Work Roles

The most prominent other social work role will be that of consultant, performing *consultation work with fellow professionals* from other disciplines. Consultation may be about psychosocial problems or psychosocial dimensions of health problems in response to the need for a comprehensive diagnosis, or about exploring and involving community resources in comprehensive treatment plans. Greene et al. (1985) listed the following areas where social work consultation can enrich a physician's diagnostic and treatment skills: (a) psychosocial aspects of the patient's functioning; (b) individual and family dynamics affecting the etiology and treatment of health problems; (c) transitions through family life stages that tend to create stress and generate problems; (d) the physician's interviewing skills with a view toward recognizing psychosocial problems masked by physical complaints, dynamics of the interactions between himself or herself and the patient, and body language signals of emotional stress by focusing on the whole person; and (e) community resources and approaches to accessing them.

SOCIAL WORK KNOWLEDGE AND SKILLS FOR ROLE-RELATED INTERVENTIONS

Here, we discuss the knowledge and skills appropriate for the various professional functions that social workers in ambulatory care settings are likely to perform as they relate to the major social work roles identified above.

Social Worker as Crisis Counselor/Manager

As pointed out earlier, two kinds of major emergencies are encountered in acute ambulatory care settings: one created by a sudden serious physical illness or injury, the other resulting from various types of person abuse that may or may not be accompanied by physical trauma. Both types of emergencies thrust the patient and his or her loved ones into a state of crisis. Even in the nonacute health care settings, patients and their families seek help when they cannot handle life's crises with their own resources.

> Poorer, less educated, more disorganized and chaotic individuals and social networks are increasingly resorting to health care providers ... to obtain problem-solving help, often for complaints which are only tangentially medical. Even when presenting complaints are emphatically medical, the psychosocial component is commonly so integral that medical attention cannot be provided without immediately addressing the nonmedical issue as well. (Wallace et al., 1984, p. 71)

In acute care settings, management of the medical aspect of the crisis is the focus and responsibility of the medical professionals, whereas its nonmedical dimensions, including emotional, social, economic, and legal, are often not given adequate attention. This unevenness in the treatment of emergencies is likely to disappear in the future. Commitment to the concepts of "comprehensiveness of care" and "treating the total patient" will result in the filling of gaps in the current system of care. Social workers will be instrumental in correcting the situation. In nonacute settings, wherever they are a part of the establishment, social workers already provide a significant part of crisis intervention services. In the future, their presence on ambulatory care teams will increase, and in taking responsibility for the psychosocial aspects of health care, they will play the role of *crisis counselors and managers.*

Knowledge of crisis theory and principles of crisis intervention is necessary for effective help in the management of crises. Because all social workers have acquired that knowledge as part of their training, it will suffice to list here the basic pieces of that knowledge and to reiterate some "shoulds" of crisis intervention. This material is drawn from several sources (Boes & McDermott, 2000; Dhooper, 1990; Golan, 1969; Morrice, 1976; Rapaport, 1967; Roberts, 2000; Shulman & Shewbert, 2000; Smith, 1977; Soskis, 1985; Wallace et al., 1984).

Social workers know that

- a crisis develops in stages, and an identifiable event precipitates the crisis;
- the normal coping abilities of the individual have either broken down or are inadequate to dealing with the situation;

- the person in crisis is more susceptible, vulnerable, and dependent than usual, and this makes him or her more accessible to intervention;
- the crisis period is time limited, and the availability of help in time is crucial—without help, the crisis may result in the individual's functioning at a poorer level;
- even a little help has a lot of positive effect—intervention is more likely to be successful if made during the acute crisis;
- the major tasks necessary for crisis resolution are (a) cognitive—viewing the situation accurately and realistically; (b) emotional—acknowledging, accepting, and discharging one's feelings; and (c) problem solving—considering and weighing the available options, developing adaptive behaviors, and seeking and using formal help and informal support.

The social worker needs to adapt whichever model of crisis intervention he or she espouses to the health care setting. The well-known Roberts' (2000) Seven-Stage model [3] is adaptable to work in medical emergencies. We present some of the important "shoulds" for social work crisis intervention in Table 5-B below.

Table 5-B Essentials of Social Work Crisis Intervention

- Believe that something positive must come out of the person's crisis experience. Hence, intervene with the purpose of enabling the patient to turn the painful life event into an opportunity for survival, growth, and improvement.
- Try to stay with the crisis (provide the maximum help as close to the precipitating event as possible). "As with any crisis, a medical crisis, especially a traumatic event, needs to be processed as early as possible before defenses have the opportunity of reconstituting" (Shulman & Shewbert, 2000, p. 426).
- Recognize and meet the patient's need for emotional support, use empathic listening, encourage expression of feelings, validate those feelings, and provide hope. Help the patient ward off feelings of powerlessness.*
- Convince and remind the patient that seeking and using help is a sign of strength, not a mark of weakness. Help only brings out the person's own innate resilience.
- Be active and direct rather than passive or neutral and indirect, without the fear of fostering dependence.
- Focus on the current situation and encourage planning and action rather than dwelling on past actions and memories.
- Mobilize for the patient the patient's own informal social supports, as well as formal sources of help inside and outside the health care setting.

---

*"Feelings of powerlessness awaken panic, which darkens one's powers to effectively cope through a crisis. Panic is like the pessimistic person who turns out all the lights just to see how dark it is. One would never attempt to drive at night down a steep, treacherous cliffside road without headlights" (Boes & McDermott, 2000, p. 408).

Although the above suggestions are worded as if the focus of social work activity were on the patient, the focus may be on the patient's family, in which case the family's understanding, needs, resources, and strengths will have to be assessed and worked with. In situations of a patient's impending death from an unexpected injury or illness, it is difficult to think of the family crisis as yielding something positive. Social workers based in acute care settings, however, know of the ever-present need for human organs and tissues for transplantation and that families who donate the organs and tissues of their deceased loved one find solace in that donation and view it as something positive coming out of their tragedy. Therefore, the social worker in ambulatory acute care settings who deals with such families should mention organ donation as an opportunity for them to make some choices and regain some control over their situation. These families have the choice of donating or not donating, and if they choose to donate, they have the option of donating all or some of the organs and tissues and deciding how the donated body parts will be used—for transplantation, medical therapy, or research.

Earlier, it was proposed that notifying the family of a seriously ill or injured, dying, or dead patient should be one of the functions of the social worker. Bearer of bad news is not a pleasant role, but the social worker is the best qualified to play that role. He or she should remember that the news may trigger a crisis for the family. Here are a few helpful suggestions based on the author's experience, the work of Soskis (1985), of Boes and McDermott (2000), and of others reported by Beder (2006). The social worker should do the following:

- See the patient before calling the family so that he or she can give a firsthand visual report to the family, if needed.
- Identify himself or herself and the place he or she is calling from.
- Explain the reason for calling briefly, clearly, and specifically, leaving no gaps for the listener to fill with his or her own imaginings.

- Ask only those questions that need to be answered immediately, such as the patient's past illnesses or present medications.
- Tell the family that the patient is critically ill (even if the patient has died) and that they should come immediately. This will give them time to prepare for the worst news.
- Assume that the shock and fear will cause many listeners to miss or distort much of what is told them and, therefore, ask the person to repeat what has been said.
- Find out whether the family can actually get to the emergency care center and whether they need assistance with transportation, directions to the center, information about parking, and so on.
- Assess the listener's ability to drive safely, and, accordingly, advise that the person either wait until emotions have settled or get someone else to drive.
- Make the call the beginning of his or her activity with the family and offer assistance with concrete needs—if they are from out of town, they may need help with lodging and long-distance communication.
- On the arrival of the family member/s, place them in a private area and share with them as much information about the patient's condition as possible, thereby reducing the element of surprise in case the patient dies. The information should be given in as simple language as possible, because wordiness and excessive use of medical terminology create confusion and increase anxiety.
- Try to refocus their anxiety by encouraging them to talk about the patient, their relationship with the patient, and other members of the family. Ask if other members need to be contacted.
- Explain the codes (internal communication within the hospital that signals emergency activity on behalf of the patient) so that the family can make a decision about the limits they want the medical team to pursue on behalf of the patient.
- If the patient has died, tell the family about hospital protocol regarding the funeral arrangements and care of the body. Tell them that they need to call a funeral home when they are able to.
- Remember that the most difficult time for most families, second to hearing of the death, is when they view the patient's body. Prepare them for what the dead body may look like. It

might have been disfigured if the patient was in an accident and may still be hooked to tubes and equipment.

- Be a source of emotional support and try to be seen as a comforting person. Offer to call other members of the family or clergy. He/she may choose to accompany the family when they go in to see the patient's body. Provide them tissues or anything else that may aid in their comfort.
- Make sure that the patient's belongings are given to the appropriate member of the family.
- If possible, make sure that the dead patient's spouse or a family member does not go home alone or to an empty house.
- Be prepared to deal with a situation in which he/she becomes the target of family members' anger toward the medical establishment for "letting the patient die."

Social Worker as Clinician and Caseworker

Even in busy and at times chaotic acute ambulatory care settings, there is room for meaningful, brief—even one-shot—clinical casework. Discussing the importance of how a patient is treated in an ER, Soskis (1985) said,

It is here that he or she receives his or her first and probably lasting impression of how the system works: helping, supporting, confusing, blaming, punishing, humiliating. . . . The social worker's attitudes and activity here may make a tremendous difference in how the patient views and copes with what is happening to him or her. (p. 53)

The social worker should remember that an acute medical condition often sets the stage for vital changes in people's lives. The old saying, "Strike while the iron is hot," represents a profound truth about human behavior. The social worker's basic assessment and intervention skills must be tailored to the realities of the acute setting. He or she should be able to do a quick psychosocial assessment and undertake an appropriate clinical activity that may involve (a) giving the patient an insight into the psychosocial antecedents or consequences of the patient's

medical problem, (b) intensifying the patient's awakened motivation to deal with the problem beyond the medical treatment, (c) sharing with the patient ideas and suggestions for help, and (d) referring the patient to an outside professional resource.

In nonacute ambulatory care settings, it is forecast that a biopsychosocial model of care will gradually replace the current biomedical model. That shift, plus the fact that a large proportion of patients seen in these settings present problems that are more psychosocial than medical, will create new opportunities for significant contributions by social workers. Their professional philosophy and skills are in tune with the biopsychosocial model, their expertise lies in dealing with psychosocial problems, and their interventions may be more appropriate for nonmedical problems. For effective clinical work, however, they will need to supplement their basic knowledge with greater understanding of biomedical and psychiatric issues—for example,

the social worker must appreciate that sexual dysfunction can be secondary to (that is, caused by) diabetes mellitus and does not always represent a "psychological" problem. Working with patients who have substance abuse problems requires a knowledge of the appropriate use of toxicology screens, symptoms indicative of withdrawal states, behavioral manifestations of different toxicotives, and so on. (Wallace et al., 1984, p. 37)

While understanding the psychodynamics of patients' problems, the social worker should also know when to seek consultation from a psychiatrist or to refer a patient to a mental health facility for specialized services. The worker should strengthen his or her assessment skills with the use of appropriate instruments for identifying patients at high risk for social, psychological, and physical problems.

The medical needs of most nonacute patients will pertain to chronic problems.

Understanding the difference between illness and disease is a prerequisite to the care of patients affected by incurable disorders. Even though many chronic conditions are incurable, the discomfort or disability they produce may be substantially modified. (Conger & Moore, 1988, p. 108)

The social worker should understand and develop sensitivity to the characteristics of chronic conditions that cannot be cured but must be managed. Buada, Pomeranz, and Rosenberg (1986) listed the following as the mandates of chronic conditions:

- Chronic conditions are long-term, and the affected patient has an ongoing need for service.
- Chronic conditions often fluctuate and thereby create the need for differing levels of services simultaneously.
- Chronic conditions involve subjectively experienced discomfort, pain, and disability, and, therefore, the measures of relief must address those subjective elements.
- Chronic conditions also significantly affect the patient's family and significant others, and the focus of service must also be on the needs of those informal caregivers.
- Chronic conditions require a service package that includes a large variety of support services, along with medical services.

Patients who are disabled because of chronic illness react to their condition in a number of ways, depending on the severity and type of disability. The pattern of reaction has such elements as (a) uncertainty, (b) anxiety, (c) depression, (d) anger expressed directly, (e) anger expressed indirectly, (f) desire for the feeling of competence, (g) helplessness and hopelessness, (h) threatened sociability, and (i) variance in good feelings (Viney & Westbrook, 1981). The social worker should be sensitive to the presence of these elements. He or she should explore and deal with them as a part of the assessment and treatment of chronically ill patients. Although it is difficult to predict a patient's reaction to disability, the more global the disabling condition, the more psychologically devastating it is likely to be (Conger & Moore, 1988).

Social workers well recognize the importance of resources for coping with stress. Those who work with the chronically ill should also remember that self-controlled resources are more effective than other-controlled resources for such patients.

Whatever the demands, ultimately, it is the individual who is constantly confronted by them, interprets them, assigns them a subjective meaning, and constantly has to respond to them. The greater an individual's control of resources, the greater will be his or her capacity to cope successfully. (Conger & Moore, 1988, p. 105)

Therefore, social work intervention should include the creation and strengthening of resources within the patient's control.

In view of the broader service missions of ambulatory care settings in the future and for dealing with the varied problems of patients and families, the social worker will have to master many skills. These should include skills in using short-term problem- or task-focused therapies, manipulating the patient's environment, and helping in the maintenance of those with chronic problems, as well as skills in using theories and techniques for behavior change in such cases as obesity, tobacco use, and substance abuse.

Among the "difficult" patients or families that all human services professionals must deal with are those who are crisis prone. Their lives seem to be a series of crises. The practice principles derived from crisis theory and other therapeutic approaches are often not effective in working with these people. Even systems theory, which guides the overall social work perspective, fails to explain their behaviors and situations. Social workers should familiarize themselves with and learn to use other potentially more useful approaches. Chaos theory promises to provide important clues to understanding and working with "chaotic" systems (e.g., see Gleick, 1987; Goldberger, Rigney, & West, 1990; Hoffman, 1988; Kagan & Schlossberg, 1989; Olson, 1989; Pietgen & Richter, 1986; Wood & Geismar, 1989). Hudson (2000) refers to chaos theory as complex systems theory and seems to agree with those who argue that the 20th century saw three major scientific revolutions—relativity, quantum, and chaos theory. He mentioned the use of this theory in psychology (particularly in the field of psychopathology), education, and sociology. Bussolari and Goodell (2009) presented an application of this theory for counselors working with clients experiencing life transitions.

There are several theories of behavior change that can be divided by the scope of their focus (i.e., intrapersonal, interpersonal, group) or the style of their focus (i.e., cognitive, behavioral, social, environmental). Social workers should understand these theories and the therapeutic approaches drawn from them and build those into their professional repertoire. Motivational interviewing is the preferred approach. Lessler and Dunn (2007) included several different theories and models under the rubric of behavior theory and discussed their assumptions and implications for promoting behavior change. Table 5-C below is based on their material.

The Stages of Change model (Prochaska & DiClemente, 1983; Walley & Roll, 2007) is considered transtheoretical. It describes the "how" of change. According to this model, behavior change is a gradual, continuous, and dynamic process. People progress through a sequence of five stages.

1. *Precontemplative:* Persons in this stage have no intention to change their behavior. They either deny they need to change or feel hopeless.

2. *Contemplative:* Persons in this stage have formed an intention to change but have no specific plan. They still may be ambivalent about change.

3. *Preparation or determination:* Persons in this stage are ready for action. They are making plans to change their behavior.

4. *Action:* Persons in this stage have begun changing their behavior, but the change may be inconsistent.

5. *Maintenance:* Persons in this stage are maintaining a consistent change. The newly acquired behavior has become a part of their lives.

Patients in the final three stages of change are less challenging for the professionals working with them. They proactively ask for advice and

Table 5-C   Theories of Behavior Change and Their Applications

Theory	Assumption/s	Theory-Based Approach
Humanistic theory	People are likely to change in the presence of those who accept them as they are.	Listen to, understand, and accept them as they are.
Health belief model	People will change if they believe they are vulnerable to risk and change will pay off.	Give them information on risks and benefits.
Self-efficacy theory	People will try to change if they believe they are able to do it.	Tell them change is possible, and emphasize their strengths.
Self-determination theory	Change is more lasting if it comes from internal reasons.	Find and emphasize their internal reasons for change.
Reactance theory	People resist advice if they perceive it to limit their freedom.	Offer them a menu of topics and change plan options.
Self-perception theory	What people hear themselves saying or see themselves doing about an issue influences their position on the issue.	Use "change talk" as a barometer of how well you are communicating.

are willing to accept it. For precontemplators, the cons for changing far outweigh the pros. For those in the contemplation stage, the importance of change is blooming, but they are pulled back by old habits. Patients in both of these stages resist exhortations for taking action with "yes, but" statements (Lessler & Dunn, 2007). Practitioners must apply different interventions at different stages of the change process, as stage-specific needs of patients are different.

Hayden (2009) views ecological models and social capital theory as the emerging theories for understanding and changing health behaviors. Social workers are familiar with the essentials of these theories. They should learn about the applicability of them in helping clients change their health behaviors.

Frankish, Lovato, and Poureslami (2007) listed a number of studies showing the effectiveness of theory-based interventions with patients who were obese, diabetic, and HIV positive, with drinking college students, and with professionals designing program activities. Hayden (2009) included in her book several published studies of theory-based interventions in such health-related areas as adolescent use and misuse of alcohol, alcohol abuse on campus, confidence in breast-feeding, fruit and vegetable consumption by low-income black American adolescents, HIV/AIDS, prevention of osteoporosis, and work-related lower back pain.

It is important to consider the appropriateness of a theory for understanding and intervening in a particular situation with a particular client/population and a particular problem. Hayden (2009) provided the following guidelines for choosing the appropriate theory:

1. Identify the health issue or problem and the affected person/population.

2. Gather information about the issue or population or both.

3. Identify possible causes of or reasons for the problem.

4. Identify the level of interaction (intrapersonal, interpersonal, or community) under which the causes or reasons most logically fit.

5. Identify the theory (or theories) that best match the level and the causes/reasons.

Lessler and Dunn (2007) gave the following tips for behavior change counseling:

1. Select one topic collaboratively with the patient.

2. Elicit the patient's view on the topic in terms of its importance and his or her confidence about the ability to change (both on a scale of 1–10).

3. Summarize the patient's view while making supportive statements to build his or her confidence.

4. Use the elicit-provide-elicit method in exchanging information or advice.
   - Elicit the patient's ideas first.
   - Provide information/advice next.
   - Elicit the patient's reaction/commitment.

Social Worker as Advocate and Broker

The need for comprehensiveness of services will, on the one hand, propel the shift of health care toward a biopsychosocial model of diagnosis and treatment and, on the other hand, emphasize the importance of mobilizing the patient's illness- or wellness-related resources inside and outside the health care setting. The mobilization of resources calls for professional roles of advocate and broker. By their history and training, social workers are the best equipped to play these roles. They have practiced advocacy at two levels: at the individual case level (*case advocacy*) and on behalf of a whole class of people (*class advocacy*). Within *case advocacy,* Wallace et al. (1984) made a distinction between social advocacy and clinical advocacy on the basis of the breadth and depth of the assessment and intervention [4]. In a health care setting, it is assumed that the need for advocacy is in response to patient deficits that have clear clinical relevance to the patient's health problem; hence, it is *clinical advocacy.* We agree with Cohen (1980) that the purpose of clinical social work is to maintain and enhance psychosocial functioning by "maximizing the availability of needed intrapersonal, interpersonal, and societal resources" (p. 30). *Class advocacy* is used to secure and protect entitlements for a group of people who share a common status and common problems (Connaway & Gentry, 1988). It is a form of social action. Freddolino, Moxley, and Hyduk (2004) identified four major traditions of advocacy in social work: (1) protecting the vulnerable, (2) creating supports to enhance functioning, (3) protecting and advancing claims or appeals, and (4) fostering identity and controls. The extent of social workers' involvement in class advocacy depends on a number of variables, such as agency goals and functions and characteristics of the worker's job. Ezell (1994) found that social workers tend to be involved in case advocacy while at work and class advocacy while volunteering. The availability of low-cost computers and user-friendly software and the development of electronic networks have opened another avenue for class advocacy. Moon and DeWeaver (2005) discussed the definition, advantages, and challenges of computer-based electronic advocacy for social workers.

Health care providers, including physicians, are also realizing the importance of advocacy. In the words of O'Toole (2007), a physician himself,

> The recent attention focused on advocacy by medical providers is an effort to restore prestige to a profession tarnished by scandal and misuse of trust. In addition, health care advocacy serves as a "call to arms" to address the growing disenfranchisement of vulnerable populations in an increasingly proprietary and market-driven health care environment. (p. 429)

He provided a typology of clinician advocacy built on the following four questions and their answers.

1. Whom are you advocating for?

   Your patient

   His or her family

   Their community

   The population

2. Whom are you advocating to?

   Your patient

   Public/public opinion

   Academic/opinion leaders

3. What are you advocating?

   Improving health services

   Affecting provider behavior

   Health system change

   Expanding access to care

   Affecting social determinants of health

4. How are you doing it?

   Interpersonal advocacy

   Organizational advocacy

   Academic advocacy

   Community organizing/coalition building

   Media strategies

He also discussed essential skills for advocacy and presented them as the following dos and don'ts.

1. Do know your issue. Always corroborate your assertions and do the necessary fact-finding before you begin.

   Don't become bigger than your issue. Don't assert expertise beyond your knowledge base or sphere of legitimacy.

2. Do know who is involved. Know who the current stakeholders are, what their stand on the issue is, what they are doing, and how you can join them in this effort.

   Don't isolate yourself or let your cause consume you.

3. Do develop your skills. Improve your communication skills. These may include writing in clear, concise, accurate, and persuasive ways,

whether you are writing for a professional journal, local newspaper, press release, issue release for legislators, or information packet. Know how policy is made, regulations are drafted, and laws are enacted.

Don't assume that your professional training is adequate.

4. Do partner, build, and organize coalitions. There is strength in numbers. The number of people and the diversity of their perspectives strengthen the advocacy effort. Involve the patients on whose behalf you are advocating, as that empowers them.

Don't be a "lone ranger" in your advocacy.

5. Do be strategic. Set benchmarks and realistic goals. Seek input from those with a vantage point on what is realistic and what the levers and pace for change are.

Don't forget what it is you want to do and why you are doing it.

Although there is a lack of consensus about the "what," "why," and "how" of advocacy within the social work profession, social workers can improve their advocacy skills by (1) purposefully applying to the advocacy task the problem-solving approach they are best at, (2) drawing helpful ideas from the relevant literature in other disciplines/professions for both understanding issues and intervening in issue-related problems, and (3) building on the existing work. For class advocacy on behalf of the elderly, for example, social workers should grasp the complexity of the reasons for the "what" and "how" of aging-related policies. Estes (1999) presented the political economy of aging as a theoretical perspective on the socioeconomic determinants of the experience of aging [5]. McGowan (1987) suggested a number of variables [6] that should be assessed for decision making in case advocacy. Connaway and Gentry (1988) included educating, persuading, negotiating, and bargaining among the strategies for case-level advocacy. Sosin and Caulum (1983) proposed a typology of strategies based on the context, which may be one of alliance,

neutral, or adversarial. Social workers should use the various strategies and techniques of advocacy purposefully and selectively. As Hepworth and Larsen (1986) put it, "In a given situation, a practitioner may employ several interventions, but a rule of thumb is to employ no more than are necessary and to cause no more disruption than is required to achieve a given objective" (p. 571). The worker should communicate his or her concerns in a factual and nonabrasive manner, try to understand the feelings and position of the other party, and consider realistic options and alternatives proposed by that party (Sheafor, Horejsi, & Horejsi, 1988).

Because advocacy is an activity on behalf of the patient, the most important "should" is to ensure that it does not undermine the patient's autonomy and sense of mastery. Such sabotage would be contrary to social work's basic belief system, as well as to the need of the health care system to treat the patient as a partner.

Social workers' broker role involves activities designed to link clients to needed resources. To perform this role effectively, the social worker should know the various resources relevant to the patient's need and how to link the patient to those resources. The resources can be classified into three categories: (1) formal health and human services in the area, (2) various self-help groups, and (3) the patient's own natural support systems.

Hepworth and Larsen (1986) grouped the formal health and human services by the following needs:

Income maintenance	Legal services
Housing	Marital and family therapy
Health care	
Child services	Youth services
Vocational guidance and rehabilitation	Recreation
Mental health care	Transportation

Examples of some self-help groups found in most communities include the following:

Al-Anon/Alateen (for families and friends of alcoholics)

Alcoholics Anonymous (for alcohol abusers)

Compassionate Friends (for bereaved parents)

Fresh Start (for smokers quitting their habit)

Gamblers Anonymous (for those with a gambling problem)

Lost Chord Club (for laryngectomees)

Mended Hearts (for heart disease patients)

Overeaters Anonymous (for compulsive overeaters and those with other eating disorders)

Parents Anonymous (for abusive parents)

Parents Without Partners (for single parents)

Parkinson's Disease Support Group

Reach to Recovery (for breast cancer patients)

Recovery, Inc. (for former mental patients)

Synanon (for substance abusers)

United Ostomy Association Group (for patients with ostomies)

Many other disease-specific self-help groups are available for patients and/or their families.

Natural support systems include the patient's family, relatives, friends, neighbors, fellow workers, and associates from school, church, and other social groups.

Most social work departments and units maintain a list of all the health and human service resources in the area, with brief descriptions of the "where," "when," and "how" of their services and eligibility requirements. The social worker should create and/or update such a resource list and add the names of specific persons to be contacted at often-used agencies and programs. It is wise to know as many of them personally as possible. Doing this will result in a smooth linking process and reduce the ill effects of the darker side of many human service organizations reflected in "complex application

procedures, needless delays in providing resources and services, discriminatory policies, inaccessible sites of agencies, inconvenient hours of service delivery, dehumanizing procedures or behaviors by staff" (Hepworth & Larsen, 1986, p. 16).

Besides knowing community resources and the people who represent those resources, the social worker should practice the principle of appropriate use of those resources.

> Many community resources are not useful with difficult-to-manage patients because the resources cannot handle them, are not equipped to make clinical interventions, and the patient has usually worn out his or her welcome there already. Inappropriate referrals often make the situation worse and, moreover, ruin the reputation of the clinician in the community where credibility in urgent situations and emergencies is crucial. (Wallace et al., 1984, p. 199)

Linking the patient with the needed resource requires selecting the resource that will match the patient's needs and referring him or her to the selected resource agency. The preconditions of a successful referral include (a) the patient's readiness for referral, (b) his or her agreement with the appropriateness of the selected resource, and (c) his or her ability to follow through with the referral. The social worker can benefit from the following suggestions for meeting these conditions:

- Reiterate his or her assessment of the patient's need for referral.
- Give information about the resource agency and its policies, procedures, and services without any false promises or unrealistic reassurances.
- Share his or her reasons why that agency would be an appropriate match for the patient's needs.
- Encourage the patient to express his or her feelings about the need to seek help elsewhere and about the resource agency itself.
- Deal with any misconception about the agency and its services and other doubts, ambivalence, and apprehension that the patient may have.

- Arrange for transportation, if lack of that is likely to be problematic.
- Suggest and arrange for someone—a family member, neighbor, friend—to accompany the patient if that would make a difference.
- Use cementing techniques (Weissman, 1976) selectively for increasing the chances of the patient continuing with the resource agency beyond the first contact. These techniques include (a) checking back—contacting the patient after the initial contact about what has been accomplished, (b) haunting—calling the patient at the resource agency after his or her initial and subsequent contact with that agency, (c) sandwiching—planning an interview with the patient before he or she goes for the initial contact with the resource agency and immediately after that contact, and (d) alternating—planning a series of interviews with the patient intermittently during his or her involvement with the resource agency.

Mobilizing the patient's own natural support system is often more difficult than approaching a formal source of help. The following suggestions are likely to be helpful in this task:

1. *Realize the complexity of people's natural social support systems.* People are the active shapers of their social networks. Those who do not reciprocate the support they receive are less likely to ask for help, and they feel guilty if they do. Those who place high value on self-reliance have difficulty asking for help. Those who have difficulty discussing their problems with others are reluctant to seek support. Those who have sought help from some of their social network members and have not received it are discouraged from asking for help from others. The effect of expecting the needed support that is not forthcoming is more upsetting than the perception that the support is not available. Potential support givers (a) may not know how the patient feels about his or her situation and need for help, (b) may feel uneasy and unsure about their helpfulness, (c) may not know how to provide appropriate help and support, and (d) may feel resentful for having to provide support (Antonucci & Israel, 1986; Brown, 1978; Dhooper, 1983, 1984;

Lehman, Ellard, & Wortman, 1986; Wortman & Lehman, 1985).

2. *Identify the patient's natural supports and analyze their potential for helpfulness.* While exploring the patient's social network, the social worker should individualize the patient's situation and give attention to the structural features of the network, the dynamic features of relationships, the patient's subjective view of the network, and significant life events that might have affected the network (Snow & Gordon, 1980). Different network structures are more or less important, depending on the nature of the need. The dynamic features of relationships indicate the positive and negative nature of interactions within the network. Significant events, such as death, retirement, and change in physical or mental health, or even change in residence of important network members, can seriously disrupt a patient's social network. Several approaches to network analysis (e.g., Dhooper, 1990; Gottlieb, 1985; Maguire, 1983) can be used. This exploring and analyzing will result in a list of potential helpers who, the patient believes, can provide the needed support.

3. *Help the patient decide how to approach the identified network members and request help and how to overcome any obstacles.* Those in greatest need are often the least able to structure their interactions to facilitate support from others (Lehman et al., 1986). This may require giving the patient suggestions or even role-playing effective ways of communication, helping him or her deal with guilt, rehearsing a backup plan, and encouraging the expression of appreciation for the help received (Dhooper, 1990).

4. *Enable the patient's helpers to be supportive.* Mobilizing the patient's social supports, at times, also involves work with the members of the social network. The distress of those in difficult situations tends to create or increase the anxiety of potential helpers. The social worker can, with the consent of the patient, give the helpers information about the patient's problem and needs, encourage them to discuss those

needs, prepare them for the patient's behavior, teach them how to manage their anxiety, facilitate communication among the helpers, and support their helping efforts. Impressive work on social network interventions has been done in mental health practice (e.g., see Biegel, Tracy, & Corvo, 1994; Tracy & Biegel, 1994), which can be a source for supplementing the worker's professional repertoire.

Closely related to advocacy and brokering is the concept of "case management," which has become prominent over the past few decades. In the field of aging, case management was identified as a basic service under the Older Americans Act of 1965 (P.L. 95-478), and the case management approach has been practiced in several other fields, such as health care, mental health, and rehabilitation (Loomis, 1988; Roessler & Rubin, 1982; Sanborn, 1983; Steinberg & Carter, 1983). Many evaluation studies of case management programs and services have shown the effectiveness of the case management approach to service delivery (e.g., see Berkowitz, Halfon, & Klee, 1992; Bond, Miller, Krumwied, & Ward, 1988; Claiborne, 2006; Goering, Wasylenki, Farkas, & Ballantyne, 1988; Macias, Kinney, Farley, Jackson, & Vos, 1994; Marcenko & Smith, 1992; Pugh, 2009; Quinn, Segal, Raisz, & Johnson, 1982).

With the general trend toward maximizing the quantity, quality, and types of community-based care, newer technologies increasingly making it possible to provide more and more services on an ambulatory basis, and the increasing number of the elderly in the population, it is likely that the importance of case management will grow in the future. In view of that importance, we discuss the social worker's role as a case manager separately.

Social Worker as Case Manager/ Service Coordinator

The commitment of ambulatory care settings to the concept of "comprehensiveness of services"

and their responsiveness to the needs of vulnerable populations, such as the elderly and those with disabilities, will bring case management services into bold relief in the future. Social workers are superbly qualified to serve as case managers because of their knowledge of community resources; their skills in communication, advocacy, and brokering; and their professional commitment to helping people obtain resources, facilitating interactions between individuals and others in their environments, and making organizations responsive to people (Hepworth & Larsen, 1986). This role will be played at two levels, depending on the needs of the individual patient. At one level, the social worker will refer the patient for case management services in the community and will use the knowledge and skills we discussed above under the advocate and broker role. At the other level, the social worker will serve as a case manager and will use many other skills, along with the advocacy and brokering skills.

New models of case management mix and match the skills appropriate for both of these levels. White, Gundrum, Shearer, and Simmons (1994) described a project in which a social worker in the role of case manager functioned as a liaison between primary care physician offices and community services. The case manager provided in-person, on-the-spot assistance and consultation to physicians and their office staff. Kramer, Fox, and Morgenstern (1992) reported on two health maintenance organizations that use social work expertise to provide access to resources, home visits, and monitoring for high-risk patients. Vourlekis and Ell (2007) described a case management program called SAFe (Screening Adherence Follow-Up) aimed at improving patient adherence to treatment recommendations. That program was tested over a period of 5 years in multiple sites with medically underserved minority women at higher risk of nonadherence.

The concept of "case management" is still evolving as it is being operationalized in serving different groups of clients with different needs in varied situations. Some basic common functions, however, are involved in all types of case management. These include assessing need, identifying and planning for services, implementing the plan (which is likely to feature linking clients with services, being an advocate for the client's best interest, and coordinating services), and monitoring and evaluating the process and result of case management. On the basis of an assessment of the individual case situation, case management may also involve significant therapeutic activities, such as emotional support and counseling. For example, case managers for families of children with both a developmental disability and a chronic health condition (Marcenko & Smith, 1992) acknowledged the chronic sorrow, social isolation, and emotional, physical, and financial stress experienced by such families and included in case management the organization of parents' support groups and informational and skill-building activities. Similarly, the case management model for serving drug-exposed infants and their chemically dependent mothers described by Berkowitz et al. (1992) included many more than the usual brokering, referring, and follow-up functions to ensure comprehensiveness, continuity, and coordination of services.

Vourlekis and Ell (2007) proposed a blueprint of theory-driven best practice case management for improved medical adherence. Their approach requires that (1) case managers be integrated into the health care setting and its routine clinical processes; (2) case managers be culturally competent; (3) case management services be individualized, interactive, and patient centered; (4) case management service plans consider all factors (predisposing, enabling, and reinforcing) that contribute to the adherence problem; and (5) case management add to the agency's quality improvement efforts. The National Association of Social Workers (1992) has established standards for social work case management.

A critical look at the basic functions of case management reveals the relevance of problem-solving skills that all social workers have acquired and practiced as a part of their training. A comprehensive psychosocial assessment of the patient will uncover all of his or her needs and the extent to which they are being met. Planning will involve discussing and exploring with the patient the available resources—formal as well as informal, the patient's own as well as the community's—relevant to the unmet needs. Implementation of the plan may involve the use of advocacy and linking skills described earlier. Wherever there is a dearth of essential resources in the community or the community lacks interagency linkages and coordination, the social worker as a case manager should also become involved in community-level groups.

> Participation in community-based advocacy groups and advisory boards supports system-level case management by broadening the potential scope of resources for the population. Participation on these boards is helpful for establishing interagency linkages and networks necessary for effective coordination and collaboration, facilitating referrals among community agencies, and enhancing community standards of practice. But ultimately, participation on community boards is a way to shape policies that are advantageous to meeting the needs of the client population. (Berkowitz et al., 1992, pp. 113, 115)

The coordination and monitoring of services are the other important functions of case management. *Coordination* involves collaboration and teamwork, and the suggestions made in Chapter 4 for sharpening social work skills for collaborative work are relevant for coordination as well. Johnson (1989) listed the following as blocks to effective coordination:

> lack of respect for or confidence in other helpers involved; lack of adequate sharing of information among the helpers; differing perspectives or values about what is to be done regarding clients; lack of capacity to share and work together; lack of time to develop cooperative relationships; and lack of agency sanctions and support for coordination. (p. 357)

In view of the need for comprehensive and coordinated services in the future, the lack of agency sanctions and support is not likely to be a major problem. Social workers as case managers will be able to negotiate the time and other resources required for effective coordination of services. For overcoming the other blocks to coordination, they will find the following suggestions helpful:

- Learn as much as possible about the perspectives, services, and skills of all the help/service providers involved in the case. This will help in knowing, accepting, appreciating, and respecting their contributions.
- While appreciating the differences among the various help providers, look for commonalities and highlight those. Concern for the patient's well-being is the central theme in everyone's activity. Highlighting that common purpose from time to time will help communication.
- Express appreciation for the commitment and efforts of all service providers, both formally and informally, and encourage the patient and/or his or her family to do likewise. Remember that communication is the soul of coordinated effort, and open many channels of communication with and among the various service providers. These channels can be formal and informal, as well as direct and indirect. Encourage and facilitate communication among all involved.
- Understand the differences in the functioning of informal helpers from the patient's natural support system and service providers from formal agencies and programs. In terms of the communication between the informal and formal systems, the balance theory of coordination (Litwak & Meyer, 1966, 1974) suggests that a midpoint be sought in the social distance between the two. If they are too far apart, they do not communicate; if they are too close, they hinder each other's functioning.
- Be conscious of the differences in the ways men and women communicate. The natural helping system seems to be more often a female system. The formal system, while staffed with both men and women, seems to function in a formalized manner that is more akin to traditional male communication. Male social workers should be particularly aware of their difference in communication styles when working with the informal helping system (Johnson, 1989, pp. 356–357).
- Appreciate the unique contributions of informal helpers to the patient's care. Do not expect them to function as formal service providers.

- Use innovation and creativity in opening new channels of communication and finding new ways of strengthening coordination among service providers.

Monitoring is the ongoing evaluation of the process and product of intervention. It is an ethical as well as technical responsibility of the social worker and refers to the periodic observations and feedback in checking and reviewing how things are going and what progress is being made (Siporin, 1975). Unlike the evaluation at the end of an activity, monitoring is a self-regulatory activity. As Egan (1990) put it,

> Appraisal that comes at the end of the process is often quite judgmental: "It didn't work." Ongoing evaluation is much more positive. It helps both client and helper[s] learn from what they have been doing, celebrate what has been going well, and correct what has been going poorly. (p. 181)

Monitoring also depends on effective communication and honest relationships among the people involved in the helping situation. The suggestions for improving communication given above are equally effective for monitoring purposes. The social worker, as a case manager, can do the following to perform the monitoring function:

- Remember that the purpose of monitoring is improvement in the service delivery, its quality, and efficiency.
- Ensure that the process and short-term goals of all service providers are clear and empirically measurable to the extent possible.
- Build into the monitoring plan as many relevant variables as possible—patient-related, problem-related, and situation-related variables.
- Concentrate on two major tasks: determining whether the service plan is being completed and whether the original goals are being met (Kirst-Ashman & Hull, 1993).
- Gather information from all available sources by using many methods of communication—formal and informal meetings, telephone calls, case records, reports, and formal evaluation devices and tools.

As in hospital-based social work, there is also room for innovation to maximize the resources and skills of the social work staff in ambulatory care settings. Some case management functions can be performed by paraprofessionals with appropriate training and supervision. In the interest of efficiency and cost-effectiveness, social workers will delegate some of their functions to others.

We discussed in Chapter 4 the necessary knowledge and skills for effective performance of the social work role of consultant. Earlier in this chapter, we briefly discussed the social worker as an educator of medical colleagues. The worker's patient-related educator role is discussed at length in Chapter 6. As in other settings, social workers will be able to make significant contributions to the efforts of ambulatory care settings to maintain quality. The "what" and "how" of continuous quality improvement approaches are discussed in Chapter 7.

RELEVANT ETHICAL CONSIDERATIONS

Ethical questions and concerns regarding the care of vulnerable patients are of tremendous importance to social workers. In this section, we discuss some of those questions and concerns.

We earlier (in Chapter 4) agreed with the definition of vulnerable patients as those wounded by social forces that place them at a disadvantage for their health (Grumbach, Braveman, Adler, & Bindman, 2007). Their vulnerability leads to their poor health status and health disparities in groups to which they belong. Health care providers and health care systems also contribute to the disparities in health for vulnerable populations.

> Studies reveal that health care workers feel ill-prepared when caring for vulnerable patients, especially those who are chronically ill, the elderly, addicted, mentally ill, victims of violence, or from minority and disadvantaged backgrounds—patients whose numbers are on the rise and patients for whom we are not currently providing adequate care. (King et al., 2007, p. xvii)

Social workers can make significant contributions to a health care facility's efforts to provide high-quality, compassionate, and ethically sound care to vulnerable patients. Social work has been ahead of other professions in its intentions, ideas, and accomplishments regarding service to the disadvantaged.

> Powerful concepts such as equality, justice, equity, human diversity, and tolerance; individual's uniqueness, inherent worth and dignity, and self-determination; and caring, competence, and professionalism are the main elements of the social work philosophy and belief system. (Dhooper & Moore, 2001, p. 5)

Social workers are trained to work with the distressed, disabled, dependent, defeated, depressed, delinquent, and deviant, as well as those who are different from people in the mainstream. They have prided themselves as being the "conscience of the corporation," and they are the health care setting's bridge to the community and its resources.

Most vulnerable patients may be educationally disadvantaged or have low health literacy and may be distrustful of the health system. A host of other factors may also prevent a fit between their needs and the health care facility's resources. There is no standard set of factors pertinent to any particular group of patients. The following example points to the variety of factors that can make the delivery of high-quality care difficult. The author explored the health care needs of foreign-born Asian Americans and found that (1) many of them had brought with them diseases endemic to their native lands, which were persisting; (2) they had acquired new diseases because of the changes in their living conditions and lifestyles; (3) they were vulnerable to the physical effects of acculturation-related stress; (4) they were holding on to their old health beliefs, non-Western theories of health and illness, and health practices; and (5) their exposure and access to the American health care system were inadequate (Dhooper, 2003). Thus, there is the need to individualize each patient; social workers can help in that important task.

Lo (2007) suggested three fundamental ethical guidelines for the clinical care of medically underserved patients: justice, respect for the person, and acting in the patient's best interest. *Justice* demands access to health care based on medical need rather than social or economic status. *Respect for the person* entails several ethical obligations. The care providers must accept a competent and informed patient's decision about care, even if it is contrary to the providers' best professional judgment. They must realize that people place different values on health, medical care, and risks. They must give patients unbiased information about the medical condition, treatment choices, expected benefits, and risks, and help them deliberate so that they can actively participate in decision making about their medical care. This also requires that patients be treated with compassion and dignity and that providers avoid misrepresentation, maintain confidentiality, and keep promises. *Acting in the best interest of the patient* requires that the patient's interests prevail over those of physicians, other providers, or third parties (e.g., health care facilities or insurers) (Lo, 2007). It also requires that a patient's refusal of a highly beneficial treatment not be simply accepted.

> Acting in the patient's best interest requires eliciting patients' expectations and concerns, correcting misunderstandings, and trying to persuade them to accept highly beneficial therapies. If disagreements persist after discussions, the patient's informed choices and the view of his or her best interests should prevail. (p. 49)

It also requires that providers be advocates for their patients and help them get the needed services, as well as advocates for systems of care that remove barriers to care.

Following these guidelines is often difficult in situations where/when

1. a patient's decision-making capacity is impaired and he/she has no surrogate or advanced directive;

2. a patient's family insists on making decisions on behalf of the patient in order to protect him/her from knowing the diagnosis of a terminal disease or to keep their cultural norm;

3. more than one ethical guideline is at play and each guides the providers in opposite ways; and

4. physicians, other health care team members, patients, and their families do not agree on the benefits and risks of intervention.

In such situations, social workers can be of help in many ways.

1. They can make the informed consent really "informed" by educating the patients appropriately. "Patients can be overwhelmed with medical jargon, needlessly complicated explanations, or too much information at once" (Lo, 2007, p. 48). Their involvement in getting patients' informed consent can serve as an opportunity for developing a relationship with those patients.

2. They can help other providers understand patients, their culture, values, and preferences.

3. They can work with a patient's family and help bring the patient, family, and care providers to an agreement on the "what," "why," and "how" of treatment.

4. They can help in understanding the values and likely choice and preference of a patient incapable of making decisions.

They can accomplish these tasks because of their understanding of the *universal* in the human condition and needs, a disciplined habit of avoiding stereotypical views of people, and interviewing skills for discovering the *unique* in the particular patient and his/her family. They will find the following suggestions helpful in understanding culturally diverse patients:

- Consider all patients as individuals first, as members of minority status next, and as members of specific ethnic groups last. This will prevent overgeneralization.
- Never assume that a person's ethnic identity tells you anything about his or her cultural values and patterns of behavior. There can be vast within-culture differences.
- Treat all "facts" about cultural values as hypotheses to be tested anew with each patient.
- Identify and build on the strengths in the patient's cultural orientation.
- Be aware of your attitude about cultural pluralism.

- Engage the patient in the process of learning what cultural content—beliefs, values, and experiences—is relevant to your work together (Royse, Dhooper, & Rompf, 2010).

Critical Thinking Question

1. Defining vulnerable patients as wounded by social forces that put them at a disadvantage for their health, identify those (economic, environmental, cultural, political, and social) forces and discuss how they contribute to patients' vulnerability. List health-related dimensions/reflections of that vulnerability that health care providers can consciously deal with.

2. Lessler and Dunn (2007) used "dancing versus wrestling" as a metaphor for behavior change counseling. Wrestling ends with a winner and a loser (or both losers), whereas "dancing" means that the patient is doing most of the talking. Imagine two encounters with a patient, one in which wrestling dominated and the other marked by dancing. List the possible elements of the process and product of the two interviews.

NOTES

1. Several hospitals across the country have such protocols. A protocol alerts the hospital staff—physicians, nurses, and the crisis clinician (social worker) to (1) provide the most appropriate clinical care, (2) make assessment of abuse, and (3) document the evidence of abuse that is reliable and court admissible.

2. The phases for debriefing groups are (1) introduction, (2) facts phase, (3) thoughts phase, (4) feeling phase, (5) symptom phase, (6) teaching phase, (7) reentry phase, and (8) postdebriefing.

3. The seven stages of the model are (1) conduct a crisis assessment, (2) establish rapport and rapidly establish relationship, (3) identify major problems (including the "last straw," or crisis precipitants), (4) deal with feelings and emotions (using active listening and validation), (5) generate and explore alternatives, (6) develop and formulate an action plan, and (7) establish a follow-up plan and agreement.

4. As an example of clinical advocacy, Wallace et al. (1984) talk about a 27-year-old married Jewish orthodox woman who presented in the ER with sleep and appetite disturbance, depressed mood, and intrusive suicidal thoughts. The social work assessment revealed a conflict between the patient's religious obligations on the one hand and her family and personal obligations on the other as the primary issue. She had been trying for 5 years to get pregnant with no success because her religious sect restricted sexual contact to a limited number of calendar days. The worker called her rabbi, who granted the patient a dispensation from her religious obligations. Her symptoms disappeared.

5. The *political economy of aging* is based on the following premises: (1) coercion and social struggles between the more and less powerful are the means of maintaining the status quo or conversely imposing change; (2) the social structure shapes how older individuals are perceived and how they perceive themselves, and that affects their sense of worth and power; (3) attributional labels applied to the elderly shape the experience of old age as well as societal decisions concerning aging-related public policy; (4) social policy and the politics of aging mirror the inequalities in social structure and outcomes of power struggle around those structural arrangements, reflecting the advantages and disadvantages of business and workers, whites and nonwhites, and men and women; and (5) social policy reflects the dominant ideologies and belief systems that enforce and extend the structure of advantages and disadvantages in society (Estes, 1999, p. 18).

6. The variables are (a) problem definition, (b) objective, (c) target system, (d) sanction, (e) resources, (f) potential receptivity of target system, (g) level of intervention, (h) objective of intervention, (i) strategy and mode of intervention, and (j) outcome of prior advocacy efforts.

6

SOCIAL WORK IN ILLNESS PREVENTION AND HEALTH PROMOTION

In the future, the health care system's current treatment orientation, which determines the point of intervention too late in the course of many diseases, will be replaced by an orientation toward disease prevention and health promotion. It will move toward the realization of health as "physical, mental, and social well-being," an idea proposed by the World Health Organization (WHO) more than 50 years ago. That movement will involve not only a vital shift in the philosophy and priorities of the health care system but also a significant change in the nature of the roles and relationships of health care providers and recipients. The system has been philosophically treatment and procedure centered and driven by incentives for costly and often excessive treatment of mostly preventable morbidity (Gellert, 1993). As the system's focus gradually shifts from illness to wellness, the patient will become a true partner of health care providers in the joint effort to stay healthy. In the past, the patient put all the faith and confidence in health care providers to keep him or her healthy. This dependence resulted in failure of the patient to take responsibility for healthy living. As Taylor, Denham, and Ureda (1982) put it,

The past generation of men and women have consumed nutritionally deficient foods, accepted increasing weight as a natural consequence of aging, used tobacco despite well-documented hazards, ingested unnecessary and sometimes dangerous drugs, failed to get necessary rest and sleep, exercised infrequently, and accepted prolonged stress as though immune to its damaging sequelae. (p. 1)

On the other hand, health care providers, particularly physicians, restricted their role to only diagnosis and treatment of disease. Illness prevention and health promotion have not been parts of their role as healers. For most of them, advising the patient in proper nutrition and exercise has lacked the professional self-fulfillment of managing a serious illness episode such as an asthmatic attack or excising an inflamed appendix (Taylor et al., 1982). All this has been a part of the larger cultural context.

Industrial societies have placed their management of health and human welfare issues into the hands of "experts," who in turn are typically associated with large, centralized bureaucracies. Thus, a relatively impersonal service takes over some of the most intimate and important human concerns—birth, death, sickness, health, education, care of the elderly and disabled, to mention just a few. (Green & Raeburn, 1990, p. 37)

This will gradually change. Besides the illogic of the way things are, the cost (in every sense of the term) to the individual and to society of waiting until problems become full-blown will become increasingly unbearable.

Conceptually, illness prevention and health promotion are distinct. Health promotion is a much wider concept than illness prevention. In *health promotion,* intervention is directed at improving the general well-being of people, and no specific disease agent or process is targeted. "Health promotion transcends narrow medical concerns and embraces less well-defined concepts of wellness, self-growth, and social betterment. Concepts related to illness prevention are more specific" (Bracht, 1987, p. 318). Health promotion is a prepathogenic level of intervention, whereas in *disease prevention,* the known agents or environmental factors are the focus of intervention, with the aim of reducing the occurrence of a specific disease (Leavell & Clark, 1965). *Illness prevention* involves actions to eliminate or minimize conditions known to cause or contribute to different diseases.

In the public health literature, all health-related activities are conceptualized as preventive and categorized as primary prevention, secondary prevention, and tertiary prevention. *Primary prevention* involves actions to keep conditions known to result in disease from occurring, thus preventing the disease process from starting; *secondary prevention* involves actions to limit the extent and severity of an illness, after it has begun, by early detection and treatment; and *tertiary prevention* involves efforts, during and after the full impact of illness, that would minimize its effects and preclude its recurrence (Barker, 2003; Watkins, 1985). In this scheme, health promotion and illness prevention are two phases of primary prevention. Together, they refer to actions and practices aimed at *preventing* physical, psychological, and sociocultural problems; *protecting*

current strengths, competencies, or levels of health; and *promoting* desired goals and the fulfillment or enhancement of human potentials (Public Health Service, 1979). These actions and practices are concerned with the total population generally and the groups at high risk particularly. To be effective, they must be comprehensive and multifocused—aimed at changing individual health behaviors, creating a positive climate for health in the community, and bringing about policy change in favor of a social and physical environment free of health hazards.

HISTORY OF SOCIAL WORK IN ILLNESS PREVENTION AND HEALTH PROMOTION

As we have seen in Chapter 2, public health has been the main actor on the illness prevention and health promotion stage. Because of the congruence between the broad goals of social work and public health, social work has been a part of public health activities and programs for more than 100 years. As Bracht (1987) put it,

Interest in health promotion and illness prevention is certainly not new, especially to social workers whose professional role has historically been targeted on the broader aspects of health and social betterment. Jane Addams engaged the first woman physician graduate of Johns Hopkins Medical School to come to Chicago in 1893 to open the country's initial well-baby and pediatric clinic. In Ohio, the Cincinnati Social Experiment, a neighborhood health center, was established by a group of social workers stressing neighborhood and environmental health. (p. 316)

In the second half of the 19th century, social workers collaborated with others in organized efforts to control communicable diseases. Their help was considered essential for the success of public health programs that required the cooperation of citizen groups. They not only collaborated with health professionals but also demonstrated the utility of social work approaches and methods for health-related work. The major social work approaches of those days were illustrated by the work of charity organizations and settlement houses. The Children's Bureau, created in 1912, had its origins in the settlement house movement. Four of the first five chiefs of the bureau were social workers. The fourth, Martha May Eliot, a physician, had worked as a social worker in the Social Service Department at Massachusetts General Hospital before entering medical school (Hutchins, 1985). During the influenza epidemic of 1918 to 1919, social workers tracked and reached out to children in the community who were at high risk because their parents had died of the flu (Harris, 1919). After World War I, the passage of the National Venereal Disease Control Act led to the development of clinics for surveillance, early diagnosis, and treatment of venereal disease. As part of those clinics, social workers educated the victims of venereal disease and their families about the cause and dissemination of syphilis (Kerson, 1979).

Social workers also participated in political advocacy, at times at great cost. They had to work against societal biases and prejudices. In the early 20th century, for their efforts to increase government's role in maternal and child health, social workers of the day were maligned by their opposition as communists, subversives, endocrine perverts, and derailed menopausics (Siefert, 1983). Nevertheless, they led a campaign culminating in the passage of the Sheppard-Towner Act of 1921. The work made possible by this law contributed substantially to the reduction of infant mortality, demonstrated the effectiveness of preventive health services, and established the principle of shared federal-state responsibility in health and social welfare (Doss-Martin & Stokes, 1989). Passage of the Social Security Act of 1935, which created the Maternal and Child Health and Crippled Children's Services, brought social workers into public health programs much more prominently. They have worked in public health and other health care organizations not only as case workers with the ill and the disabled but also as case finders, planners of outreach services, prevention workers (in maternal and child health, family planning, alcohol and drug abuse, and mental health programs), health educators, advocates for and planners of comprehensive health projects, consultants, researchers, and trainers of paraprofessional personnel (Bracht, 1978).

Social workers have believed in the widest definition of *public health.* In 1981, the National Association of Social Workers adopted, with minor modifications, Winslow's definition of public health (given in Chapter 2) as part of its official policy statement on social work in health settings and laid down the standards for social work practice in public health. Others (e.g., Morton, 1985) have built on those ideas. Table 6-A below provides a list of general objectives of public health social work.

These objectives have demanded that social workers assume different and varied roles, such as provider of direct services, case manager,

Table 6-A General Objectives of Social Work in Public Health

- Ensuring the provision of psychosocial services for individuals and families
- Providing information and knowledge about community service networks to consumers and health linkage care providers
- Collaborating with professionals from other disciplines in delivering comprehensive care coordination of care
- Promoting social work values, such as self-determination, within the health care system
- Encouraging consumer participation in the planning and evaluation of services
- Discovering systemic factors that prevent access or discourage use of services ex. transportation
- Documenting social conditions that interfere with the attainment of health and working for program/ policy changes to address those conditions ex. poverty, early pregnancy, Ard use

administrator of a program, coordinator of services, program planner, consultant, and program evaluator. Social workers work in all kinds of illness prevention settings/programs, such as prenatal and postnatal clinics, health centers, health maintenance organizations, clinics for children with developmental or physical disabilities, and special programs for genetic counseling, bereavement work, prevention of child abuse, teenage pregnancy, teenage suicide, AIDS, and substance abuse.

Social work also has contributed to the theory and technology of illness prevention and health promotion. While incorporating the principles of epidemiology into social work practice, social workers have applied the philosophy, principles, and methods of their profession to public health work. The work of social work theoreticians such as Bloom (1981), Bracht (1990), Germain (1984), and Germain and Gitterman (1980) is noteworthy. Basic social work philosophy, theory, and techniques have significant relevance for the illness prevention and health promotion field, and social workers can enter this field with a high degree of confidence in their abilities. The major elements of their professional repertoire are highlighted below.

The philosophy of social work is based on democratic values, as well as the values of science. In the words of Weick (1986),

> The profession has developed an intellectual heritage based on two separate but related intellectual approaches: a commitment to scientific inquiry spawned by the rise of an empirical, technical world view and a commitment to philosophical principles motivated by humanistic, democratic beliefs. (p. 551)

This philosophy, on the one hand, generates the belief that people can change if given the reason and the wherewithal, and creates such practice principles as self-determination, individualization, and participation of people (as individuals, groups, and communities) in the change efforts. On the other hand, it emphasizes the need for rationality, objectivity, and a nonjudgmental attitude, and the study and assessment of people and their situations for professional intervention. This philosophy is essentially optimistic and strength oriented, as is reflected in the social work axioms "Let people determine the course of their own lives," "Work with people's strengths," and "Consider people within their social environment." In illness prevention and health promotion work, whether the emphasis is on increasing personal strengths, decreasing personal weaknesses, increasing social environmental resources, or decreasing social environmental stresses, the overall social work philosophy will keep the worker on the right professional path. Moreover, this theme blends well into the philosophical basis of health education practice, which is founded on democracy as a political philosophy and citizen participation as a professional principle (Steckler, Dawson, Goodman, & Epstein, 1987).

Because the focus of social work is on person in environment, systems theory provides a useful model for conceptualizing social work practice. This theory offers a holistic view of people and their problems and situations; it (a) helps social workers perceive and better understand the social environment, (b) helps in identifying practice principles that apply across different contexts, and (c) can help in integrating social work theories and unifying the profession (Martin & O'Connor, 1988). Therefore, social workers engaged in illness prevention and health promotion work can apply the systems perspective to their assessment, planning, and intervention, yielding significant results at all levels of their activity. This perspective fits into the ideal health promotion approach, the ecological perspective that seeks to influence intrapersonal, interpersonal, institutional, community, and public policy factors. This approach adds to educational activities "advocacy, organizational change efforts, policy development, economic supports, environmental change, and multimethod programs" (Glanz & Rimer, 1995, p. 15). Other social work concepts effective in this work include "enabling," "empowerment," and "community organization."

FUTURE SOCIAL WORK ROLES IN ILLNESS PREVENTION AND HEALTH PROMOTION

In Chapter 3, we discussed the *lack of resources* jeopardizing the ability of state and local public health departments to perform effectively even their basic functions. The Institute of Medicine (1988a) study on the future of public health found that

> public health functions are handicapped by reductions in federal support; economic problems in particular states and localities; the appearance of new, expensive problems such as AIDS and toxic waste; and the diversion of resources from communitywide maintenance functions to individual patient care. (p. 156)

The study recommended the following: (a) Federal support of state-level health programs should help balance disparities in revenue-generating capacities through "core" funding, as well as funds targeted for specific uses, and (b) state support of local-level health services should balance local revenue-generating disparity through "core" funding. In the future, the wellness movement will gradually improve the legitimacy of the claim of public health departments for a greater share of resources, but the claim will not automatically translate into the availability of more resources.

> Without major health reform in the interim, projections of the Health Care Financing Administration, based on continued inflation of costs, indicate a national expenditure by 2030 of 15,969 trillion dollars, with 206 billion dollars remaining for preventive programs. This will represent a further reduction in the public health share of expenditures to 1.29%, or about half of the current proportion. (Koplin, 1993, p. 400)

Even if a greater share of the national dollar for health activity is allowed for illness prevention and health promotion, public health departments will be competing with many other public and private entities providing illness prevention and wellness services.

In the future, more and more hospitals will expand their activities to include illness prevention and health promotion work, and most of them will expect that work to generate profit or at least be self-sustaining financially. Similarly, other agencies involved in such work are likely to need greater financial resources to improve the extent and quality of their efforts.

Besides the paucity of funds, one major hurdle to the effectiveness of the local health department is organizational. Most of such departments are too small to have adequate resources for effectiveness and efficiency; they lack the necessary infrastructure. The large number of local departments can be traced to a necessity valid in the horse-and-buggy days of transportation. More than 60 years ago, Emerson (1945) saw the small size of local health units as a problem and proposed their restructuring, but the then-prevailing local home-rule philosophy would not allow for any sacrifice of the local unit's autonomy (Koplin, 1993). The consensus about the core functions of public health departments is sufficient, and the Institute of Medicine (1988a) study suggested a number of significant attainable courses of action for public health units at all levels. The focus of planning must be on the removal of barriers to the effective and efficient functioning of these units. Creating greater resources and convincing politicians of the need for reorganization would break most of those barriers.

Beyond that, *planning* community-based health promotion and illness prevention programs would involve a bifocal approach that considers and provides for activities that help modify health-risk behaviors *and* the conditions and environments that support those behaviors. These activities include communitywide health education, risk-factor interventions, and efforts to change laws and regulations in areas that affect health (Wickizer et al., 1993). Planning for a hospital's illness prevention and health promotion program would involve deciding on the "what," "where," and "how" of its activities. Planning in agencies devoted to the prevention of a specific illness or problem would involve the same process but would be much more focused. At the national level of these organizations, planning also would be guided by the particular focus/foci of the agency's activity. Ganikos et al. (1994) identified the following four roles that a national health education and promotion organization can take: (a) a broker of knowledge, information, and communication strategies and skills; (b) a producer of educational strategies, messages, and materials; (c) an energizer, through sponsorship of market research, educational model development, and demonstration programs; and (d) a catalyst, serving as the consensus builder and coordinator of a national strategy.

Even *service provision* activities in the area of illness prevention and health promotion must be bifocal—focused on individuals and groups as well as the community at large. Individuals must be educated and encouraged to change their health-related behaviors directly, as well as through the community's reinforcing atmosphere, pressure, and sanction. This would be true whether the agency was the public health department, a hospital, or a voluntary nonprofit organization. While recognizing that the two important components of a public health program are enforcement and education, even the public health department would rather convince than coerce people.

> Even though police power exists and can be used as necessary, public health workers recognize their inability to be in all places at all times to enforce good health practice in public and private sectors. It is necessary, therefore, to concurrently emphasize health education to enhance voluntary compliance with recommended health practices. (Brecken, Harvey, & Lancaster, 1985, p. 37)

In the future, in every illness prevention and health promotion organization—public health departments, hospitals, and disease-specific agencies such as the American Cancer Society—social workers will be able to assume roles that have relevance to the organization's major needs. In different combinations, these needs are (a) generation of financial resources, (b) planning for appropriate service programs, and (c) provision of effective services.

Social Work Role in Creating and Mobilizing Financial Resources

Social workers can make significant contributions to all agencies engaged in illness prevention and health promotion in exploring and generating financial resources. Despite the commitment to the idea of general welfare, as a nation, the United States generally has been reluctant to provide for those with special needs—the disabled, disadvantaged, distressed, defeated, dependent, and deviant—which are people of special concern for social workers. Social workers, therefore, have been forced to be creative and skillful in generating and mobilizing resources. Generating future funds for the three types of agencies will require different approaches. For augmenting the resources of state and local public health departments, applying for grants from the federal government will be the major strategy. For hospitals, marketing their wellness activities both as part of their health maintenance package and as an independent program will be the preferred approach. For other organizations, streamlining their fundraising efforts will be the focus of the social worker's contributions. Social workers will play the role of the *creator and mobilizer of financial resources.*

Social Work Role in Program Planning

Planning involves specifying objectives, evaluating the means for achieving them, and making deliberate choices about the appropriate courses of action (Barker, 2003). This process is applicable at all levels and is relatively easy for social workers to practice and perfect because of their understanding of and expertise in problem solving. The different needs of the three types of agencies will dictate differential emphasis on the various steps of the planning process.

The possibilities of "what" activities to include in a health promotion program are countless. For example, Longe and Wolf (1983) listed six categories of health promotion activities offered by hospitals: (a) *community patient education* in such areas as living with arthritis, management of asthma, and parenting a child with diabetes; (b) *behavior change* for smoking cessation, stress reduction, and weight control; (c) *wellness and lifestyle* involving aerobic exercises and walking, communication and conflict resolution, and low-calorie, low-sodium, and low-fat cooking; (d) *medical self-care,* providing knowledge and skills about choosing a physician and understanding medications; (e) *lifesavers,* including babysitting certification, cardiac crisis program, cardiopulmonary resuscitation (CPR), and first aid; and (f) *workplace-related activities* such as employee assistance programs, organizational safety or hazard assessments, safety education, and worksite chronic disease control programs.

The question of "where" a hospital's health promotion activities should be offered can also have numerous possible answers. These activities can be offered at the hospital, its clinics in the community, community centers, churches, libraries, recreational sites, schools, workplaces, and conferences and fairs. Similarly, the "how" of these activities is limited only by the imagination and resources that can be devoted to them. Basic social work skills, with some focus and refinement, are relevant for these functions. Social workers can easily play the role of *program planner* in all agencies engaged in illness prevention and health promotion work.

Social Work Role in Program Implementation and Service Provision

Illness prevention and health promotion agencies also will offer social workers opportunities in areas other than resource generation and program planning. Social workers can significantly contribute to the implementation of an agency's program and provision of its services. Their major roles will be as *educator* and *community activator.* Community activation is a means to public education. These roles involve planning, conducting, and evaluating the necessary activities.

Other Social Work Roles in Illness Prevention and Health Promotion

Social workers have special sensitivity for, understanding of, and expertise in the problems of child abuse, intimate partner violence, AIDS, and old age. They should, therefore, take on leadership roles appropriate for illness prevention and health promotion in these areas. They also have something special (in terms of professional attitude and skills) to give in the area of health promotion in multicultural populations. Moreover, in the future, illness prevention and health promotion organizations will be required by policymakers and third-party payers to show that their efforts lead to the desired health status outcomes and are cost-effective. Social workers will be able to contribute to the needed research activities pertaining to this requirement.

SOCIAL WORK KNOWLEDGE AND SKILLS FOR ROLE-RELATED INTERVENTIONS

As in earlier chapters, our discussion of social work knowledge and skills necessary for illness prevention and health promotion work is organized in relation to the roles identified above.

Social Worker as Generator of Financial Resources

The social worker should know that the possible sources of funds for illness prevention and health promotion programs are likely to be different for different agencies. On the one hand, for most local public health departments, the local government is not likely to be a resource beyond the minimal funds it already allocates for public health activities. Social workers must seek more resources from the federal and state governments. Similarly, state public health departments must look to the federal government and the state legislature for extra resources. On the other hand, voluntary organizations engaged in illness prevention and health promotion work must raise funds from the general public and supplement those with grants from government and charitable foundations. Social workers can bring their skills for grant writing, fundraising, and political advocacy to bear on the agency's efforts to increase its financial resources. They will find the following information and suggestions helpful in enriching and refining those skills.

Grant Writing

The federal government makes money available to local governments and nongovernmental agencies by contract and by grant. By contract, the government buys the effort of someone to do specifically what the government wants done. A grant provides the money for the recipient to do something he or she wants to do that also is in the government's area of interest. Thus, a grantee has much more freedom of action than a contractor. The various kinds of grants can be broadly grouped as formula grants and project grants.

A *formula grant* is money distributed to a class of entitled agencies (e.g., state or local governments, universities). All members of the class are entitled to receive a portion of the total sum appropriated as long as they meet the conditions governing entitlement to the money. The money is distributed on approval of the application on the basis of some mathematical formula, which, with state government, typically is weighted according to population and per capita income. . . . *Project grants* are not entitlement. These are grants awarded on a competitive basis. The applicant develops a plan or proposal stating what is to be done if money is awarded. The applications are

reviewed competitively, though, in fact, the government is sensitive to the need to spread the awards around. (Raffel & Raffel, 1989, p. 308)

Block grants and capitation grants are kinds of formula grants. Some grants, both formula and project, require that the applicant match the government grant. Local and state public health departments should seek formula grants and insist that these grants be based on need. "Project grants and those requiring matching local funds are not recommended because they favor the better-established entities and are therefore disadvantageous for the poorer, rural, and otherwise underserved areas" (Koplin, 1993, p. 396). Project grants can supplement the resources of local and state public health departments. Similarly, hospitals and other voluntary organizations should seek project grants to add to their funds from other sources.

Other sources of grants include foundations of various kinds—community trusts (e.g., Cleveland Foundation), special-purpose foundations, corporations (e.g., General Electric Foundation), family foundations, and general-purpose foundations (e.g., Rockefeller Foundation). A foundation may fall into more than one category. The appropriate foundation can be located in the latest edition of the *Foundation Directory,* which has a double listing—alphabetical by state and by field of interest. Foundations are likely to fund demonstration projects more easily than ongoing programs. All federal invitations/requests for grant applications are published in the *Federal Register.* Another source of information about federal funds is the *Catalog of Federal Domestic Assistance.* The following suggestions about grant writing are based on workshops on fiscal resource development that the author attended over the years and on his experience as a grant reviewer for the U.S. Department of Health and Human Services.

Elements of grant proposals submitted to the government or private foundations are essentially the same, although foundation requests are generally shorter. A summary of the proposal is followed by these detailed sections: (a) introduction,

(b) problem statement or assessment of need, (c) project/program objectives, (d) methodology, (e) evaluation, (f) budget, and (g) future support for the project/program. While writing a grant proposal, the social worker should give special attention to the following suggestions:

- Learn as much as possible about the funding source and its expectations of the grant seeker; study the material about the grant, call and talk with the appropriate officer in the funding department of the government or contact the grantmaker at the foundation—"discover what that source is interested in supporting, and figure out how your organization can help the source meet its funding priority" (Nickelsberg, 1988, p. 126). In the proposal, address what the funding organization wants to fund.
- In the introduction, build the agency's credibility as one that deserves to be supported.
- Be specific about the problem and the target population; document the need for the project/program. Be truthful about the population being served by the agency or the number of potential beneficiaries of the project.
- Do not mix project objectives and methodology; list specific objectives that are realistic and measurable.
- Be innovative in the approach to the problem, but justify the proposed methodology; do not make assumptions that cannot be backed; describe the "how" of the methods; and show how the agency has the capacity to carry out the project/program, particularly in terms of the experience and skills of its personnel. Most funding sources are also interested in the replicability of the projects they fund. Show how yours can be easily replicated.
- Build in an evaluation design for ongoing and final evaluation, both in terms of the project implementation process and its impact on those served.
- Make sure the proposed budget is appropriate, reasonable, and adequately justified; describe the fiscal control and accounting procedures to be used.
- Present a plan for the continuation of the program beyond the grant period.
- Overall, be clear, concise, and logical; avoid unsupported assumptions and the use of jargon;

and package the proposal so as to make it attractive in terms of proper typing, spacing, margins, tabs, and correctness of spelling.
- Read, review, and rewrite the proposal as many times as necessary to make it as good and strong as possible. Have someone who knows nothing about the project read the proposal and point out which parts are confusing or unclear. Also, in this process of refining the document, consult the appropriate officer in the government or the grantmaker at the foundation, if needed.
- Mail the proposal in plenty of time; let your proposal be among the first to arrive, and after a week or so, call your contact and ask whether any other information is needed.
- Do try to know the people who make decisions about funding proposals or those who influence the decision makers. Some authors are of the opinion that, in the case of an application for a federal grant, copies of the proposal should be sent to one's congressperson and senators. "Get to know either the members themselves or, more important, one of their key staff people who might be interested. That staff person could go with you to your interview with the grantmaker or could help his or her boss follow up with letters and phone calls" (Nickelsberg, 1988, p. 129).

Fundraising

Social workers in voluntary organizations are likely to be involved in all major functions of the agency, including fundraising. With their professional expertise, particularly communication and problem-solving skills, they can easily assume leadership in this activity as well. The literature on different aspects of the "how" of fundraising is vast and rich. For example, Bakal (1979) described at length the various techniques of fundraising [1]. Most of these require elaborate planning in terms of "what," "where," "when," and "how." The "how" part invariably involves skills appropriate for communication, persuasion, and motivation.

Social workers should realize that their basic communication skills are as applicable in approaching people for charity as they are in problem-oriented assessment and intervention with individuals, groups, and larger entities. Persuasion strategies involve giving information that influences the recipient to feel, think, and act in a new way. The attributes of successful persuaders are expertise, trustworthiness, and likability. An effective persuader is perceived as possessing one or more of these (Simon & Aigner, 1985). The social worker should make conscious efforts to conduct himself or herself well and to come across as an expert and trustworthy. This task can be accomplished by (a) a thorough grasp of the agency's mission, programs, and activities, and the material being shared with people, and (b) an unwavering commitment to social work values. Likability depends on many factors, and the individual may have no control over some of these. However, "individuals are more likely to like, or be attracted to, workers whom they view as genuine, understanding, and accepting" (p. 120). People have differing reasons for giving; they are guided by their philosophies, upbringing, religious attitudes, and social desirability of the people giving, as well as their experience with the particular cause. In general, giving is considered more blessed than receiving, and giving may also enhance an individual's social and self-esteem.

For motivating people to give, the approach must be both generalized and special. The generalized approach is based on answers to the question, "What does everyone need to know about us and our cause?" The special approach builds on assumptions about "what the particular person needs to know about us and our cause." Nickelsberg (1988) is of the opinion that making people feel good about giving will stimulate them to give. Appreciate their giving by giving them something tangible—a little gift (with your logo on it) that people cannot get any other way, something they can show off. This possibility will make them feel good about it. Nickelsberg's other advice: "Set up categories of support to make people feel they are joining an elite club. Finally, always publish lists of joiners because it's nice to have personal recognition—and testimonials encourage joiners" (quoted in N. M. Davis, 1988, p. 125).

To motivate organizations to give, the approach should be directed at appealing to their self-interest, pride, and social values. With his focus on large corporations, Nickelsberg (1988) proposed several tenets of fundraising: (a) People give only to people, (b) people give only to people they know, (c) people who give want visibility, (d) people love to support a winner, and (e) people want to invest in the future.

These tenets can be turned into techniques for fundraising. "People give only to people, the people they know" suggests that fundraisers should be people-people and should try to know the prospective givers before approaching them. Social workers are people-people by training and can thus provide one basic ingredient of a successful fundraising program. Knowing the potential corporate giver may require talking with the agency's board members (who are generally businesspersons with contacts and connections) and requesting one of them to accompany the worker while approaching for funds. The worker should approach corporate givers with the aim of establishing common interest between them and his or her agency, showing them how the agency's programs are likely to bring about improvement in the community, and explaining how contributing to the cause is an investment in the community's future. Therefore, the worker should be armed with facts when approaching a corporate executive.

Most social workers are creative and resourceful. They should let those qualities inform their fundraising work as well and just be themselves. A social worker with the Salvation Army in a large Midwestern town conceived the idea of approaching the corporate office of the area's largest chain of food stores and suggesting that the chain give its shoppers the option of donating to the Salvation Army any change less than a dollar that was due to them. The corporation agreed and thereby became a proud partner in the raising of thousands of dollars on a regular basis for a local charity.

Social workers should always remember and remind others in their organizations that accountability is an absolute necessity for fundraising.

They all can learn an important lesson from Canada. A poll of Ontario hospital foundations showed that 96% of them published audited financial statements and made these available to their donors and community. Members of the Association for Healthcare Philanthropy made presentations to an Ontario government committee in support of legislation requiring disclosure (Locke, 1993).

Political Advocacy

In Chapter 5, we discussed the concept of "advocacy" and its application at the case and class levels—that is, advocacy in micro as well as macro social work practice. Here are a few suggestions that social workers will find helpful in sharpening their political advocacy skills. More are presented later in the section on community organizing.

1. *Be proactive.* Proactivity involves being on top of the issues pertaining to the cause one is advocating. It requires gathering facts and formulating a clear position on the issues.

> It means generating a social view of oneself as someone who is prepared and has to be dealt with, rather than as someone who is reactionary and who comes to confront well after the fact of a decision having been made or action having been taken. (Flynn, 1995, p. 2177)

Proactivity creates credibility with those who have authority, influence, and power.

2. *Know the local, state, and federal legislative systems and understand the legislative processes.* To influence legislation appropriately, besides expert knowledge of the issues, one must know how the system works and keep abreast of changes in policymaking bodies—for example, the membership of various legislative committees.

3. *Remember that influence can result from several approaches, such as provision of information on the issues, personal persuasion, negotiation, and constituency support* (Checkoway, 1995). Lawmakers and their staffs welcome valid

information on issues, but persuasion has limits. It is often wiser to concentrate on reinforcing the opinions of those who are in basic agreement with one's stance. Negotiation and compromise go hand in hand. Politicians are sensitive to the support of their constituents. Combining these and other approaches in a systematic and pragmatic strategy will yield greater results.

4. *Build on basic social work communication skills for approaching and educating policymakers and program administrators, mobilizing clients and community groups, and forming alliances with other groups and organizations.* Many human service organizations and groups have tried and tested different approaches to influencing sources of power. Their examples (e.g., see Douglass & Winterfeld, 1995; McFarland, 1995; Myers, 1995; O'Toole, 2007) can also guide advocacy work.

Social Worker as Program Planner

The term *planning* refers to both a process and an outcome. The planning *process* deals with the movement from problem definition to problem solution along the various stages between the two points. The planning *outcome* is a plan, a design for action that specifies the essential elements of the program. It spells out *what the objectives* of the program (short-term as well as long-term) will be; *what targets* will be influenced or changed; *how the change* will be brought about in terms of the tasks, tactics, and procedures to be used; *who will perform* the required tasks and procedures; *where and when* the services will be provided in terms of the facilities and timing for the use of personnel and their procedures; *what fiscal and other resources* will be needed to implement the program; and *how the program will be monitored and evaluated.*

There are several planning models. The PRECEDE-PROCEED model (Green & Kreuter, 1991) is a noteworthy one because it has been widely applied in illness prevention and health promotion programs and tested in research and evaluation projects with more than

1,000 published applications (Frankish, Lovato, & Poureslami, 2007). It has nine phases, the first five of which are diagnostic: (a) *social diagnosis* of the self-determined needs, wants, resources, and barriers in a community; (b) *epidemiological diagnosis* of health problems; (c) *behavioral and environmental diagnosis* of specific behaviors and environmental factors for the program to address; (d) *educational and organizational diagnosis* of the behavior-related predisposing, enabling, and reinforcing conditions; and (e) *administrative and policy diagnosis* of the resources and barriers within the organization and community. The remaining four phases pertain to implementation and evaluation: (f) *implementation,* (g) *process evaluation,* (h) *impact evaluation,* and (i) *outcome evaluation.* Process evaluation begins as soon as the program implementation starts, and impact evaluation begins as the implementation proceeds. The impact evaluation is done when enough time has passed, as specified in the program objectives. Rainey and Lindsay (1994) divided the community health promotion program planning process into eight stages: (a) epidemiologic assessment, (b) needs assessment, (c) analysis of behavior, (d) working through social institutions, (e) goals and objectives, (f) political groundwork, (g) implementation, and (h) evaluation. They listed 101 questions that a planner should ask to ensure that nothing of importance has been left out. The planning-related suggestions, listed below, elaborate on some of these stages. Social workers can enrich their knowledge and skills by taking these suggestions to heart:

1. *Take the task of developing program objectives seriously.* This may be the single most important part of the job as a planner. Many plans fail because the objectives are too loose, too subjective, too narrow, or too difficult to measure. Build the objectives on a thorough analysis of all relevant factors, such as the problem, policy, program, and environment. An understanding of the nature, origin, and scope of the problem or need is an absolute necessity for this task.

2. *Know the various approaches to problem analysis and needs assessment.* The major strategies include (a) review of the literature; (b) interviews with key informants—the people with special knowledge or expertise about the problem or the people with the problem; (c) use of focus groups made up of agency staff members and potential program beneficiaries, with the aim of learning people's preferences regarding community health promotion and the reasons for their choices (Longe & Wolf, 1983); (d) study of statistical documents on the problem and the people affected by it, as well as reports of the local and regional health planning agencies; (e) surveys of prospective program participants; and (f) community forums where interested community members can express their opinions about the proposed program. Similarly, an analysis of the policy relevant to the problem and the proposed program is important for specifying program objectives.

3. *Know the various models of policy analysis.* Policies determine major approaches, priorities, and funding for programs. Various models *of policy analysis* learned in basic social work courses are appropriate for this purpose. A *program analysis* of either the agency's past efforts regarding the problem or similar other programs would help in developing the appropriate objectives. Particular attention should be paid to the organizational, budgetary, and cost-benefit aspects of the programs being analyzed. For example, the design and implementation of a hospital's community health promotion program would depend on the hospital's mission, scope of the program, and decision about where the program would fit into its organization and what kind of personnel and resources would be allowed for it. Longe and Wolf (1983) discussed three organizational structures for hospital-based health promotion programs. Such a program can be operated as a function of an existing department or division, as a department in itself, or as a separate corporate entity. All of these can be either for-profit or not-for-profit. In cases of multi-institutional hospital systems, again, there

are several possibilities. Each hospital may have its own health promotion program, one hospital may have the program that provides health promotion services for the entire system, or the program may be part of the corporate management entity separate from individual hospitals (Longe & Wolf, 1983).

4. *Include in an environmental analysis the study of factors likely to help and hinder the program being planned, as well as the major trends that may affect it positively or negatively.* A hospital that wants its illness prevention and health promotion program to make a profit or at least pay for itself may also need a market analysis along with a needs assessment. A *market analysis* shows who the actual and potential consumers of community health promotion activities will be, which offerings they will participate in, and how they will determine their satisfaction with an offering (Longe & Wolf, 1983).

5. *Let the carefully selected realistic objectives lead to the specification of other elements of the program, such as the appropriate technologies, staff functions, personnel policies, and procedures.* Make sure the program will have the necessary tools for its implementation; these are economic, informational, management, legal, and political. For health promotion, make sure the program allows for multilevel integrated interventions. Elder, Schmid, Dower, and Hedlund (1993) categorized a community heart health program's interventions as (a) social marketing; (b) direct behavior change efforts that include health education, skills training, and contingency management; (c) screening; and (d) environmental change efforts that include changes in policy, as well as in physical environment.

6. *Build into the program a strong evaluation element with the appropriate needed information system.* Evaluation of the program—ongoing, periodic, and final—is as important as its implementation. In this age of accountability and scarce resources, an agency's ability to document

the effectiveness and efficiency of its program determines the program's continued existence. All kinds of designs—pre-experimental, quasi-experimental, and experimental (Campbell & Stanley, 1966)—can be used for evaluating programs. Similarly, an evaluation can have many foci, such as the program's acceptability, accessibility, adequacy, comprehensiveness, continuity, cost-effectiveness, efficiency, effort, impact, integration of services, performance, and process (Attkisson & Broskowski, 1978; Suchman, 1967). Choose a design and the focus according to the purpose of the program and the need and resources of the agency. Select evaluation measures that quantify the extent to which the program objectives would be met and even capture the qualitative aspects of the program consequences.

Social Worker as Educator and Community Activator

The social work educator role involves giving new information and helping in the acquisition and practice of new behaviors and skills. It is one of the oldest professional roles, sometimes standing out as the major thrust of social work activity and often embedded in a worker's total practice. Social workers have played this role not only in their work with individual clients but also in community programs, in family life and consumer education, and in the training of volunteers for community service (Siporin, 1975). In the words of Connaway and Gentry (1988),

> Social workers helped Asian and European wives of returning servicemen learn how to shop, cook, and negotiate social institutions in their adopted country. We taught budgeting and food commodity preparation to financially struggling families. We taught members of youth clubs how to make decisions. We assisted immigrants to learn how a democratic society works. We helped unemployed persons practice filling out job applications. We designed learning opportunities for persons with specific developmental lags and disabilities to acquire skills to master environmental tasks. (p. 114)

Social workers traditionally have engaged in the educator role in two contexts: with one person at a time and with groups of persons. Most social workers today come out of their training programs adept at playing this role. Social workers in illness prevention and health promotion will be expected to play this role not only with individuals and groups but also at the larger community level. The importance of the community cannot be minimized. We agree with the view of Green and Raeburn (1990):

> The most effective vehicle for health promotion activity, whether it be directed at policy, environmental change, institutional change, or personal skills development, is the human group, a coalition with all its aspects of social support and organizational power. Community groups can exist to set priorities in health promotion, to run programs, to advise public officials, and to help each other in a wide variety of ways. These groups are perfect vehicles for an enabling approach. (p. 41)

Community organization has been an area of social work practice throughout its history, and social work has made significant contributions to the development of the theory and technology of community organization. Earlier, we alluded to the role of social workers in public health who functioned both as caseworkers and community organizers. The significance of their contributions is reflected in the judgment of Rosen (1974) that "the roots of social medicine are to be found in organized social work" (p. 112).

Before suggesting effective approaches to individual-, group-, and community-level illness prevention and health promotion work, we discuss the concepts of "enabling," "empowerment," and "community organization" relevant for this work.

Enabling is to make able, to provide the means or opportunity, and to help in the improvement of capacity. Enabling traditionally has been viewed as a social work role. As an enabler, a social worker helps individuals, groups, and communities articulate their needs; identify and clarify their problems; explore, select, and apply strategies to resolve those problems; and develop their capacities to deal with their problems more effectively (Zastrow, 1985). Skills for this role include conveying hope, reducing ambivalence and resistance, recognizing and managing feelings, identifying and supporting strengths, breaking down problems into solvable parts, and maintaining a focus on goals (Barker, 2003). WHO's (1986) Ottawa Charter defined *health promotion* as "the process of enabling people to increase control over and improve their health." To be effective, illness prevention and health promotion work has to be bifocal. Green and Raeburn (1990) called these foci theoretical and ideological perspectives:

> The first emphasizes political and sociological or "system" factors in health. The second emphasizes personal and small group decision making, psychological factors, and health education methods. An integration of these viewpoints appears to prevail in actual policies and practice, though some advocates and practitioners continue to defend or push for one of the more polar views on the health promotion spectrum. (p. 30)

The principle of "enabling" is not only applicable at both these levels but also can be used to merge the two perspectives into an integrated, total, person-environment approach in which the responsibility for health is shared between individuals and systems. This enabling approach involves "returning power, knowledge, skills, and other resources in a range of health areas to the community—to individuals, families, and whole populations" (Green & Raeburn, 1990, p. 38).

Empowerment refers to the process of gaining, developing, facilitating, or giving power. Because the history of social work is essentially the history of its work with the poor and the powerless, empowerment has been a part of the social work approach to serving its clients. Simon (1994) identified the following five components of the empowerment approach that have existed across every period of social work history since 1893: (a) the construction of collaborative partnerships with clients; (b) the emphasis on their strengths rather than their weaknesses; (c) the focus on both individuals and their social and physical environments; (d) the recognition of the clients' rights, responsibilities, and needs; and (e) the direction of professional energies toward helping historically disempowered individuals and groups. Despite this history, some questioned the ability of social workers to empower their clients because of their own powerlessness. Others considered power to be a central theme in social work practice and wanted client empowerment to be made the cornerstone of social work theory and practice (e.g., see Calista, 1989; Hasenfeld, 1987; Heger & Hunzeker, 1988). Over the past 40 years, social workers have been making significant contributions to the development of a theory of empowerment and formulating empowerment-related practice principles and techniques (e.g., Gutierrez, 1992; Hasenfeld, 1987; Kieffer, 1984; Parsons, 1988; Pinderhughes, 1983; Soloman, 1976; Staples, 1990). Others (for our purpose, those in the fields of health, education, and community psychology) also have recognized the importance of empowerment and explored this concept and ways of operationalizing it (e.g., Bernstein et al., 1994; Flynn, Ray, & Rider, 1994; Israel, Checkoway, Schulz, & Zimmerman, 1994; Schillinger, Villela, & Saba, 2007). Now there is a consensus regarding empowerment processes and outcomes in social work practice. "Building on empowerment theories of the 1980s and 1990s, social work has moved the concept of empowerment from value and philosophical levels to practice principles, frameworks, and methods" (Parsons, 2008). Empowerment-based practice is used in work with vulnerable populations such as women, minorities, people with mental illness, those with disabilities, and the aged (Parsons, 2008). Neighbors, Braithwaite, and Thompson (1995) hold that empowerment operates on multiple levels and suggest that personal empowerment and community action must go together. Social workers should keep themselves abreast of new and emerging empowerment-related knowledge and skills.

Community organizing means helping people understand and join together to deal with their shared problems and build social networks for collective action (Rubin & Rubin, 2001). Community can be defined in many ways: It can refer to geopolitical, geocultural, or interest communities. Various entities and ideas such as race, ethnicity, faith, gender, age, physical or mental disability, and sexual orientation can be the focus of organizing. Examples of community organizing abound in arenas such as

> labor, agrarian reform, racial justice, neighborhood improvement, welfare rights, the women's movement, senior power, immigrant rights, the LGBT movement, housing, youth-led organizing, environmental justice, education, tax reform, health care, transportation, public safety, city services, and disability rights. (Mondros & Staples, 2008)

There are several models of community organization practice. For example, Rothman (1970) proposed the following three models, which he has further revised and elaborated on (Rothman, 2001): locality development, social planning, and social action. *Locality development* seeks to bring about community change through broad participation of citizens in identifying goals and selecting actions. The emphasis here is on the process of generating self-help and improving community capacity and integration. *Social planning* emphasizes the use of technical processes to solve substantive community problems by rational, deliberate, and controlled efforts. *Social action* seeks basic changes in the institutions and/or community practices by shifting power relationships and resources. "Innovation and creativity are the norm in this dynamic field of practice, which goes to the heart of social work values such as justice, empowerment, participatory democracy, self-determination, and overcoming all forms of oppression" (Mondros & Staples, 2008). Community organizing draws from many different disciplines and includes both "conflict" and "consensus-building" approaches to social action. The "conflict" approaches assume that people can organize to force power holders to acquiesce to community demands, whereas "consensus-building" approaches encourage partnering with power holders in an effort to produce community improvements (Mondros & Staples, 2008).

New models and strategies of community organization incorporating advances in information and communication technology are being developed. For example, campaign organizers can now use cell phones, conference calls, video teleconferencing, faxes, transmittance of images, video streaming, text messaging, organization of webpages, webcasting, e-mail discussion lists, chat rooms, Internet information or resources, and computer programs to produce flyers, letters, PowerPoint presentations, and videos (Hick & McNutt, 2002; Roberts-DeGennaro, 2004). The strategies and techniques of the various models can be mixed and matched for different purposes. We discuss more of the "what" and "how" of community organizing in Chapter 8.

Bracht and Kingsbury (1990) proposed an extensive five-stage model of community organizing for health promotion. They discussed the key elements of each of the stages: (a) community analysis, (b) design initiation, (c) implementation, (d) maintenance-consolidation, and (e) dissemination-reassessment. On the basis of experience from the community heart health programs, Elder et al. (1993) offered the following helpful ideas that can serve as practice principles: (a) Community participation in planning, designing, and evaluating the program promotes its adoption by the community; (b) feedback to the community is essential; (c) primary prevention should be given priority over secondary prevention; (d) interventions using multiple strategies and promoted through multiple channels are more effective; and (e) policy and environmental interventions should be preferred over direct behavioral change efforts.

Different approaches to education may be taken when the target is an individual or small group rather than the community. For their role as educators of individuals and groups, social workers will find the following suggestions helpful:

1. *Strive for a match between the educational strategy and the characteristics of the system (individual, group, or community) to be worked with in terms of its composition, demographics, and culture.* Answers to the question, "Given what is to be learned and the characteristics of the system, how best can it learn the needed information and skills?" will guide in ensuring the needed communication fit.

2. *Remember that different people learn in different ways.* Some learn primarily by doing (enactive learners); others by summarizing, visualizing, and organizing perceptions into patterns and images (iconic learners); and still others by abstracting and conceptualizing (symbolic learners; Jerome Brunner, mentioned in Gitterman, 1988). Social workers should try to respond to different learning styles by using the appropriate teaching methods, which may include (a) the *didactic* method, which involves sharing information and ideas; (b) the *discussion* method, which allows for much more interaction between the worker and the client system; (c) the *visual* method, which uses graphs, diagrams, pictures, films, and other aids for learning and understanding; and (d) the *action* method, which emphasizes learning through experiencing and allows for role-modeling and coaching.

Beyond the above general educational methods, Gitterman (1988) listed the following specific educational skills and strategies for social workers in health care: (a) providing relevant information, (b) clarifying misinformation, (c) offering advice, (d) offering interpretations, (e) providing feedback, (f) inviting feedback, (g) specifying action tasks, and (h) preparing and planning for task completion.

3. *Be sensitive to such system characteristics as intelligence, verbal ability, and self-respect in choosing an educational strategy.*

In general, the most effective strategies are those that partialize information and tasks into manageable units applied to real problems or tasks. Some system members who do not tolerate stress well can benefit from learning opportunities arranged in a clear, step-by-step manner to fit their needs. (Connaway & Gentry, 1988, p. 123)

For health promotion aimed at behavioral change, the educational strategy must include skills training and contingency management. The components of skills training are "instruction, modeling, practice during training sessions, feedback, reinforcement, and practice between sessions," and "contingency management involves altering consequences for behavior to change the probability of the behavior in the future" (Elder et al., 1993, p. 470).

4. *Carefully select the context of educational activity.* Again, an understanding of the system's characteristics will help in selecting the context that promises a high degree of success. Any context has room for mixing and matching the various educational approaches and techniques mentioned above. Similarly, the social worker should determine the degree of structure for the educational activity, with an eye toward maximizing the impact of that education.

Degree of structure is the extent to which a technique determines what information is presented and how persons interact about this information. We determine degree of structure imposed by examining precisely what the technique requires people to do. A paper-and-pencil test has different behavioral requirements than watching a film or participating in a discussion or role-playing (Connaway & Gentry, 1988, p. 126).

Social workers are able to engage in the educational role at the larger community level without much difficulty. Nolte and Wilcox (1984) considered two sets of abilities essential for success in reaching the public: personal characteristics and skills. Their list of personal characteristics includes awareness, courage, creativity, curiosity, diplomacy, empathy, judgment, speed, and thoroughness; these are not at all uncommon in social workers. The required skills are essentially the same as the problem-solving skills that all social workers have learned and practiced. In organizing community-level educational activities, social workers will be able to benefit from the following suggestions:

- *Supplement knowledge and skills with ideas and strategies from the literature on health education and social marketing.* Social marketing is a methodology that applies profit-sector marketing techniques to the task of increasing the acceptance of social ideas and practices and thereby changing people's attitudes and behaviors (see e.g., Hastings, Devlin, & MacFadyen, 2005; Kotler, 1982).
- *Use existing resources in the community.* Various disease-specific organizations, such as the American Heart Association, American Lung Association, and National Kidney Foundation, are doing impressive illness prevention and health promotion work. "They have produced publications, public service announcements, and programs which have frequently been both sustained and effective" (McGinnis, 1982, p. 413). Other groups are engaged in more generic wellness activities. Social workers should reach out to these organizations, collaborate with them, and coordinate their own educational activities with theirs.
- *Target specific groups and populations for intensive education and use audience-appropriate educational strategies.* A multipronged approach involving several strategies is likely to produce the maximum impact. Social workers should remember that the goal of their activities is not merely imparting information but being instrumental in bringing about behavioral changes.
- *Let knowledge of the target population and its need, agency's resources, other resources in the community that can be mobilized, and imagination create a package of appropriate strategies.* (This suggestion is given because there is no standard list of educational strategies for illness prevention and health promotion work.)
- *Treat the local mass media—both print and electronic—as a special resource.* Attract their attention, gain their support, and cultivate an ongoing positive relationship with them. The media are moving toward what Joslyn-Scherer (1980) called "therapeutic journalism"; that is, besides being sources of information, they want to become active shapers of helping trends. Helping the media with their need would serve the social worker's public education purpose well. Flora and Cassady (1990) defined three roles that media organizations can play in community-based health promotion: (a) media organization as a news producer, (b) media organization as an equal partner, and (c) media organization as a health promotion leader.

These authors discussed ways of integrating those media functions into the health promotion process. Several books on how to make the media work for you (e.g., Brawley, 1983; Klein & Danzig, 1985) can help in improving workers' know-how.

- *Master the media advocacy approach.* In the literature on health education, *media advocacy* refers to the use of mass media (including paid advertising) for influencing individual behavior, stimulating community action, and changing public policies. Wallack (1994) considered it a strategy for empowering people and communities. According to him, whereas the traditional media approaches seek to fill the "knowledge gap," media advocacy addresses the "power gap." "Social, economic, and political determinants of health have been largely ignored by the most pervasive media. Media advocacy tries to change this by emphasizing the social and economic, rather than individual and behavioral, roots of the problem" (p. 421). The primary strategy is to work with individuals and groups to claim power of the media for changing the environment in which health problems occur.

- *Remember that much planning goes into media advocacy.* The major steps are (a) establishing the policy goal, (b) deciding the target, (c) framing the issue and constructing the message, (d) delivering the message and creating pressure for change, and (e) evaluating the process and its outcome. Social workers, well versed in the problem-solving process, should not have much difficulty in mastering the media advocacy approach. Wallack, Dorfman, Jernigan, and Themba (1993) provide several examples of media advocacy works.

- *Stay abreast of technological advancements and enrich activities and programs from the same.* Emerging technologies, such as CD-ROM, interactive videodiscs, and virtual reality programs, are providing newer media with tremendous possibilities for illness prevention and health promotion programs. "Enter-education" or "edutainment" is a concept that combines entertainment and education for changing attitudes and behaviors. Its operationalization as an approach to health promotion has great potential for success because "the entertainment media are pervasive, popular, personal, and persuasive" (Steckler et al., 1995, p. 320).

The social work educational role may need to be directed toward educating politicians and policymakers. Social workers should sharpen their class advocacy skills, which are appropriate for educating and influencing policymakers. There are many time-honored methods,

> including one-to-one lobbying; collecting and presenting signed petitions; initiating and managing letter-writing, telephone call, and telegram campaigns; mobilizing groups to appear at public hearings; preparing and presenting statements at public hearings; and suggesting the wording of the proposed law. (Dhooper, 1994a, p. 159)

They should make sure that their cause and point of view are presented in a forceful, dignified, and polite manner.

Facts, arguments, and demonstrations of power are the tools for influencing policymakers. Therefore, social workers should use a strategy that includes presentation to the policymakers and their staffs of accurate and unbiased information on their cause, rational and nonemotional argument in favor of that cause, and subtle hints about the backing of an organized voting block whenever possible.

Social workers should keep in mind that all politicians want to stay popular, desire to be viewed as sensitive and responsive to the needs and situations of their constituents, and need to give the impression of being tough-minded and responsible public servants. Social workers should try to meet these needs by keeping in touch with them, providing them information and opinions on important issues, sending them reports of their agency's work, inviting them to its events, and being involved with their offices.

This section ends with two sets of principles of health education, one focusing on the "what" and the other on the "how." Freudenberg and his associates (1995) drew the first list from relevant theories, practice, and research. Although presented as hypotheses, these can guide social work activities. We present these principles in Table 6-B below.

In Chapter 5, we presented theories of behavior change. Frankish et al. (2007) reviewed the various theories of behavior change and health

Table 6-B Principles of Health Education

- Effective health education interventions should be tailored to a specific population within a particular setting.
- Effective interventions involve the participants in planning, implementation, and evaluation.
- Effective interventions integrate efforts aimed at changing individuals, social and physical environments, communities, and policies.
- Effective interventions link participants' concerns about health to broader life concerns and to a vision of a better society.
- Effective interventions use existing resources within the environment.
- Effective interventions build on the strengths found among participants and their communities.
- Effective interventions advocate for the resource and policy changes needed to achieve the desired health objectives.
- Effective interventions prepare participants to become leaders.
- Effective interventions support the diffusion of innovation to a wider population.
- Effective interventions seek to institutionalize successful components and to replicate them in other settings.

and identified a number of common elements. They presented the following principles of behavior change and health education based on that work. These principles are relevant for multicultural health promotion activities as well.

- *Principle of educational diagnosis:* This involves identification of the causes of health behavior in specific groups. An intervention linked to a diagnosed problem in its social and cultural context has the greatest chance of success.
- *Principle of hierarchy:* This states that there is a natural order in the sequence of factors influencing health behavior. Predisposing factors must be dealt with before influencing enabling factors, which in turn must be dealt with before focusing on reinforcing factors.
- *Principle of cumulative learning:* Experiences must be planned in a sequence that takes into account the person's prior learning experiences and the concurrent incidental learning experiences or opportunities.
- *Principle of participation:* Persons must be involved so that they can identify their own need for change and select a method or approach that they believe will enable them to change.
- *Principle of situational specificity:* There is no "magic bullet" approach to health education. The effectiveness and efficiency of a method depend on circumstances and characteristics of people—both the target audience and the

change agent. Success lies in the application of an approach to the right audience, at the right time, in the right way.

- *Principle of multiple methods:* A comprehensive program should employ different methods in consideration of the interaction of person-specific and situation-specific factors.
- *Principle of individualization:* The program method should be tailored to persons, their need, and their situation so that they can be actively involved in their learning experiences.
- *Principle of relevance:* The contents and methods of the program should be relevant to the learner's interest and circumstances.
- *Principle of feedback:* The program should provide feedback on participants' progress and effects of their health behaviors. It allows them to adapt to both the learning process and behavioral responses within their own situation and at their own pace. This principle is relevant to both program participants and health professionals.
- *Principle of reinforcement:* Build into the program an activity or feedback that is designed to reward a person for the desired health behavior, because a behavior that is rewarded tends to be repeated. Reinforcement may be intrinsic or extrinsic in nature.
- *Principle of facilitation:* Make the intervention provide the means for people to take the desired action or reduce barriers to health behavior.

Social Work Role in Work With Special Populations/Problems

In this section, we discuss the knowledge and skills appropriate for social work with problems and populations for which social workers are likely to be looked to for leadership. These problems include (a) health promotion for AIDS prevention, (b) prevention of child abuse, and (c) illness prevention and health promotion among the elderly. Involvement in these will require social workers to assume several professional roles simultaneously.

Health Promotion for AIDS Prevention

AIDS will continue as a major health and public health concern for the foreseeable future. More than a million Americans are living with HIV or AIDS (Centers for Disease Control and Prevention [CDC], 2007), and there are 40,000 new HIV infections each year (Kaiser Family Foundation, 2007). Despite the high rates of prevalence and incidence of the disease, society has been reluctant to respond to it in the past. Because the majority of those affected by AIDS belonged to groups viewed as socially marginal (e.g., gay men, intravenous drug users, Hispanics, and blacks), society let bigotry, racism, homophobia, and elitism dictate its responses. On the one hand, these attitudes promoted ignorance and antipathy, delayed recognition of the disease, and obstructed development of effective prevention efforts (Altman, 1987); on the other hand, they allowed most U.S. citizens to believe that they were not at risk of contracting HIV (House & Walker, 1993). Even after 20 years, these opinions have not lost their validity.

As mentioned earlier, social workers have been among the pioneers in creating programs and activities to serve AIDS patients. They have much to offer to the prevention efforts as well. Some impressive medically oriented preventive work has been done—for example, antiretroviral treatment, which reduces the risk of transmission of HIV from a woman to her baby to less than 2%,

has reduced the rates of mother-to-infant transmission of HIV (Kaiser Family Foundation, 2007). All efforts to prevent the infection of children are welcome, but prevention of infection of women is the ideal strategy. That will require combining and integrating birth control, family planning, HIV testing, and counseling services. Social workers engaged in AIDS prevention programs will find the following facts and suggestions helpful.

1. *Most people at risk of AIDS are not a cohesive community.* Despite the decline in the incidence of the disease among gay men, they—particularly rural gays and younger gays who do not see themselves at risk—must be given special attention. Men who have sex with other men and do not openly identify themselves as gay are another hidden population. Similarly, most intravenous drug users are at high risk for AIDS, but they are an invisible minority. Adolescents are also at great risk for the spread of HIV. Other populations of concern are runaways, prostitutes, the homeless, older persons, and those with disabilities. Racially, Hispanics and blacks continue to be at greater risk.

2. *Identifying and reaching out to most of these high-risk groups is difficult.* Even after they are identified, each of these groups poses special problems for reaching out to, educating, and influencing them. It is difficult to educate those under the influence of drugs. Adolescence is characterized by a sense of immortality and invulnerability, experimentation, confusion, and challenging of authority (Gray & House, 1989). Merely giving adolescents information is not sufficient to change their behaviors. Cultural and religious factors discourage Hispanics from being open about sex and drugs. The belief that it is wrong to touch their own bodies and that spermicides may hurt them is widespread (Lewis, Das, Hopper, & Jencks, 1991). The taboo against homosexuality is strong in the black population. Dalton (1989) listed reasons why blacks resist AIDS education, including their reaction to larger society's blaming of race as a reason for the origin and spread of the disease, their general

mistrust and suspicion of whites, and their resentment about being dictated to once again.

3. *Overall, AIDS education has been underfunded, erratic, uncoordinated, confusing, and timid* (Levine, 1991). Numerous AIDS education programs, many of them quite innovative and targeted to specific at-risk populations, have been tried with varying degrees of success, but they often have been implemented without community input or formal planning (House & Walker, 1993). This observation is true not of the past alone.

Social workers should use their community organizational skills for designing top-down community AIDS-prevention programs. They should refine and strengthen those skills with ideas and suggestions from the literature on community assessment, coalition building, community involvement, and service coordination, and tailor these to the specific task at hand. The following is an impressive design for a blueprint to organize an HIV education program:

- Obtain political commitment from community members.
- Establish a community education task force.
- Review existing education information and materials.
- Identify the high-risk groups targeted for education in your community.
- Develop, implement, and evaluate a short-term plan of action.
- Develop and implement a long-term plan of action.
- Evaluate the program results. (House & Walker, 1993, p. 286)

4. *AIDS prevention work involves challenging and changing social norms, and, therefore, community institutions must be made a part of the effort.* As Wolfred (1991) put it, "AIDS educators must be prepared to push social norms and community leaders to new limits in order to stop the spread of HIV infection" (p. 135). Most institutions can be involved somehow, directly or indirectly, in some aspect of the effort. Social workers should try to make the task force (Item 2 in the above suggestions) as broad-based as possible. They should educate the task force about

what has been learned from past efforts in this area. The major lessons are as follows:

- A long-term commitment to inform and motivate people to change behavior is needed.
- Programs must be designed to reach all at-risk populations with their specific needs.
- It is necessary to slant messages toward members of specific high-risk groups.
- All AIDS education programs must be culturally and community sensitive.
- Educational programs that merely provide information are not likely to be effective.
- Programs that provide specific tools and techniques for behavioral change are most effective.
- Peers teaching peers will have positive results in both attainment of knowledge and behavioral change (Ostrow, 1989).

5. *Planning of an AIDS prevention and control program should involve the following elements*:

- Establishing goals. These may be (a) to prevent HIV infection, (b) to reduce the personal and social impact of HIV infection, or (c) to reduce the AIDS-related fear and stigma.
- Doing an initial assessment of people's AIDS-related knowledge, behavior, culture, and sources of information.
- Defining the target audiences by demographic indicators, reference groups, organizations, or risk-prone behaviors.
- Setting objectives and performance targets on the basis of information from the assessment.
- Developing (a) messages and materials appropriate for target audiences and (b) channels of communication, institutional networks, and activities that can best attract the attention of target audiences.
- Promoting and ensuring support services such as counseling, HIV testing, promotion of condoms and spermicide, development and distribution of educational materials, and training of health educators.
- Deciding monitoring and evaluation procedures and process.
- Establishing a schedule and budget for the different components of the plan.
- Reassessing on the basis of any new data on changes in the program, audiences, program impact, and so on (WHO, 1989).

6. *Both primary and secondary prevention efforts should appropriately target different groups.* Primary prevention focuses on (1) increasing education regarding transmission of HIV/AIDS facts, (2) improving risk reduction skills, (3) reducing high-risk behaviors such as drug use, (4) building social and peer normative support for risk-reduction behavior change, (5) increasing self-efficacy, and (6) encouraging positive intensions and attitudes regarding the individual's ability to change behavior (Kelly & Kalichman, 2002). High-risk populations that should be differentially targeted are youth under age 25, drug users, men who have sex with men, and heterosexual women. They are the most vulnerable to HIV exposure groups. The CDC (2001) has released a Compendium of HIV Prevention Interventions with Evidence of Effectiveness, which consists of descriptions of programs targeting high-risk populations. Secondary prevention attempts to reduce the damage for those who are already infected and living with HIV/AIDS by focusing on early detection, medication adherence, risk reduction, and quality of life. Through the Replicating Effective Programs initiative, the CDC is identifying and replicating evidence-based successful programs. Partnership for Health project (Richardson et al., 2004), the Healthy Relationships project (Kalichman et al., 2001), the CLEAR (Choosing Life: Empowerment, Action, Results) program (Lightfoot, Rotheram-Borus, & Tevendale, 2007), and CHAMP+ (Collaborative HIV/AIDS and Adolescent Mental Health Project–Plus) (McKay, Block, Mellins, & Traube, 2005) are some of the population-specific programs.

7. *The importance of assessing, mobilizing, and creating the needed resources cannot be minimized.* The local mass media are a vital resource for any educational endeavor. Social workers should keep in mind that awareness and education also create expectation for services. A health promotion program for AIDS prevention, for example, cannot simply educate people about the risks of unsafe sex. It must ensure that people have access to the wherewithal for safe sex, that testing services are available, and that

those who are HIV-seropositive but asymptomatic, those who have AIDS-related complex symptoms, and those who have full-blown AIDS have the necessary counseling, health, and social services. In providing services, targeting the setting should also be considered important. Latkin and associates (1994) examined the relationships between HIV-related injection practices of drug users and injection settings. They found that injecting at a friend's residence, in shooting galleries, and in semipublic areas, and the frequency of injecting with others were significantly associated with the frequency of sharing unclean needles. Social workers' grant-writing skills would be helpful in exploring financial resources. Myers, Pfeiffle, and Hinsdale (1994) described the building of a community-based consortium for obtaining federal funds for the treatment of AIDS patients.

8. *Understanding the psychosocial barriers to behavioral change is extremely important.* The relevant barriers include (a) a person's perceived vulnerability to HIV infection, (b) perceived benefits of changing behavior, and (c) self-efficacy (Hayes, 1991). Social workers should address these barriers by convincing the targets of their efforts that they are vulnerable, highlighting for them the benefits of change, and helping them become competent and comfortable in trying new behaviors. Similarly, given the significance of cultural and religious values pertaining to sex-related behaviors, workers should try to understand and work with those values.

9. *Social work values should guide the selection of intervention strategy.* Workers should eschew scare tactics and even hints of moral condemnation. Their strategy should incorporate techniques of education, motivation, and enabling for responsible behavior. While working with adolescents for education and behavioral change, social workers should treat them as grown-ups and at the same time use their propensity for influence by their peers to reinforce their learning and efforts to change. Treating them as responsible grown-ups demands

that, beyond giving them information and facts, they are engaged and encouraged to discuss those facts and to learn about the "what" and "how" of the desired behavioral change.

10. *Social workers as health promoters for AIDS prevention should observe the following "dos" that WHO (1989) called the health promoter's responsibility*:

- *Be informed:* Remain abreast of fresh knowledge.
- *Be bold:* Challenge their assumptions about sexuality, find new resources, and work with people previously considered unimportant.
- *Be clear:* Speak plainly, honestly, and directly, and avoid ambiguous language, half-truths, and technical jargon.
- *Avoid stereotyping and blaming:* HIV is a virus with no racial, ethnic, or sexual preference.
- *Concentrate efforts on changing the behavior of target groups.*
- *Act on a broad front:* Under people's reasons for maintaining their behavior, find acceptable alternatives and provide the resources and support required to introduce the alternatives.

Child Abuse Prevention

The problem of child abuse will persist in the future, both as part of the overall violence in society and because of changes in the family. Families will become more complex and unstable in their structure and weaker in their social supports and other resources. Both these sets of factors will likely increase the risk of abuse and neglect for children, and the need for efforts to deal with the problem will continue. Two decades ago, the U.S. Advisory Board on Child Abuse and Neglect concluded that child abuse and neglect in the United States represented a national emergency and that the country's lack of an effective response was a moral disaster. It presented 31 recommendations organized into the following eight areas: (a) recognizing the national emergency, (b) providing leadership, (c) coordinating efforts, (d) generating knowledge, (e) diffusing knowledge, (f) increasing human resources, (g) providing and improving

programs, and (h) planning for the future (U.S. Department of Health and Human Services, 1990). The validity of these recommendations has not diminished and is not likely to diminish in the future. Social workers always have been a significant part of the efforts to deal with the problem of child abuse and will continue to contribute to all the above areas of activity.

Earlier, we introduced the concepts of "primary prevention," "secondary prevention," and "tertiary prevention."

> In the area of child maltreatment, primary intervention efforts aim to completely avoid the onset of parenting dysfunction; secondary intervention efforts attempt early detection of parenting problems so remediation procedures can be applied; and tertiary interventions are treatment-oriented services designed to rehabilitate maltreating parents. (Kaufman & Zigler, 1992, p. 271)

The primary prevention of child abuse has been the most overlooked dimension of the work done in the field of child abuse and neglect. From the beginning, the focus has been on "child rescue," preventing child abuse from recurring. "Although the definitive intellectual history of child abuse has yet to be written, it appears to have taken nearly 50 years before primary prevention was actually embedded in child abuse and neglect program designs" (Rodwell & Chambers, 1992, p. 160). Given the enormity and complexity of the problem, interventions at all levels will continue to be needed, and prevention of recurrence through secondary and tertiary interventions is also of vital importance.

Gordon (1993) proposed a different system of classifying preventive interventions in behavioral/mental health problems, with the focus on who receives the intervention. According to his system, interventions are "universal," "selected," and "indicated," with universal interventions targeted to all segments of the population, selected interventions targeted at high-risk populations, and indicated interventions directed at those already affected by the disorder. The following discussion of social work contributions to the prevention of child abuse includes primary and secondary or universal and selected interventions.

How can social workers intervene at the primary prevention level? The first requirement is knowledge of the predictors of child abuse. The utility of the available knowledge is questionable. Winton and Mara (2001) listed 12 theories of child abuse and neglect and classified those into the following three groups.

1. *Psychiatric/medical/psychopathology models:* (1) medical (biological) model, (2) sociobiological/evolutionary theory, and (3) psychodynamic/psychoanalytic theory.

2. *Social/psychological models:* (1) social learning theory, (2) intergenerational transmission theory, (3) exchange theory, (4) symbolic interaction theory, and (5) structural family systems theory.

3. *Sociocultural models:* (1) ecological theory, (2) feminist/conflict theory, (3) structural-functional/anomie/strain theory, and (4) cultural spillover theory.

However, no theory is adequate to explain the complex problem of child abuse, and as Rodwell and Chambers (1992) concluded, "No set of variables, or combination, does a good enough job of early identification to allow those committed to child protection to speak thoroughly about the efficacy of primary prevention because accurate targeting is practically impossible" (p. 173). They recommended that priority be given to secondary prevention or treatment programs that are effective in limiting the damage of the first abuse incident and/or preventing recurrence.

Although it is true that social work does not have and is not likely to have an empirically validated grand theory of child abuse, considerable work has been done in studying its etiology, and various conceptual frameworks have been presented. Belsky's (1980) ecological framework is the most comprehensive and akin to the social work perspective. It conceptualizes child maltreatment as a psychosocial phenomenon determined by multiple forces across four levels: the individual (ontogenetic development), the family (the microsystem), the community (the exosystem), and the culture (the macrosystem).

On the ontogenetic level, Belsky gave characteristics of parents who mistreat their children, such as a history of abuse or experience of stress. On the microsystem level, he discussed aspects of the family environment that increase the likelihood of abuse, such as having a poor marital relationship or a premature or unhealthy child. On the exosystem level, he included work and social factors, such as unemployment and isolation; and on the macrosystem level, he depicted cultural determinants of abuse, such as society's acceptance of corporal punishment as a legitimate form of discipline. (Kaufman & Zigler, 1992, p. 269)

Kaufman and Zigler extensively reviewed the literature on intervention programs and delineated strategies appropriate for each of the four levels in the Belsky model.

1. The *ontogenetic level* strategies include (a) psychotherapeutic intervention for abusive parents, (b) treatment for abused children, (c) alcohol and drug rehabilitation, (d) stress management skills training, and (e) job search assistance programs.

2. The *microsystem level* strategies include (a) marital counseling, (b) home safety training, (c) health visiting, (d) parent-infant interaction enhancement, (e) parents' aids, (f) education for parenthood, and (g) parenting skills training programs.

3. The *exosystem level* strategies involve the development/establishment or facilitation of (a) community social and health services, (b) crisis hot lines, (c) training for professionals to identify abuse, (d) foster and adoptive homes, (e) informal community supports, (f) family planning centers, (g) Parents Anonymous groups, (h) respite child-care facilities, and (i) a coordinating agency for child abuse services.

4. The *macrosystem level* strategies include (a) public awareness campaigns; (b) formation of National Commission on Child Abuse and Neglect grants for research; (c) establishment of a National Commission on Child Abuse and Neglect; (d) the requirement that states adopt

procedures for the prevention, treatment, and identification of maltreatment; (e) a legislative effort to combat poverty; (f) establishment of laws against corporal punishment in schools; and (g) research on incidence of maltreatment and effectiveness of prevention and treatment.

Guterman and Taylor (2005) mentioned the following among prominent efforts to prevent child abuse and neglect that are being tried across the country.

1. *Home visitation services* for at-risk families identified via the health care system at the point of birth of a child. Home visitors provide parenting guidance and link those families with the necessary resources and supports.

2. *Nurse home visitation program* aimed at improving the outcomes of pregnancy, quality of maternal caregiving, child health and development, and maternal life course development.

3. *Social support interventions* focused on helping at-risk parents overcome social isolation; tap informal support networks for emotional, informational, and material help; and link with mutual aid groups such as Parents Anonymous.

There is also a movement toward universal prevention strategies addressing the problem of child abuse, analogous to other universal preventive health strategies such as child immunization. On the other hand, Daro and Donnelly (2002) highlighted the difficulty of the preventive work by identifying mistakes made by the field, such as oversimplifying the problem of child abuse, overstating the potential of prevention, ignoring significance of partnership with child protective services, sacrificing the depth and quality of programs for the breadth and quantity of coverage, and failing to fully engage the public through multiple ways.

Despite the complexity and multidimensionality of the problem, comprehensive child abuse prevention programs can succeed with an extensive coordination among health and human service agencies such as hospitals, clinics, child protective services, schools, and public health departments. The social work profession historically has been involved in the design and delivery of child protective services as well as in addressing the social conditions that perpetuate the problem (Wells, 2008). Social workers' training makes them superbly qualified to take the lead in this work. Depending on their work setting, they can contribute to primary and secondary prevention. Those working in hospitals can exploit the special advantage that hospitals provide in this respect. As Kaufman, Johnson, Cohn, and McCleery (1992) put it,

> The hospital's influence can be viewed at a number of levels. Educational efforts, such as prenatal classes, postnatal instruction, and parental skills workshops, are directed toward the community as a whole. In-service trainings provide medical and psychological updates necessary for community physicians and community mental health providers to offer high-quality educational, diagnostic, and treatment-oriented services. Finally, prenatal visits, well-child visits, annual physicals, and specialty clinics for chronically ill children represent opportunities for hospital personnel to intervene at the individual level. (p. 193)

Despite their emphasis on tertiary care, hospitals have been involved in primary and secondary prevention activities, and these can be further strengthened. Altepeter and Walker (1992) mentioned several relatively short-term parent-training programs that can be made available to parents of all socioeconomic levels. Social workers can be instrumental in institutionalizing such programs. They can easily help other health care professionals sharpen their basic interviewing skills to screen parents of infants and children seen in the hospital outpatient departments using criteria across the four areas included in the Belsky model. Belsky (1980) conceptualized child abuse as a psychosocial phenomenon determined by many forces at work across the four levels mentioned above. He drew from diverse theories, including psychological disturbance in parents, abuse-eliciting characteristics of children, dysfunctional patterns of family interaction, stress-inducing social forces, and abuse-promoting cultural values. A follow-up system for families at high risk can be built into outpatient services. These programs should be directed at meeting parent-child needs.

Social workers, whether based in hospitals or working as a part of other agencies, should take a lead or significantly collaborate with others in building a systematic evaluation of program outcomes in child abuse prevention efforts.

> In addition to ongoing quality improvement, addressing public perceptions regarding funding of social services and preventive efforts could be tackled through the conducting and use of cost-effectiveness studies to show how much financial and societal cost can be saved by early intervention. (Wells, 2008)

There are strong reasons for targeting school-age children and their families for child abuse prevention work. The developmental period spanning the ages of 6 to 12 years represents the highest risk period for at least one type of abuse: sexual abuse (Finkelhor & Baron, 1986). Moreover, most abused or potentially abused children come to the attention of authorities when they start school. Planning preventive interventions at this time also takes advantage of the child's (and, thereby, the family's) expanding connection with the community. "Even the most isolated families will need to contend with the myriad changes brought on by their child's increased involvement with school and other community settings" (Rosenberg & Sonkin, 1992, p. 79). Social workers in public health and those in hospitals with strong community-oriented health promotion programs can organize school-based child abuse prevention programs. Although school-based programs are only part of the answer, and parents, other adults, and potential abusers must also be the focus of preventive efforts, these programs have been found to be helpful. They clearly prompt many victimized children to disclose their abuse. On the basis of a review of evaluation studies of sexual abuse prevention education programs, Finkelhor and Strapko (1992) said that

> they certainly rescue many children, who would not have otherwise been rescued, from extremely troublesome situations, and they short-circuit situations

which might otherwise have continued for an extended period of time at much greater ultimate cost to the child's mental health. (pp. 164–165)

The prevention and treatment of abuse of adolescents has been a particularly neglected area. "Adolescent maltreatment tends to be associated with problematic acting-out behavior of the teenager or dysfunction with the family, and tends to be dealt with as such by agencies other than protective services" (Garbarino, 1992, p. 105). Garbarino proposed several hypotheses about adolescent maltreatment and found support for them in the available research literature:

- Prevention programs should target adolescents, because the incidence of adolescent abuse equals or exceeds the incidence of child maltreatment.
- These programs should give special attention to female adolescents and the issues they face.
- Some adolescent abuse is the continuation of abuse and neglect begun in childhood; other abuse represents the deterioration of unwise childhood patterns or the family's inability to meet new challenges of adolescence. Programs should take account of these different etiologies.
- Programs in general should reach families across the board, regardless of their socioeconomic resources.
- Families with stepparents should be special targets.
- Less socially competent adolescents are at high risk and should be given special attention.
- Programs should adopt a broadly based approach to supporting and redirecting families that tend to be at high risk on the dimensions of adaptability, cohesion, support, discipline, and interpersonal conflict.

These recommendations can be woven into family preservation approaches that are being tried all over the country and are likely to become more popular in the future. Social workers can also help in incorporating these recommendations into school health programs.

The area of child sexual abuse is particularly difficult for preventive work. Determining targets for intervention is all the more difficult because sexual abuse is not strongly linked to demographic factors and because knowledge about the characteristics of offenders is insufficient (Melton, 1992). Finkelhor (1979) conceptualized four preconditions—at the individual and societal levels—for sexual abuse: (1) factors related to motivation to abuse sexually; (2) factors predisposing to overcoming internal inhibitors; (3) factors predisposing to overcoming external inhibitors; and (4) factors predisposing to overcoming a child's resistance. Most prevention efforts so far have focused on the last precondition. Social workers should keep themselves abreast of the latest research and programmatic work in the field and enrich their interventions with lessons from that work.

Whatever setting they are working in, social workers should engage in larger systemic change efforts aimed at effective coordinated involvement of the various societal systems in child abuse prevention. That will require the use of their lobbying skills.

Illness Prevention and Health Promotion Among the Elderly

In the future, the elderly will constitute a substantial proportion of the population, and their health care needs will demand special attention. Social workers will realize more and more the importance of preventive work with the elderly as well. Illness prevention and health promotion work focused on the elderly is quite new. For example, public health has turned its attention to older persons only lately. "The Gerontological Health section of Aging and Public Health Association was founded in 1978" (Kane, 1994, p. 1214). Several reasons have been proposed for the past neglect of this work [2], including the following: (a) The focus of health promotion programs is on extending life, and the elderly are not perceived as having a future; (b) the goal is usually prevention of premature death, and the elderly are considered to be beyond that point; (c) the programs often promote looking youthful and preventing signs of aging; and (d) their focus is on avoidance of

chronic disease, which is irrelevant for older adults because almost 85% of them have one chronic disease (Minkler & Pasick, 1986).

This picture is slowly changing. Realization is increasing that people of all ages can benefit from health promotion activities, although the progress of illness prevention and health promotion activities for the elderly is impaired by a lack of scientific data. The need for health promotion in the elderly is, however, obvious. The circular pattern of unhappy and unhealthy aging that results *in* and *from* poor nutritional intake, lack of physical and social activity, depression, and chronic disease (Fallcreek, Warner-Reitz, & Mettler, 1986) needs to be broken. Social workers have the skills to create and implement illness prevention and health promotion programs, as well as to contribute to the generation of much-needed knowledge.

Arnold, Kane, and Kane (1986) divided the preventive strategies into two groups: those focused on conditions or disease states, and those focused on specific behaviors that are likely to have beneficial or adverse effects on the disease states. They showed that the elderly have generally been excluded from studies of both these types of preventive strategies.

In planning illness prevention and health promotion programs for the elderly, social workers should do the following:

- Realize that needs of the elderly are manifold and that no agency's own resources are likely to be adequate to meet all needs. Take stock of what and how much their own agency can do.
- Design the program to meet the unique needs of the target population. For identifying and specifying the target population and its needs, do a systematic assessment. We have discussed elsewhere the various approaches to needs assessment. These efforts should be aimed at a twofold purpose: (a) an assessment of the needs and (b) a survey of the relevant community resources. In looking for resources, include both the current and potential resources and define the concept of "resources" broadly. These should include (a) funder service providers and volunteers; (b) use of space and facilities

and other in-kind contributions; (c) special-interest groups such as the Heart Association and Cancer Society, and service clubs such as the Lions Club; (d) local newspapers and other mass media; and (e) experience, skills, and knowledge of the target population itself (Fallcreek et al., 1986).

- Take advantage of existing programs for the elderly. For example, nutrition programs have become a central and permanent part of services under the Older Americans Act. These provide hot, nutritious meals to millions of elderly on a daily basis. These can be used for surveying the needs of the elderly, imparting information about illness prevention and health promotion programs, and motivating them for participation.
- Strive for the best possible match between the identified needs and available resources. Within the overall goals of the program, involve the participants in setting its specific objectives that reflect their existing health status and motivation for change.
- Mix and match the preventive strategies and, in general, aim at the prevention or minimization of functional impairment, rather than the cure for particular ailments. Select general health promotion activities on the basis of an assessment of the realistically achievable improvements. A multifaceted health promotion program may address physical fitness, safety, nutrition, appropriate use of medication, stress management, and communication skills. Choose a mix of educational approaches and strategies. We discussed several earlier in this chapter. Again, try to match the educational strategies to the audiences.
- Use imagination and creativity in planning illness prevention and health maintenance and promotion activities. In Japan, "health notebooks" have been used to aid the aged in managing their health (Gotou et al., 1994). The elderly are given notebooks in which they record their concerns, questions, and health data, as well as health professionals' advice, recommendations, and suggestions.
- Make sure that appropriate measures have been taken to legally protect the agency's assets and employees, as well as program participants. These measures include screening participants (through such tools as preprogram

health-screening examination), having appropriate liability insurance, and using appropriate release forms. "All participants are required to sign a program release-from-liability form; physician release forms are obtained when possible. Although such measures are not always legally binding, they demonstrate that care and precaution have been taken to provide for participants' safety" (Fallcreek et al., 1986, p. 232).

- Build into the program a strong evaluation component that captures its process, as well as its impact, so that the experience gained adds to the knowledge and skills of the service community.

Social Worker as Researcher

Evaluation of illness prevention and health promotion programs for their effectiveness and efficiency on a continuing basis will become an absolute necessity in the future. In Chapter 7, we discuss at some length social work's contribution to the various approaches to quality assurance. Here, we briefly discuss areas of health promotion work that should be subjected to systematic research not only for quality assurance purposes but also for building theories and testing intervention models.

Health promotion approaches and strategies can be categorized by the level of intervention—individual, community, and policy. These are based on different theoretical assumptions and models. At the individual level, strategies that deal with both intrapersonal and interpersonal dimensions are based on theories of *social learning and self-efficacy* (Bandura, 1986), *learned helplessness* (Seligman, 1975), *coping* (Lazarus & Folkman, 1984), *social support* (Cassel, 1976), and *consumer information processing* (Bettman, 1979), as well as models such as the *stages of change model* (Prochaska, DiClemente, & Norcross, 1992) and the *health belief model* (Rosenstock, Strecher, & Becker, 1988). Some impressive work has been done on individual-level strategies, but much more needs to be learned.

Steckler and his colleagues (1995) suggested that future research should further explore the role of social support and the mechanism of its action, the most effective combinations of strategies in comprehensive interventions, approaches to long-term adherence to changed health behaviors, ways of adapting what we already know works to the needs of new and diverse groups, and the impact of emerging learning technologies on individuals.

At the community level, strategies have been built on ideas from theories of *community organization, organizational change,* and *diffusion of innovation,* and interventions have included mediating social structures (e.g., through community coalition building), linking agents (e.g., through network interventions), empowerment, and ecological approaches (Steckler et al., 1995). More research is needed to discover the effectiveness of these strategies in various combinations for health promotion.

At the policy level, there is an obvious neglect of research into effects of the sociopolitical environment on health behavior and health status. As Wallack (1994) put it,

> Even though 30% of all cancer deaths and 87% of lung cancer deaths are attributed to tobacco use, the main focus of cancer research is not on the behavior of the tobacco industry, but on the biochemical and genetic interactions of cells. (p. 429)

Even researchers in health education, while acknowledging the importance of sociopolitical environmental factors for health-related behaviors, have focused most of their work on factors at the individual level. Future research should be aimed at enhancing the understanding of the nature of social, economic, and political power, and ways of influencing the policy processes.

Social workers could use their research-related knowledge and skills to contribute to this dimension of their agency's work. They should strive to design research studies that not only evaluate the efficacy and effectiveness of particular strategies but also test the validity of the underlying theoretical assumptions.

We end this section with Table 6-C, which recaps future social work roles in illness prevention

Table 6-C	Future Social Work Roles in Illness Prevention and Health Promotion

- Social work role in creating and mobilizing financial resources
- Social work role in program planning
- Social work role in program implementation and service provision
- Social work role as educator and community activator
- Social work role in work with special populations/problems
- Social work role as researcher
- Other social work roles in illness prevention and health promotion

and health promotion and appropriate role-related skills.

RELEVANT ETHICAL CONSIDERATIONS

Individuals and groups that are culturally different from mainstream Americans have many more barriers to health care in all sectors of the health care system. These are demographic, cultural, and health care system barriers. This reality raises several ethical questions. In this section, we discuss the ethical problems, issues, and dilemmas in illness prevention and health promotion programs.

Although significant cultural differences exist among as well as within the various minority groups, there are clear differences between Anglo-American and other ethnocultural groups in their worldviews as well as their theories of illness and approaches to health care and wellness [3].

The terms *ethical problem, ethical issue,* and *ethical dilemma* denote three different ethically challenging situations. Kachingwe and Huff (2007) provided the following examples of these situations:

Ethical Problems. A client comes to his or her appointments 10 minutes late on four consecutive occasions, perhaps because in that client's culture, the perception of time is different. If so, this is a cultural problem. Such problems are easy to resolve. The practitioner can make the appointment time more flexible or discuss with the client the significance of his or her coming on time because the clinic schedules depend on everyone coming on time.

Ethical Issues. A health promoter wants to organize an AIDS awareness workshop for students at a local high school, but parents of those students have a number of issues with the holding of such a workshop based on their religious and cultural values and traditions. Such situations are harder to deal with and require much imagination and work. It may be necessary to conduct a focus group or a survey of parents to identify the issues in clear and concrete terms. That may be followed by an open discussion with a sample of parents in order to get their input and support. At this step, their agreement on the topics to be covered in the workshop can be sought. Finally, it may be appropriate to conduct a workshop for parents first in order to gain their support for the workshop for their teens.

Ethical Dilemmas. A health promoter is faced with an ethical dilemma when the situation allows for two equally favorable or unfavorable options. An ethical dilemma also occurs when two moral reasons come into contact and the course of action is not obvious (Gabard & Martin, 2003). Searight and Gafford (2005) gave the following example of an ethical dilemma: A practitioner is asked by the family of a newly diagnosed cancer patient not to disclose the diagnosis to the patient. In their judgment, disclosure will cause unnecessary stress to the patient, which may lead to the patient giving up hope of recovery. That judgment might be culturally conditioned. Ethical dilemmas occur when a client's views on health and health care delivery conflict with those

of the health practitioner. These are also likely to occur when a client's cultural behaviors and practices appear to violate the ethical and moral definitions of human rights and obligations. Kachingwe and Huff (2007) offered female circumcision and wife beating as examples of such violations. Ethical dilemmas can be resolved through culturally proficient practice.

The term *cultural proficiency* denotes a higher level of ability than denoted by terms such as *cultural awareness, cultural sensitivity,* and *cultural competence.*

> Cultural competence is a process of possessing the knowledge to appreciate and respect the cultural differences and similarities within and between cultural groups, acknowledging and incorporating the importance of culture, and working within the cultural context of an individual in an unbiased manner to meet the client's needs. (Kachingwe & Huff, 2007, p. 46)

The aim is the provision of *culturally congruent* care. *Culturally proficient* practice involves not only culturally competent care at the individual level but also reaching out to the community to meet its needs through advocacy and other community-level activities.

We present here the Kachingwe-Huff model of culturally proficient and ethical practice. The model involves the following five steps:

Step 1: Cultural Awareness. This begins with practitioners reflecting on their personal and professional cultures. This reflection makes them cognizant of their own personal identity and helps them assess how their personal beliefs, attitudes, and behaviors affect their views of others. This also makes them realize that they were socialized into the culture of their profession, with its set of beliefs, practices, and rituals. This realization shows how their views, attitudes, and actions are affected by their professional values and commitments. This model also acknowledges the fact that individuals are innately ethnocentric, and ethnocentrism tends to lead to distorted perceptions of others' behaviors and unfounded judgments and stereotyping of others. Therefore, authors have suggested a series of questions that can help in getting in touch with one's own ethnocentric attitudes.

Step 2: Cultural Knowledge. Practitioners should increase their understanding of various cultures. This will enable them to acknowledge and respect similarities and differences among cultural groups. They can increase their knowledge by learning about the cultural beliefs and practices of their clients, including differences in communication, variations in personal space, and differences in the perception of time. They can learn from their clients as well as through reading the relevant literature and visiting their communities. Going to these communities to shop and eat or attend cultural events makes it possible to interact with cultural groups outside the confines of practice settings. They should grasp the differences within cultural groups, because people sharing a common culture are likely to be at different levels of acculturation and differ in their adherence to cultural beliefs and practices. Nevertheless, generalization about cultural groups is necessary in order to build further enquiry or initiate program activities, but generalization should be done carefully. Kachingwe and Huff (2007) point to one pitfall in generalization: "When cultural generalizations relate more to the motive behind a behavior than to the actual observed behavior, the generalization may be oversimplified—leading to stereotyping" (p. 48). Stereotyping can lead to a lack of respect for and stigmatization of a culture.

Step 3: Interpersonal Communication Skills. Practitioners should improve their communication skills, as these are an absolute must for effective interviewing at the individual client level and for designing and implementing health promotion programs. Conducting a cultural assessment should be the aim of first interviews with culturally diverse clients. Effective communication with those who cannot speak English adequately will involve working with an interpreter. Practitioners should make sure that the interpreter is well trained and is not a member of the client's family, particularly his or her child. "It is also important to realize any potential discrepancies between the interpreter's ethical code of conduct mandating objectivity and neutrality and the realities of the client-interpreter cultural interaction" (Kachingwe & Huff, 2007, p. 49). In addition to effective verbal communication, practitioners should be cognizant of nonverbal communication, particularly touching the client. A touch considered inappropriate by the client can lead to misinterpretation of intentions, whereas an appropriate and respectful touch can help build trust with the client.

Step 4: Cultural Collaboration. This involves working as a practitioner-client team that formulates goals and a mutually agreed-on plan of care. It is often possible to come up with a plan that combines the Western medical and folklore healing practices, leading to better client compliance and outcomes (Lattanzi & Purnell, 2006). This may involve practitioners of conventional medicine working with the practitioners of traditional healing techniques. Cultural collaboration is also critical for planning programs at the community level. It involves connecting with organizations and individuals who represent the targeted population and seeking their insights, suggestions, and support at all stages of program planning and implementation.

Step 5: Cultural Experiences. This step emphasizes practitioners enriching their professional repertoire with cultural experiences. These experiences can be gained through immersion projects or other approaches. However, these should have an important self-reflection component so that, along with the experience of another culture, practitioners become aware of their ethnocentrism. These experiences will heighten their ability to provide culturally proficient care. No model can help practitioners provide culturally proficient and ethical care unless they have a personal conviction in the fundamentalism of culture. Conviction is a belief, held as a truth, that becomes an ideology compelling one to action (Kachingwe, 2000). Practitioners' ability to act on their convictions is enhanced if those convictions are backed by their professional codes of ethics. The National Association of Social Workers (2000) Code of Ethics clearly mandates culturally competent practice. Section 1.05 ("Cultural Competence and Social Diversity") under "Social Workers' Ethical Responsibilities to Clients" requires the following:

a. Social workers should understand culture and its function in human behavior and society, recognizing the strengths that exist in all cultures.

b. Social workers should have a knowledge base of their clients' cultures and be able to demonstrate competence in the provision of services that are sensitive to clients' cultures and to differences among people and cultural groups.

c. Social workers should obtain education about and seek to understand the nature of social diversity and oppression with respect to race, ethnicity, national origin, color, sex, sexual orientation, age, marital status, political belief, religion, and mental or physical disability (National Association of Social Workers, 2006).

We end this section with a list of "shoulds" for ethical health promotion by social workers. These are taken from Kline and Huff (2007).

- Be aware that there is a high likelihood of encountering health promotion issues that contain an ethical component because of the vast differences among multicultural groups.
- Recognize that within and outside multicultural settings, the most important ethical principles for health promotion practitioners are (1) autonomy that allows an individual to make his or her own decisions, (2) beneficence—the duty to do good in the best interest of the client or the community, (3) confidentiality in respecting the privacy of information, (4) nonmalfeasance—causing no

harm to the client or the target group, (5) respect for people and their rights, and (6) justice—equity or fair treatment for all.

- Be attentive to the influences of a client's or target group's culture when working within ethnically diverse communities.
- Recognize that in order to resolve an ethical dispute, cultural collaboration may necessitate working in partnership with traditional forms of medicine and healing.
- Remember that ethical practice requires cultural competence, which involves having appropriate knowledge and relevant skills.

Appropriate knowledge includes

- concepts of culture, ethnicity, acculturation, and ethnocentrism and how these may affect their ability to assess, plan, implement, and evaluate an illness prevention and health promotion program;
- many ways of perceiving, understanding, and approaching health and disease processes across cultural and ethnic groups that can present barriers to effective health care intervention;
- perceptions of target groups about their agency, as these may not be positive and may impede the health promotion process;
- possible barriers that may be encountered when a program is targeted to a community primarily composed of first-, second-, or even third-generation Americans;
- communication style of the target group and the rules governing the communication process;
- the typical Western medical model of communication (which seeks to quickly establish the facts of the case and often relies on the use of negative and double-negative questions) and how it may be seen as cold, too direct, and otherwise in conflict with the target group's traditional beliefs, values, and ways of communicating;
- health concepts about the locus of control for disease causality (being outside the individual) held by many cultural groups that may result in those groups choosing not to seek Western medical intervention;
- differences between the biomedical model and lay model of illness—the more disparate the differences, the greater the likelihood the

patient will resist the Western illness prevention and health promotion program; and

- various health promotion and health behavior theories that can guide their thinking about devising effective approaches to planning interventions.

Relevant skills include

- appreciation and respect for cultural differences within and between cultural groups and work in an unbiased manner to meet the client's or target group's needs;
- care in assessment, intervention, and evaluation processes that do not overlook, misinterpret, stereotype, or otherwise mishandle encounters with those who are different from them;
- assessment of the degree of acculturation in the target group, as there is a tendency in many to resist acculturation;
- reframing of the term *race* to *multicultural ethnic* or *culturally diverse* in order to promote greater sensitivity to the challenges, potentialities, and awards of working with culturally diverse groups;
- stepping out of their current frames of reference and risking the discovery of their biases, stereotypes, and ethnocentrism;
- using strategies that have been demonstrated to be effective in overcoming barriers to illness prevention and health promotion work with culturally diverse groups;
- using appropriate assessment instruments, including acculturation scales; and
- flexibility in the design of programs, policies, and services to meet the needs and concerns of target groups.

 # Culturally competence

Critical Thinking Questions

1. Interview a member of your immediate or extended family who is at least two generations removed from you, and explore his or her concepts of health, illness, and disease. Compare and contrast those with the present-day Western biomedical explanations.

2. Based on your exposure to culturally different clients/people, make a list of a group's cultural values and religious beliefs that are totally different from yours. Identify from that list beliefs and values that can be used as positive elements in working on a disease prevention and health promotion program for that group.

NOTES

1. These techniques include (a) advertising appeals, (b) street and door-to-door collections, (c) silent salespeople (coin-collecting devices in stores and restaurants), (d) "something" for the money—special events, (e) selling services and things (e.g., Girl Scout cookies), (f) secondhand chic (charity-run thrift shops), (g) auctions—live and televised, (h) art shows, (i) fashion shows, (j) other people's homes (showing outstanding homes with such treasures as rare paintings), (k) movie and theater benefits, (l) fun and games, (m) gambling—leaving charity to chance, and (n) walk-a-thons and other "thons" (Bakal, 1979).

2. Reasons given by Arnold, Kane, and Kane (1986) include (a) difficulty in applying the traditional taxonomy of prevention—primary, secondary, and tertiary prevention—to the chronic diseases that the elderly suffer (a condition may be at once a preventable disease and a risk factor for another disease); (b) lack of adequate understanding of the propensity of the elderly to change their behavior for reducing the risk factor; (c) uncertainty of effectiveness of an altered risk factor for preventing the disease; (d) issues of cost and efficacy, which are often hard to demonstrate; (e) the long past-time horizon of the elderly posing questions such as when to intervene, especially when time of exposure to risk is a significant factor; and (f) difficulty in distinguishing between the possibilities of doing good and doing harm.

3. Commonalities among groups culturally different from mainstream Americans include the following:

- *Meaning of the family*—family has a special meaning and place in their lives. Family members are socialized to consider family's needs, prestige, stability, and welfare as more important than the individual's aspirations, comfort, and well-being.

- *Extended family ties*—great importance is placed on maintaining a wide network of kinship.
- *Place of religion*—religion affects their attitudes and practices regarding food, medical care, mental health, recreation, and interpersonal relationships both within and outside the family. Religious faith and institutions influence their ability to deal with their problems.
- *Experience as Americans*—these groups have a history of being the victims of racism. Their experiences include hostility from the mainstream community in the form of prejudice, economic discrimination, political disenfranchisement, immigration exclusion, physical violence, and social segregation.
- *Poverty and lower economic status*—large proportions of these groups live below the poverty line.
- *Level of acculturation*—all these groups have concerns, needs, and priorities related to their level of acculturation.
- *Culture-related disorders*—many of these groups experience culture-related disorders and syndromes. Many discourage owning mental and physical problems, and in some, psychological problems are expressed as somatic complaints (Dhooper & Moore, 2001).

7

SOCIAL WORK IN LONG-TERM CARE

*L*ong-term care, as the term suggests, is care provided over a sustained period of time. It may be continuous or intermittent. Besides the length, the name does not reflect other characteristics of this type of care. It is generally understood, however, that long-term care is not of an acute nature. It differs from acute care not only in its duration but also in the intensity and expected outcome of service. It is not concerned with curing disease or preventing mortality (Weiner, 1994).

Long-term care is concerned with individuals' functional incapacity for self-care, and this incapacity may never be completely overcome. The functional incapacity or impairment might have resulted from any combination of physical, cognitive, emotional, and social factors (Kane & Kane, 1981). Therefore, the need for this type of care cannot be predicted by the presence or absence of a particular medical problem (Malone-Rising, 1994). The care is aimed at reducing the degree of functional impairment and enabling the person to attain the highest level of health and well-being by improving his or her functional ability.

Functional ability is defined in several ways. The general areas of function are physical, cognitive, emotional, and social. *Physical functioning* is frequently viewed as a person's ability to perform activities of daily living and instrumental activities of daily living. Basic activities of daily living include ambulating, bathing, dressing, toileting, and eating; instrumental activities of daily living are those necessary to maintain independent living, such as preparing meals, shopping, housekeeping, telephoning, and managing finances. A person's ability to perform these functions is rated as either full, partial, minimal, or nil. It is affected by physical, mental, and social conditions and economic status. The person may be (a) independent, (b) requiring mechanical assistance, (c) requiring personal assistance, or (d) unable to do specific activities (Evashwick & Branch, 1987). Measures of the ability to perform these activities are diverse.

Recipients of long-term care are both the old and the young. They can be categorized into three groups: the elderly, nonelderly adults, and children. The elderly, being at greatest risk of functional disability, form the majority of the users of long-term care. Nonelderly adults needing this type of care are those with long-term disabilities resulting from (a) accidents such as spinal-cord injury, (b) heart attacks and strokes, (c) multiple sclerosis, (d) cerebral palsy, (e) developmental disabilities, and (f) chronic mental illness.

affect dis

215

Disability for nonelderly adults is generally defined in terms of their ability to perform income-producing work. Most children requiring long-term care are those with developmental disabilities.

It is difficult to determine precise numbers of those who need long-term care; different sources of data use different definitions of functional disability and employ different data collection methodologies. Here, we mention the rising number of older adults in the United States, most of whom live in noninstitutional settings. Depending on the number of functional disabilities they experience, however, the number of those needing community-based long-term care varies. According to the AARP Public Policy Institute (Houser, Fox-Grage, & Gibson, 2006), 40% of older adults in 2005 had a disability. Currently, 4 out of 5 adults over age 50 (or 70 million individuals) have been diagnosed with at least one chronic condition. In 2005, about 10 million Americans received long-term care (Komisar & Thompson, 2007), which cost almost $207 billion (Burman & Johnson, 2007).

The settings for long-term care are numerous and varied: (1) institutions such as nursing homes; (2) "quasi-institutions" such as boarding homes and various other kinds of living arrangements, including foster homes, shared housing, and Elder Cottage Housing Opportunity units; (3) community-based ambulatory program sites; and (4) the care recipients' own apartments in retirement villages and life-care communities, as well as their own homes within the regular community. It is unclear what the "institutional" long-term care settings are and how they differ from one another. The following statement from Brody (1977), made almost 35 years ago, is still true:

Distinctions are blurred, and different institutional names mean different things to different people in different places at different times. A few of the names used in referring to institutions that provide long-term care are homes for aged, homes or hospitals for chronically ill, nursing homes, geriatric centers, rehabilitation hospitals, county homes, veterans' homes, and psychiatric hospitals. (p. 29)

On the other extreme, ambulatory sites for long-term care include physicians' offices; outpatient clinics; comprehensive assessment clinics—both pediatric and geriatric; day-care centers for adults and children with disabilities; day hospitals; mental health clinics; alcohol and substance abuse rehabilitation centers; and senior centers providing wellness, informational, educational, recreational, and social group programs, transportation, and congregate meals. In-home care may include home health; homemaker and personal care services; high-technology home therapy (e.g., kidney dialysis, respiratory care, tube feeding); use of durable medical equipment; hospice, home visiting, and telephone contact services; respite and attendant services; and home-delivered meals. A set of financial programs such as home equity conversion, reverse annuity mortgage, and sale/lease-back programs make more cash available to elderly homeowners and thereby allow them to continue living in their communities.

As is evident from the above discussion, long-term care includes health and social services. Experts do not agree about the boundaries between this type of care and many other service sectors, such as primary health care, mental health, and adult social services (Kane, 1987). This type of care, however, differs from acute care in that it involves such "life choices" as where to live and how to live (Merrill, 1992). As stated above, other than one's own home, living arrangements may include retirement communities, senior housing, congregate care facilities, and adult family homes.

We have included in this chapter a discussion of hospice care even though only a few of the ideas about and attributes of long-term care presented above apply to it. Like other forms of long-term care, hospice care is not concerned with curing disease or preventing mortality. It is aimed at making the last stage of a person's life pain-free and peaceful. Whereas the need for other forms of care cannot be predicted by the presence or absence of a particular disease, the presence of a terminal illness creates the need for hospice care. Whereas other forms of care are aimed at improving the care recipient's functional ability, the aim of hospice care is to deal with the needs of a person beyond the relevance of functionality. Like the recipients of other forms of care, those receiving hospice care are both old and young, but the old dominate the scene. Unlike the lack of clarity about who needs the different kinds of long-term care and the settings where that care can be best provided, there is a consensus about who needs hospice care and the venues for its provision.

HISTORY OF SOCIAL WORK IN LONG-TERM CARE SETTINGS

As pointed out earlier, long-term care is provided in many settings—institutions, quasi-institutions, outpatient centers, and clients' own homes. The history of social work involvement in long-term care is different in different settings. Because we have focused on the care provided through nursing homes, community residential care settings, and home-based/near home-based programs, we look at the history of social work in these separately. Because of the special nature of hospice care, a separate section is devoted to social work in that area.

Social Work in Nursing Homes

The history of social work in nursing homes is not long. Social workers, like other health care professionals, were rarely involved in nursing homes prior to 1965. The Social Security Act amendments of 1965 led to many changes. The law required hospitals to enter into transfer agreements with extended care facilities, and the provision of social services was included as a requirement for certification for an extended care facility (Clark, 1971). Nevertheless, nursing homes continued to be on the periphery of the medical establishment. Not only did the health care provided to nursing home residents remain of questionable quality, but the psychosocial needs of those residents also continued to be given minimal attention. Legal requirements were met in many ways. Some nursing homes valued social work education and employed social workers with appropriate professional degrees;

others hired a "social work designee," someone often without any social work training and experience. These nursing homes contracted with a professionally trained social work consultant to guide the social work designee in attending to the psychosocial needs of residents. Many nonprofit sectarian nursing homes employed qualified social workers, even those with master's degrees, whereas many private for-profit nursing homes tried to do without them (Greene, 1982). This situation continues. The federal government requires all nursing homes with more than 120 beds to employ a full-time qualified social worker who may or may not have a degree in social work [1]. The federal regulations do not clarify if facilities with 120 or fewer beds need to hire a social worker but can do so on a part-time basis. This is important because 70% of the nursing homes in the country have fewer than 100 beds. States have the option of extending or strengthening the federal regulations. State requirements for qualifications of nursing home social workers greatly vary (Bern-Klug, 2008).

Social work roles and functions in nursing homes have varied vastly. At the one extreme, nursing home social workers may deal mainly with admission-related financial arrangements and coordination of services, organization of recreational activities for residents, and attendance to a resident's obvious social needs. At the other extreme, social workers' professional skills may significantly affect most dimensions of the nursing home's functioning. They may provide services to (a) residents, (b) families of residents, (c) nursing home staff, (d) nursing home policymakers, and (e) the community in relationship to the nursing home. In the nursing home industry as a whole, social workers in the latter group have been more an exception than the rule. In their study of skilled nursing facilities, Pearman and Searles (1978) identified the above five areas of unmet social service needs. As a conceptual road map for exploring the social work territory in the nursing home world, their findings have as much relevance today as they did 30 years ago. Since then, the psychosocial needs of nursing home residents have been reviewed as part of the quality-of-life issue.

Nursing home reform legislation (Omnibus Budget Reconciliation Act of 1987 [P.L. 100-203]) made the goal of enhancing the quality of life of nursing home residents a part of the national policy. Regulations under that law, implemented in October 1990, require all nursing homes to identify the medically related social and emotional needs of their residents and assist them in the adjustment to the social and emotional aspects of their illness, treatment, and stay in the facility. Every nursing home of more than 120 beds is also required to provide social work services. Variance in the degree and nature of social work as practiced in nursing homes, however, persists. Simons, Shepherd, and Munn (2008) reviewed the research-based literature on social work in long-term care settings, including nursing homes, and found evidence of social work's contribution to meeting the needs of nursing home residents. The studies they mentioned include (1) Malench (2004), which found that nursing homes employing qualified social workers are more likely to provide family support groups; (2) Osman and Becker (2003), which discovered positive influence of social workers in the implementation of advanced directives; and (3) Newcomer, Kang, and Graham (2006), which found that residents in the intervention group (receiving social work case management) had a higher rate of discharge and shorter median length of stay than the usual care group.

Social Work in Community Residential Care Settings

Most information about the involvement of social work in community residential care settings comes from the Department of Veterans Affairs' residential care programs; community residential arrangements for deinstitutionalized persons with mental illness, mental retardation, and developmental disability; models of care designed to keep older adults out of nursing homes in the state of Oregon; and foster care for children who cannot live with their natural families. Community residential care serves persons who

are less impaired than those in nursing homes and more impaired than those who are still living in their homes. It gives residents more privacy and autonomy than is available in nursing homes and is economically more efficient than providing services in individual homes (Lehning & Austin, 2010). However, there is not much in research-based literature on the evaluation of community residential care, partly because of the lack of uniformity in the definitions of this type of care (Wilson, 2007). Social workers have played many roles and performed many functions in these programs. On the one hand, they have identified, trained, supervised, and monitored foster care providers. On the other hand, they have created, organized, and supervised foster care and other living arrangements. They are also involved in the working of group homes, sheltered residential facilities, and life-care communities in different capacities.

Social Work in Home-Based/ Near Home-Based Care

Given the complexity of home-based/near home-based care, it is difficult to talk definitively about the extent of social work involvement. It has varied considerably. In some settings and programs, social workers have occupied center stage; in others, they have been on the periphery; and in still others, they have been hardly visible. In social service programs for the elderly, social workers have functioned as program planners and organizers; case workers and case managers; and supervisors and pacesetters for paraprofessional and volunteer service providers. In health clinics and mental health centers, they have functioned as psychosocial therapists and service coordinators. In agencies serving people with disabilities, they have provided such services as psychosocial assessment and intervention; case management and coordination; environmental manipulation; and protection from physical abuse, neglect, and financial exploitation. They have helped families of people with disabilities deal with the physical, emotional, and social stress of caring. They have worked with multidisciplinary teams serving people with disabilities and the community at large on their behalf.

Social workers have played these varied professional roles despite the constraints on social work activities imposed by reimbursement rules of various funding sources. In home health care agencies, the social work role has been secondary. Although Medicare conditions for home health agencies mandate that social services be made available to patients, they do not require that a social worker see these patients or be involved in the planning for their care. A nurse usually determines the need for social work intervention. Medicaid-funded programs are even less clear about the role of social workers. There is no uniform requirement that social work services be available to patients, and even when needed, payment for these services is not reimbursed by the program (Cox, 1992). The review of research-based literature by Simons et al. (2008) found several studies of social work in home health care, primary care, and modality-specific programs such as community-based case management programs. Some of these explored the impact of the setting and payment systems on social work practice, and others focused on the efficacy of social work.

Social Work in Hospice Care

Hospice care for the terminally ill and their families is a recent development. It represents an approach to caring based on a philosophy that emphasizes quality of life of the dying patient. The core belief is that the terminally ill should die pain-free and with dignity and that their families should be supported to ensure that happens. Dame Cicely Saunders started the hospice movement in England in 1967, when hospice care was first provided in the inpatient setting of St. Christopher's Hospice in London. The movement brought about a change in the way we think about dying (Brooks, 2010). Saunders had a rich and varied professional background. She had been trained as a nurse, physician, and social

worker (Raymer & Reese, 2008). Hospice is a form of palliative care, which is defined by the World Health Organization (2011) as

> an approach that improves the quality of life of patients and their families facing the problems associated with life-threatening illness, through the prevention and relief of suffering by means of early identification and assessment and treatment of pain and other problems, physical, psychosocial, and spiritual.

However, there are differences between hospice and palliative care [2]. Hospice is a philosophy of care more than a place of care or a subset of service (Beder, 2006). As the movement spread to other parts of the world, the local conditions and needs influenced the actual delivery of services. The first American hospice was started in Branford, Connecticut, in 1974, and others that followed developed a character of their own. They grew as grassroots community movements against such faults of the American health care system as its focus on technology and cures, and its tendency to view many terminally ill individuals as "failures" and subsequently "abandon" them because nothing more could be done (Raymer & Reese, 2008). Hospice focused on aggressive palliative care provided in a patient's own home. In 2009, there were about 5,000 hospice programs in the country, and an estimated 1.56 million terminally ill patients (and their families) received hospice care (National Hospice and Palliative Care Organization [NHPCO], 2010).

Hospice embodies (1) social work values of self-determination, dignity and empowerment of patients, service, and social justice, and (2) social work focus on patient and family as a unit of service, interdisciplinary care, and comprehensive services that deal with all dimensions of life. Social workers have been a part of the hospice scene from the beginning. They play several professional roles—most as social work clinicians, some also as bereavement counselors and coordinators of volunteer services, and a few as administrators.

In all sectors of long-term care, social workers currently play many professional roles and perform important functions. Some roles and functions are likely to persist although they may have to be reemphasized and asserted. Others will have to be assumed in view of the changing situation and needs of long-term care facilities.

FUTURE SOCIAL WORK ROLES IN LONG-TERM CARE SETTINGS

Chapter 3 identified the major needs of the long-term care sector as (a) *nursing homes* improving their public image, becoming a part of an integrated continuum of services, and extending themselves into the community; (b) *community residential care settings* increasing their visibility, increasing their resources, and improving their service performance; (c) *home-based/near home-based program agencies* improving the overall quality of their care (so their services are appropriate, comprehensive, well-coordinated, and sensitive to the unique situations of their clients); and (d) *hospice organizations* reducing barriers to the utilization of their services by minority patients and their families, and improving their access to people living in rural areas. Table 7-A below lists the social work roles geared to meeting these needs. A discussion of these roles follows the table.

Social Work Roles in Nursing Homes

It is likely that as more and more educated, assertive, and hitherto politically active elderly enter nursing homes, emphasis on quality of life will increase. These elderly will demand improvements in services. Hubbard, Werner, Cohen-Mansfield, and Shusterman (1992) described the development of "seniors for justice," a political and social action group of nursing home residents in the greater Washington, D.C. area, and how this not only gave a group of cognitively intact nursing home residents a sense of empowerment and enhanced self-esteem but also resulted in many other positive changes. In the future, nursing homes will realize the importance of social work skills for dealing with the psychosocial needs of their residents, as well as for intervening at the system level for positive changes. Social workers' involvement with the community on behalf of their nursing home will be like icing on the cake. That involvement will enable them to use their professional skills for, on the one hand, more comprehensive and meaningful work with and on behalf of their clients and, on the other hand, a more effective integration of the nursing home with community health and human services. Such integration would enhance the public image of the nursing

---

Table 7-A   Future Social Work Roles in Long-Term Care Settings

- Social worker as a helper with adjustment to the nursing home
- Social worker as a sustainer of resident-family relationships
- Social worker as a contributor to the nursing home as a therapeutic community
- Social worker as a community liaison and community organizer
- Social worker as a recruiter of community residential care providers
- Social worker as a trainer of community residential care providers
- Social worker as a provider of support and monitor of quality of care
- Social worker as a contributor to the agency's continuous quality improvement
- Social worker as a case manager and service coordinator
- Social worker as a contributor to improving hospice access to people living in rural areas
- Social worker as a helper in reducing barriers to hospice services for minority patients

home. Hence, social workers will play many roles vital to nursing homes in the future.

Social Work Role in Helping Residents Adjust to the Nursing Home Environment

Even now, most nursing home social workers view helping residents adjust to the nursing home as one of their most important roles, although the time devoted to it is inadequate for the residents' psychosocial needs and the workers' professional satisfaction. They know that the decision about placement and the actual entry into a nursing home are difficult experiences for most people. Feelings of loss with the potential for depression, helplessness, and hopelessness are common (Solomon, 1983).

Vourlekis, Gelfand, and Greene (1992) compared the views of nursing home social workers and administrators on (a) psychosocial needs of residents and families and (b) functions performed and expected to be performed by the social worker. Both groups agreed on three of the five top-ranked needs. These three needs were for support/help with (a) transition to the home, (b) feelings of loss throughout the stay in the home, and (c) relatedness and intimacy issues. This finding may reflect the beginning of convergence of different opinions on the appropriate roles and functions of nursing home social workers. In the future, adjustment to the nursing home environment will have many more implications, with more end points of placement than is currently the case. Nursing home residents move back and forth between nursing homes and acute care hospitals until they die either in the nursing home or at the hospital. In the future, they will have many more options.

Social Work Role in Improving Residents' Relationships With Their Families

The warmth and meaningfulness of human relationships are among the ingredients of quality of life. As the enhancement of residents' quality of life becomes an important goal of nursing homes, social workers will assume this role with the aim of increasing meaningful involvement of families in the lives of nursing home residents. Families do not necessarily abandon members who are old and disabled when they can no longer care for them at home. The decision regarding the placement of a family member in a nursing home is often as painful for the family as it is for that member. Even if nursing home placement is not abandonment by the family, feelings of abandonment are part of the reality of institutionalization. Beyond the initial crisis of placement, families need help staying involved in the lives of their institutionalized family members. Families in the future will become increasingly more diverse structurally and weaker in their emotional and social resources. Consequently, they will need more assistance, encouragement, and professional direction in sustaining mutually fulfilling relationships with their loved ones in nursing homes.

Social Work Role in Making the Nursing Home a Therapeutic Community

For maximum impact of the social work presence in nursing homes, social workers should go beyond work with individual residents and their families and contribute to the conversion of the nursing home into what Jones (1953) called a therapeutic community. Social workers are generally involved in dealing with "difficult" residents and families, admissions and discharges, and institutional "crises," and are able to use their professional skills effectively in the resolution of these problems. They can easily add another dimension to that role and make significant contributions to the organizational health of nursing homes and the quality of their services so that these homes do not breed difficult residents and problem situations. This contribution requires addressing three sets of variables: (a) the organizational policies, procedures, and routines; (b) staff attitudes, opinions, relations, and perceptions of organizational climate; and (c) meaningful involvement of residents and their families.

Social Work Role in Improving the Nursing Home–Community Relationship

For nursing homes to become important elements in the coordinated and comprehensive continuity of health care in the future and also to improve their public image, they must do some creative and proactive reaching-out work in the community. No other nursing home professional is as well acquainted with the community's health and human services network and as used to coordinating services as the social worker. Besides knowledge of the community's formal and informal resources and of case management skills, he or she also possesses basic community organizational know-how. With little extra imagination and creativity, nursing home social workers can take on this role and make significant contributions to the field of long-term care, as well as to the viability and healthier public image of their institutions.

Social Work Roles in Community Residential Care Settings

In view of our earlier discussion of the needs of community residential care settings, the following social work roles will attain prominence in the future.

Social Work Role in Recruiting Community Residential Care Providers

The search for noninstitutional approaches to the needs of people requiring long-term care will continue and likely will become more essential as families are less able emotionally and financially to care for their aged members with disabilities. Identification, recruitment, and retention of individuals and families willing to provide this type of care will become an important social work function. With the advantage of their experience in the fields of child welfare and mental health, social workers will be able to take on this role with creativity.

Social Work Role in Training Community Residential Care Providers

Appropriate training, supervision, and support of those caring for children; adults with emotional, mental, and physical disabilities; and the elderly are necessary for the success of community residential care programs. Most care providers have the desire to serve their fellow human beings and the ability to relate to them warmly, but they often lack an understanding of (a) needs and problems, general as well as specific, of those under their care; (b) appropriate responses to those needs and problems; (c) community resources relevant to those needs and problems; and (d) approaches to accessing those resources.

Social Work Role in Supporting and Monitoring Community Residential Care

The technical knowledge and know-how of community residential care is important for effective service, but care providers also need appreciation, encouragement, and support from their sponsors, organizers, and employers. Very often, those they serve cannot show their appreciation for the services provided. This is particularly essential in view of the fact that society generally tends to value and reward the least those who perform the most difficult and unpleasant tasks. Social workers will be able to fill that important gap.

Social Work Roles in Home-Based/ Near Home-Based Care

Social workers will have opportunities to demonstrate their unique skills in response to the needs of the in-home and near-home health care organizations identified earlier. No other professionals are more suited by their training, philosophy, and experience to make significant contributions to the quality-of-care efforts or to deal with such problems as the (a) lack of a holistic view of human problems, (b) inability to devise comprehensive approaches to those problems, and (c) difficulty in providing coordinated services. The following are some ways that social workers can serve these organizations.

Social Work Role in the Organization's Continuous Quality Improvement

The total quality management (TQM) philosophy demands total organizational commitment to continuous improvement in quality of care; an organizational culture that encourages participation by all who use the organization's services; and ongoing feedback from patients, families, and health care practitioners. This patient-inclusive approach, when compared with traditional provider-centered approaches, is one of the greatest challenges presented by the Joint Commission on Accreditation of Health Care Organizations' Agenda for Change (Lehr & Strosberg, 1991). The challenge becomes awesome when one considers the nature and structure of in-home care (which make monitoring of quality difficult); the lack of regional, state, or national norms for such care; and the problems encountered in in-home care agencies. These problems include unprofessional conduct on the part of service providers, which takes the form of disregard for dignity, autonomy, and independence of the client; tardiness and absenteeism; inappropriate service and inadequate records; drug and alcohol abuse; and theft and fraud. Social workers will be able to contribute positively to the efforts for quality improvement.

Social Work Role in Case Management and Service Coordination

In the future, the recipients of health and human services will be more educated and avid consumers of health care information, aware of their rights, and vocal in their demands. They will not tolerate services that are not appropriate, adequate, comprehensive, and culturally sensitive and proper. That stance will increase the importance of case management and service coordination. Their professional philosophy and training give social workers a holistic view of human problems and comprehensive approaches to those problems. They will have opportunities to demonstrate their superior abilities to perform this role.

Social Work Roles in Hospice Care

A national survey of 66 hospices by Reese and Raymer (2004) found that increased social work involvement in hospice care was significantly associated with lower costs; better team functioning; more patient and family issues being addressed; reduced levels of pain, medication, and other costs; fewer visits by other team members; and enhanced client satisfaction. This indicates that at the micro level of intervention, social workers are doing impressive work. They have the necessary knowledge and skills to do equally well at the mezzo and macro levels. The needs of hospice organizations that we have identified require social work intervention at those higher levels. The pertinent social work roles will include (1) *improving hospice access to people living in rural areas* and (2) *reducing barriers to the utilization of hospice services by minority patients.*

SOCIAL WORK KNOWLEDGE AND SKILLS

Before we discuss the knowledge and skills needed for social work practice in long-term care in relation to the identified roles, we make a few general observations and list general principles proposed by the Institute of Medicine (2001) that should guide efforts to improve the quality of long-term care.

Earlier, we referred to the person in environment as the unique social work perspective and to systems theory as providing a useful model for conceptualizing this perspective. Similarly, the concepts of "enabling" and "empowerment" are operationalized as important elements of social work practice. These are useful for practice in long-term care settings as well. The helping world is discovering the validity of the social work perspective and practice principles. A comprehensive perspective on the client's reality, encompassing the person and the environment as well as a life span view, is becoming popular. Other professionals are adopting the social work client-worker relationship, marked by equality, as the principle of equal partnership between clients and helpers.

Because the major recipients of long-term care services are the elderly and the disabled, social workers should understand the laws—federal, state, and local—that reflect the various policies and service programs for these populations. They should judge these policies and programs by the underlying value that people have a right to services designed to maximize their capacities to meet basic human needs (Brody, 1977). Maslow's conceptualization of human needs can be used to determine, for example, the extent of a nursing home's work toward the improvement of its residents' quality of life in compliance with the Omnibus Budget Reconciliation Act of 1987 (Umoren, 1992).

Social workers should recognize that despite the fundamental rights that the elderly and the disabled have as citizens and the government policies addressing their special needs, society tends to view and treat these people as less than equal. Often, society's negative view of the aged and the disabled is accepted and believed by the aged and the disabled themselves. They need to be treated as populations at risk.

Within the overall needs resulting from their old age or disability, there are tremendous variations among individuals. Old age or disability does not affect all individuals and their families in a standard way. Numerous variables in myriad ways result in peculiar reactions, situations, and needs of these people. Social workers should be sensitive to the universal as well as the unique elements of their realities and build those into plans for intervention, whether in the form of case-level therapeutic work or class-level advocacy.

Although disability affects an individual in many ways, it does not define his or her total being. Social workers should consciously desist from making or accepting such assumptions as the following: (a) Disability is located solely in the biology of persons with disabilities; (b) when a person with a disability faces problems, the impairment causes the problems; (c) the person with a disability is a "victim"; (d) disability is central to the self-concept, self-definition, social comparisons, and reference group of the person with the disability; and (e) having a disability is synonymous with needing help and social support (Fine & Asch, 1988).

Social workers should also be in tune with major developments and philosophical shifts in the fields of chronic physical disabilities, chronic mental illness, and developmental disabilities. Overall, movement has been away from the traditional psychotherapeutic models in favor of educational models (Hirschwald, 1984).

The professional development work in the areas of palliative and hospice care is quite impressive. Not only has the NHPCO (2005) produced the Hospice Standards of Practice, but the National Association of Social Workers (NASW, 2004) also has created the NASW Standards for Social Work Practice in Palliative and End-of-Life Care. Several journals publish material of educational value for social workers. These include *American Journal of Hospice and Palliative Medicine*, *Hospice*, and *Journal of Social Work in End-of-Life and Palliative Care*. Other social work journals such as *Health and Social Work*, *Social Work in Health Care*, and *Journal of Gerontological Social Work* are also sources of new ideas and information. *Living with Dying: A Handbook for End-of-Life Health Care Practitioners* (Berzoff & Silverman, 2004) is an impressive addition to the field. Social workers have the basic knowledge and skills for direct practice, interdisciplinary and multidisciplinary teamwork, organizational work, and community-level interventions. They can refine their professional abilities to take on the roles we identified earlier to meet the current and future needs of hospices.

The following are the general principles recommended by the Institute of Medicine (2001):

1. Long-term care should be consumer centered rather than solely provider centered.

2. A system of consumer-centered long-term care should be structured to serve people with diverse characteristics and preferences.

3. Reliable and current information about the options available and the quality of care provided should be easily accessible to allow people to make informed choices about long-term care.

4. Access to appropriate long-term care services is both a quality-of-care and a quality-of-life issue.

5. Measures of the quality of long-term care should incorporate its many dimensions, especially quality of life.

6. Providers should be held accountable for their performance in providing high-quality long-term care, including the outcomes of care they could affect.

7. A motivated, capable, and sufficient workforce is critical to quality long-term care.

8. Improving the quality of long-term care requires sustained government commitment to develop and implement fair, effective regulatory and financing policies.

9. Improving quality of care must be an ongoing objective. Building the capacity for high-quality long-term care depends on improved knowledge of the practices and policies that contribute to the well-being of people using that care. (pp. 31–33)

Social Worker as Helper With Adjustment to the Nursing Home

The nursing home reform law (P.L. 100-203) requires, among other things, that nursing homes assist their residents in adjusting to the social and emotional aspects of their illness, treatment, and stay in the facility. Because improving their public image is the major need of nursing homes, meeting the needs of residents and acquiring a reputation for that will simultaneously benefit both clients and the institutions. Social work skills are superbly appropriate for both purposes. Here are a few suggestions for social work with new residents adjusting to the nursing home environment:

1. *Anticipate the possibility that the cognitively intact elder or person with a disability entering the nursing home has a negative image of the place as a setting for long-term care.* Whether the resident comes from a hospital or from home, the decision about placement in a nursing home is always painful. He or she may also experience a sense of being abandoned by the family. The decision to enter can trigger feelings of loss, which without intervention often result in depression with concomitants of helplessness and hopelessness. This can happen so easily because the decision to enter is an acknowledgment to self and others of diminished capacity to care for oneself (Solomon, 1983, pp. 86–87).

2. *View this as a stressful event for the individual and plan on reducing the stress.* Because most nursing home social workers are involved in preadmission planning, it will be comparatively easy to build some stress-reduction elements into the preadmission and postadmission protocol. These elements can include a preadmission visit to the family member with a twofold purpose: (a) giving information about the institution, answering questions, giving the person a good feel for the institution in terms of both its pluses and minuses, and suggesting ways of preparing the individual for the move, and (b) obtaining information about the individual and his or her modes of functioning.

3. *Use the information about the person to develop creative ways of making the institutional environment congruent with his or her previous modes of functioning* (Solomon, 1983). Use crisis intervention skills in dealing with the person's transition to the nursing home. Make sure that attention is given to such issues as privacy, possessions, display of family pictures, and decorations in the room. This will give the individual a sense of control. A general demonstration of warmth, interest, and concern on the part of the staff will convey the message that he or she is welcome and is among caring and concerned people. These simple and inexpensive gestures will yield positive results in assisting the person's adjustment.

4. *Stimulate or support aggressive mobilization of psychological resources so that the person does not withdraw and fall prey to depression.* The mastery of adjustment is dependent on the person's ability to mobilize his or her aggressive feelings and to remain active (Solomon, 1983). The "how" of this stimulation will depend on an assessment of the individual's personality, style, and resources. Therefore, do a thorough psychosocial assessment.

5. *Encourage family and friends to visit often and spend more time with the newly placed individual, at least during the first few days and weeks.* The importance of these visits is reflected in a quote from a nursing home resident who asked a friend to visit often "so I will know I am alive" (Williams, cited in Kane, 2001). Explore family conflict, guilt, feelings of abandonment, and other effects of placement on the family; help them deal with these; and encourage open communication between them and the resident. The aim of this extra effort is to remove psychological hurdles from the path of the institutionalized member's adjustment, to sustain the family's positive involvement in that member's life, and to win allies in the nursing home's efforts to improve its public image.

6. *Encourage the resident to join group activities.* It is likely that the nursing home already has some organized group work going on. If not, be instrumental in starting groups that can benefit residents. The therapeutic effects of group experiences are being increasingly realized, and group approaches will become even more popular in the future. Groups are believed to be particularly suitable for work with the elderly because of the advantages of economy, socialization, and emotional validation. Nursing homes can be appropriate settings for innovations in group modalities of social work intervention. Dhooper, Green, Huff, and Austin-Murphy (1993) tested the efficacy of an eclectic group approach to reducing depression in elderly nursing home residents and found the approach effective. Other models have been tried with different groups of nursing home residents. For example, Hyer and associates (1990) applied a cognitive behavioral model to two groups of older people with stress-related problems: recent (adjustment reaction or grief) and remote (posttraumatic stress disorder). Capuzzi, Gross, and Friel (1990) discussed five types of groups: (a) reality orientation, (b) remotivation therapy, (c) reminiscing, (d) psychotherapy, and (e) topic-specific and support groups. Group approaches are being tried even with those who are cognitively impaired, the goal being reminiscence, reorientation, and rehabilitation (Salamon, 1986). The gerontological literature is growing richer in ideas and suggestions for effective group work (e.g., see Abramson & Mendis, 1990; Chung, 2005; Fernie & Fernie, 1990; Greenberg, Motenko, Roesch, & Embleton, 2000; Ng & Chan, 2008; Stones, Rattenbury, Taichman, Kozma, & Stones, 1990).

Here, we reiterate the age-old social work practice principles. Social work activity guided by these principles will effectively help a resident deal with the transition and adjustment to the nursing home environment:

- *Be honest and open* with the client; people respond to authenticity and genuineness.
- *Start where the client is;* begin with the client's definition of the problem.
- *Maximize the client's choices and options;* there is always room for reducing the "institutional effects" of nursing homes—increasing the degree of privacy, independence, and convenience, and decreasing the rigidity of schedules and controls and the extent of isolation from the outside world.

Social Worker as Sustainer of Resident-Family Relationships

Although the family in the future will change in its structure and resources, its meaningfulness for its members will not diminish. Variations based on ethnic, racial, and regional differences will occur in that meaning, however. For most elderly, the family will continue to be a crucial reference point. We have discussed admission into a nursing home as a stressful event for the person concerned. It is also a serious and painful crisis for the family (Dobrof & Litwak, 1977). Even when care for the person at home is stressful and draining emotionally, physically, financially, and socially (Dhooper, 1991), many familial caregivers continue to experience considerable emotional stress and subjective burden after the loved one's institutional placement (Colerick & George, 1986; Pratt, Schmall, Wright, & Hare, 1987; Townsend, 1990; Zarit & Zarit, 1982). Families need help dealing with the emotional and other consequences of placement of a loved one and sustaining mutually fulfilling relationship with him or her. Social workers may benefit from the following suggestions:

1. *Keep abreast of the emerging literature on family involvement in long-term care settings.* A book edited by Gaugler (2005) presented and discussed several programs for and approaches to family involvement, including the Family Visit Education Program, Family Involvement in Care, Partners in Caregiving, The Eden Alternative, Family Councils, participation of certified nursing assistants in family involvement, support group intervention for family members, story sharing between families and staff, and web-based interventions.

2. *Keep in mind that, in general, the visibility and concern of the family have a positive effect not only on the mental health of the institutionalized person but also on the quality of care he or she receives.*

3. *Be instrumental in establishing and supporting institutional practices/facilities that encourage family visits.* These may include open visiting hours, coffee shops and lounges for family members to spend time with the resident, encouragement for bringing special food treats, and many open channels of communication between nursing home staff and families (Solomon, 1983).

4. *View the person's admission as a crisis for his or her family.* Explore the crisis and provide

necessary assistance. "The developmental task which accompanies the crisis of admission is that of maintaining close family ties while feeling angry, hurt, afraid of rejection and abandonment, and most of all feeling deeply sorrowful" (Solomon, 1983, p. 90). Depending on a host of factors, the nature and extent of the crisis for each family varies. For families with a history of severe relationship problems, maintaining closeness may be complex and challenging. Such families are becoming more the rule than an exception, partly because people are living longer and have more time for experiences that are sources of conflict and alienation.

> In some cases, they [schisms] are about property disputes, with the elderly believing they have been financially mistreated in some business arrangement with their children or grandchildren. In other cases, the conflicts may result from disapproval either by the parents or their children of the other's marriages, divorces, child-rearing practices, career pursuits, smoking, alcohol and other substance abuse, religious choices—the lists are endless. (Harbert & Ginsberg, 1990, p. 136)

In general, family members may feel an element of guilt, whereas the reactions of the person being placed may reflect anger, rejection, and separation.

5. *While assessing the family's situation, reactions, coping style, and resources for adjustment, look for their potential and capacity for sustaining ongoing family relationships* (Greene, 1982). At the same time, acknowledge and validate the enormity of the task before them. Provide and/or procure for family members the needed help from within the nursing home or from outside in the community. The help the social worker can provide may include brief casework, education and consultation, mediation between family members and the resident, and an offer of membership in an ongoing family-support group, if available.

Families of patients with dementing illnesses such as Alzheimer's disease have special problems of transition when the patient must be placed in a nursing home. Most families have cared for their member at home for 5 to 7 years after the diagnosis (Cheek, 1987) and have experienced and adjusted to numerous burdens caused by the member's progressively worsening condition. Morgan and Zimmerman (1990) identified factors that made the transition from in-home care to institutional care less stressful for spousal caregivers. They clustered these factors into five categories: (a) emotional support, (b) control of situation, (c) acceptability of nursing home, (d) acceptance of situation, and (e) permission/command by an authority figure. Transform ideas from such findings into the strategies for intervention with these families.

6. *Encourage the family to reminisce together.* Since Butler (1963) first described the therapeutic value of reminiscing, life review therapy has been found to be a viable approach to helping the elderly maintain self-esteem, reaffirm a sense of identity, and work through personal losses. Family reminiscing can also be a powerful method of bringing families together. As Solomon (1983) put it,

> The elderly relative is given the opportunity to be valued in her entirety with strengths as well as weaknesses and dependencies. Younger people are given the chance to learn from the struggles of the past and to preserve those struggles. And for the family, reminiscence becomes the family legacy; it can ensure family continuity; it is the preservation of the past, which ensures the future. (p. 94)

Reminiscence is particularly helpful if family members seem not to know what to talk about during their visits.

7. *Take on the responsibility of coordinating activities for all the staff and helping them incorporate family involvement into the resident's care.* This involvement will add another meaningful dimension to the family's visits. This can be done through regular participation in patient care conferences and sharing the family's needs and concerns, interpreting the behavior of the family and resident, and suggesting ways of involving the family in the resident's life (Dobrof & Litwak, 1977; Greene, 1982).

8. *Attend to the special needs of families whose members are becoming disoriented and confused.* Such families may find it increasingly more difficult to maintain their interest in visiting. They can be taught basic reality orientation techniques. Families thus trained can make their visits with the resident meaningful and also supplement the nursing home staff's efforts to keep the patient alert and oriented. Explore and assist in this form of family involvement.

Family members whose relatives are severely disoriented need help. If they come to visit, they experience emotional frustration, pain, and upset, and if they do not come to visit, they feel guilty. On the one hand, they need to know that their visits are important and to hear that keeping their visits short or less frequent is OK. On the other hand, family members visiting a demanding, talkative relative can use help setting limits without feeling guilty (Greene, 1982).

Social Worker as Contributor to the Nursing Home as a Therapeutic Community

Helping the nursing home provide a therapeutic environment essential for the optimal quality of life and independent functioning of the residents is one of the social work responsibilities under NASW standards. This can be done through a multipronged approach that includes (a) advocating on behalf of all residents, with the aim of easing stringent organizational routines, policies, and procedures; (b) advocating for and helping residents create and maintain a mechanism for their active involvement in the working of the institution, with the aim of ensuring that their voices influence the organizational policies and practices; and (c) educating staff and administrators, with the following goals:

1. Sensitizing them to the importance of the residents' cultures for their well-being, with the aim of incorporating aspects of their culture into care

2. Making them aware of the rights of residents and their social and emotional needs, with the aim of individualizing planned programs for residents

3. Training them, with the aim of improving their (a) attitudes toward residents, (b) knowledge of the needs of residents, (c) understanding of roles of all involved in caregiving, (d) cooperation and communication, and (e) integration of care of residents (Pearman & Searles, 1978).

The following suggestions are likely to be helpful for social workers in operationalizing the above approach:

1. *Consider themselves the best suited for this role of contributor to the nursing home as a therapeutic community because of the social work belief system and training.* Social workers believe in individuals' right to self-determination and self-direction. They have learned how to clearly communicate that belief and to generate a desire to exercise that right. They have been trained to offer people choices, encourage decision making, and stimulate active participation in problem solving. Hence, they should take the responsibility of providing leadership in the facility's efforts to become a therapeutic community.

2. *Share with administrators the emerging literature on the benefits of changing the nursing home's milieu for the residents, staff, and institutional image in the community.* We mentioned culture change in nursing homes in Chapter 1, and Misiorski (2003) described the process of changing nursing home culture. Help administrators realize that residents who are involved in decisions about their care and caregiving policies and procedures reveal healthier and happier attitudes (Blair, 1994–1995). When residents are a part of the decisions concerning themselves, their autonomy and self-worth are upheld (Lindgren & Linton, 1991), and that has a positive effect on their motivation. That, in turn, makes the work of the staff worthwhile. It is satisfying to work with those who are actively involved in their care, are motivated to benefit from the service, appreciate the work being done, and are intent on drawing the best out of the service providers. The residents' participation in the running of the institution further benefits the staff because it leads to a more smoothly run facility (Grover, 1982). Similarly, the interest and energy of families can

be a tremendous resource if channeled into the care of their institutionalized members and the needs of the nursing home.

3. *Use advocacy skills to motivate or reinforce the support of administrators and staff in favor of changes.* Share with them the relevant principles and approaches, seek ideas and input, and neutralize resistance. The following are a few examples of helpful strategies:

- The hospice ideology has a special appeal for those who work with the dying, and nursing home staff also experience death often. The hospice approach is based on principles that include a *total needs emphasis, increased resident autonomy, a community ideology,* and a *multidisciplinary team orientation* that cuts across levels of staff hierarchy. These principles can be relevant for humanizing nursing home environments (Munley, Powers, & Williamson, 1982).
- The health promotion movement has generated principles and techniques that can be applied to the task of motivating and involving the nursing home residents in their care and the life of their "home." Health promotion emphasizes the residents' responsibilities and incorporates their abilities into the management of their disabilities. The social work concepts of "enabling" and "empowerment" have significant relevance for health promotion work.
- Resident councils or committees are a popular approach to encouraging the involvement of residents and the creation of a community spirit in a nursing home. Helpful information about how to form these councils and encourage reluctant residents is becoming available (e.g., see Blair, 1994–1995; Grover, 1982; Miller, 1986).
- Group work is used not only for therapeutic purposes with nursing home residents but also for converting nursing homes into therapeutic communities. Whereas therapeutics may be the main purpose of many groups such as activity, art therapy, exercise, humor, movement therapy, music therapy, poetry therapy, reality orientation, reminiscence, and psychodrama groups, these also enrich the lives of residents and thereby change the atmosphere of the place. Various types of discussion, governing, and activities groups can also be organized to create an integrated therapeutic milieu. Johnson, Agresti, Jacob, and Nies (1990) described the

history of group work in the nursing home unit of a Veterans Affairs medical center that culminated in an ongoing weekly video program. That program, over time, created *therapeutic persona*—characters that are "outrageous, funny, and ridiculous, yet which represent some unacknowledged common experience of the residents. These characters then serve as the basis for an ongoing series of video skits" (p. 209). These authors hold that "the collective awareness of these characters provides an endless source of jokes and kidding during the week and serves to support an environment of intimacy among staff and residents" (p. 216), and that contributes to the building of a therapeutic community.

- Adelman, Frey, and Budz (1994) described the process of creating and maintaining the community spirit in a residential facility for persons with AIDS. During the entry phase, the newcomer is assisted through several formal strategies, including a buddy system, an orientation packet, support group meetings, and postentry interviews. The full participation of residents is facilitated through such strategies as weekly house meetings, a three-member elected residents' council, private meetings between residents and the director of the facility, support group meetings, in-house seminars, cultural events, assigned house duties, and the availability of counselors for substance abuse problems and pastoral care. During the last phase, the resident is offered practical, psychological, and spiritual assistance in preparing for death, and others (residents and staff) go through elaborate community coping rituals.

4. *To encourage families as active members in the lives of residents, a multifold approach is effective.* We earlier discussed approaches to involving families in the planning and implementation of individual care programs, as well as those to help them sustain meaningful relationships with their institutionalized member. Family members can also function as volunteers, performing important chores within the nursing home or in the community on behalf of the nursing home. It is not uncommon for family members to offer assistance, for example, in such group activities as outings and trips for residents. Volunteers add an important element to the community spirit of the facility. Maximize communication between families and the nursing home. This should be done both formally and informally. One nursing home created a family information center in its main lobby (Conroy, 1994), where official communications, notices of upcoming events, health and welfare service announcements, and appeals for volunteers were displayed. Orientation and ongoing support groups serve several purposes. These enable family members to know the place, get acquainted with the staff, contribute to the care of their loved one, and understand how they can add to the quality of the place and its services. Devise arrangements whereby the contributions of families as volunteers are publicly recognized and appreciated.

Wildon (1994) discussed going beyond "home" and creating a hometown to generate a sense of community in the facility. Her nursing homes participate in July 4th festivities. Their efforts yield impressive results. "More than 20,000 fellow community service members take part in an old-fashioned Independence Day complete with car shows, kid games, local radio and television personalities and dignitaries, and fireworks—all on our campus" (p. 9). They also have an elaborate holiday gift-giving program and other Christmastime activities. Their presents-for-patients program matches residents without families with people in the community, who visit them at Christmastime and bring gifts ("Conference," 1994). These activities give nursing home residents and their families a touch of the holidays to which the whole community has contributed.

There are also other ways of involving the community and expanding the world of nursing home residents. Identify the community ties that existed before their admission and reestablish those ties.

> Many residents had group associations such as church or synagogue, veterans' organizations, Golden Age Clubs, fraternal orders, and charitable or service organizations. Identifying those links to the community can lead to invitations for them to visit or to arrange for the resident to attend their meetings. (Brody, 1977, p. 268)

Social Worker as Community Liaison and Community Organizer

The strategies of community work we discussed in Chapter 4 are equally applicable for helping nursing homes extend themselves into the community. Here, we focus on the social worker's role in helping the nursing home improve its image in the community. Starting with the assumption that a good image of an entity depends on its doing good, looking good, and letting the world know it is good, the social worker as a nursing home's liaison with the community can adopt a multipronged approach. The following are a few suggestions on the "what" and "how" of that approach:

1. *Help the nursing home in the provision of the best possible care that is resident centered, family involved, and community conscious.* We have already discussed some ways of incorporating into their care the wishes and preferences of residents and involvement of their families. Attending to the total needs of residents, understanding and accommodating the needs of families, and involving families meaningfully in the care of their loved one impresses the families, who carry their positive impression into the community.

2. *Mix and match the various strategies to make families believe that the nursing home cares about them and their need to maintain family integrity despite the placement of a member.* Mintz (1994) recommended assessing needs, establishing a "buddy system," starting a support group, establishing a caregiver resource center, inviting families to social events, suggesting a family council, encouraging family involvement with other residents/activities, designating family-staff liaisons, involving families in care planning, and making visiting easier. Build into the admission protocol a requirement for (a) asking every family about its greatest need and expectation for help, (b) processing that information, and (c) planning an appropriate intervention. The answers to most families' needs lie in already existing services or arrangements.

3. *Survey families of nursing home residents semiannually about their satisfaction with the nursing home services and their suggestions for improvement.* Sample survey forms are available from the American Health Care Association Quest for Quality program (Wood, 1994). Also, institute a program for regular follow-up of discharged residents to see how they are doing and whether they are getting the needed community-based services. This follow-up can be done through telephone calls by volunteers. Share the findings of these family surveys and follow-up contacts with care providers at all levels, seek their reactions and suggestions for improvement, and urge management to take the same seriously.

4. *Identify the unmet community needs for which the nursing home has the resources and initiate activities to meet those needs.* The identification of needs can be accomplished informally through ongoing contacts with human services professionals and organizations, contacts regarding the coordination of services for specific clients or problems and issues of interest to the local professional community, or through formal needs assessment. In Chapter 4, we discussed approaches to needs assessment. Several areas of need can be explored. The combined efforts of the American Association of Homes for the Aging and the Catholic Health Association of the United States produced a document, *Social Accountability Program: Continuing the Community Benefit Tradition of Not-for-Profit Homes and Services,* that suggests a number of activities for responding to community needs (Trocchio, 1993):

- *Services that can improve quality of life,* such as offering intergenerational recreation programs, providing respite care, becoming part of a communitywide recycling program, and encouraging residents to volunteer in community charitable projects
- *Services that can improve health status,* such as screening blood pressure and other health conditions and teaching sessions on health promotion and disease prevention at health fairs, providing immunization services, helping with meals-on-wheels programs, and making space available for various self-help and support groups

- *Services that can improve accessibility to needed services,* such as providing information and referral services for such vulnerable groups as AIDS patients and the elderly, opening an adult day care, offering comprehensive assessment services to the elderly, initiating a physician referral program for physicians who participate in Medicaid, and working with other community groups to provide primary care for the homeless
- *Services to help contain the cost of health care services,* such as offering free or discounted services to those unable to pay for them, donating unneeded equipment or food to homeless shelters and other programs, and becoming part of telephone reassurance programs for shut-ins or latchkey children
- *Services that reach out to minorities, the poor, persons with disabilities, and other underserved persons,* such as opening child-care programs for families unable to pay full cost, teaming up with community schools to develop self-esteem programs for children with learning disabilities, providing internships for persons with disabilities from sheltered workshops, making facility vans available to disability groups, establishing an "adopt-a-grandchild" program with children of single-parent families, and operating a legal clinic for the community elderly
- *Services that demonstrate leadership and the role of the facility,* such as offering rotations for medical, nursing, and other health professionals; participating in research on innovative ways of caring for patients; participating in efforts to reduce such problems as overmedication among the elderly; sponsoring radio and television talk shows on important issues; and sponsoring such events as a volunteer opportunities fair

5. *Share with the nursing home administration the information about community needs, their extent, and the potential for the home to extend itself into the community.* The initiation of a new program requires consideration of many variables, including its financial viability and marketing. Provide meaningful input on many of these variables. Impressive literature is available on the establishment of long-term care services. For example, Henry (1993) described some important dos and don'ts of opening an adult day-care center.

Wood (1994) is of the opinion that, to enhance their image, nursing homes should choose one or two charity groups (e.g., Alzheimer's Association, Arthritis Foundation, feeding the homeless) and assist them by raising money or donating staff time. Many such groups can use the services of social work professionals and the resources of local human service agencies. Be instrumental in the nursing home's involvement in such groups.

6. *Let the public know about the agency's efforts and accomplishments.* This can be done by (a) developing and distributing an annual community benefit report; (b) incorporating community benefit efforts in all the facility's communication tools—newsletters, calendar of events, advertisement, bulletin boards, speeches to community groups, and other reports to the board and the public (Trocchio, 1994); and (c) taking advantage, for publicity, of opportunities that make the facility newsworthy and cultivating an ongoing relationship with the local media. Its innovative programs, community involvement, human-interest stories, and special celebrations make a nursing home newsworthy. Make the staff mindful of events that may be of interest to the general public and the media ("Conference," 1994). Create an information file that lists the media (all newspapers, magazines, radio stations, television stations), appropriate contact persons, and requirements (e.g., formats for news releases, preferred types of stories, length restrictions, lead times, and deadlines for submitting items). Invite reporters to cover events or send news items and stories followed by notes of appreciation, provide them with accurate information in usable format, and help them meet their deadlines (Chapman, 1989).

7. *Undertake outreach educational programs targeted at families of potential nursing home residents.* Since the passage of the Patient Self-Determination Act of 1991, nursing home residents (and their families) are playing a larger role in decisions about their care. By encouraging the use of advance directives, the 1991 act extends the autonomy of patients into the period when they can no longer communicate. In most places, social workers are responsible for giving patients

information about the law, telling them about advance directives, inquiring about their choices, and having them sign the necessary papers. However, this is done at the time of admission.

> Unfortunately, the sheer volume of paperwork involved in an admission meant that patients and family members often may not devote enough attention to such crucial question as who could serve as proxy decision makers if the resident cannot communicate. (Stoil, 1994, p. 8)

Although social workers implement this law, the community education part of its provisions is neglected. The lack of public education and inadequate attention given to this issue at the time of admission results in the family being forced into making a difficult decision in a crisis situation and experiencing conflict with the nursing home. Social workers can minimize these problems and enhance the image of the nursing home by undertaking outreach educational programs targeted at families of potential nursing home residents.

Social Worker as Recruiter of Community Residential Care Providers

Community residential care facilities are the best solution for those who have no families or whose families can no longer care for them at home and who do not belong in a hospital or a nursing home. The availability of these facilities can also be reassuring to elderly parents unable to continue caring for their middle-aged child with mental retardation. "The knowledge that family life and a sense of stability will go on without a need for institutionalization can also alleviate fears held by the disabled person" (Sherman & Newman, 1988, p. 171).

The prospect of going to a family-like environment is also reassuring to the elderly who are ready for discharge from a hospital but cannot go home and do not want to go to a nursing home. For many old and disabled persons, foster care can at least postpone, if not prevent, nursing home placement. In view of the advantages of this type of care, there is the need to create more foster care settings for the frail elderly and persons with mental illness, mental retardation, and developmental disability. Although foster care has a long history, the general public does not know of adult foster care. Social workers in hospitals, social service departments, and agencies serving the elderly and persons with mental illness and mental retardation must consider the development and promotion of this type of care as an essential part of their professional responsibilities. Here are a few helpful suggestions:

1. *Explore ways of educating the public about the need for families and individuals willing to provide this type of care and to receive the satisfaction of providing care.* Approaches to public education can range from mass media communication to word of mouth. Discussing New York State, Sherman and Newman (1988) stated that recruitment is primarily by television and radio public service announcements (PSAs), newspaper advertisements, transit cards on subways and buses, and word of mouth. Lawrence and Volland (1988) recruited foster home caregivers through advertisements placed in the classified sections of city and suburban newspapers.

Although newspaper advertisements are not very expensive, PSAs on radio and television are free of cost, and the audience reached is large. Under the Communications Act of 1934, radio and television stations licensed by the Federal Communications Commission were required to give free time to PSAs, and the time devoted to this public service was taken into consideration when their licenses came up for renewal. During the Reagan administration, that requirement was changed so that radio and television stations are no longer required to air PSAs. Most stations, however, still provide this service. If their agency does not have a public relations department, social workers can take on the job of preparing and having a PSA aired. This involves a twofold action: (a) preparing a statement, rehearsing it, and tape-recording it, and (b) calling the radio station newsroom, identifying oneself, and giving the statement.

If the station airs the announcement, send a letter of thanks. If it does not, write and ask why (Klein & Danzig, 1985).

Besides the use of mass media, selling the idea of adult foster care and recruiting of foster families can be done through talks and presentations at churches, offices for the aging, and parent-teacher association meetings (Talmadge & Murphy, 1983). Use creativity and imagination in deciding the "what" and "how" of these presentations so that they are audience appropriate. Stress the benefits of such care for both the provider and the receiver.

> Foster family care doesn't require extensive outlays of money for bricks and mortar; rather, it takes advantage of the spare bedrooms of empty-nesters, widows and widowers, and others who can so usefully contribute to the lives of the less fortunate, and in the process enhance their own. (Heckler, 1984)

2. In response to the PSA, newspaper advertisement, or talk given at a meeting or from an acquaintance, some potential care providers will contact the worker's agency for more information. *Express an appreciation for their interest and arrange for an in-person interview with them at their home.* Use the visit to their home for a threefold purpose: (a) giving information about foster care and expectations from the caregiver, (b) assessing the person's values and nurturing skills, and (c) determining the appropriateness and adequacy of the home for accommodating persons with special needs. Give them information about the range of people needing care, the needs of these people in general, the efforts made to match persons needing care and the caregiving family, and the type of support that will be available from the worker's organization and what can be expected from other local health and human service agencies.

The general consensus is that no particular set of demographic variables combines to make an ideal foster care provider. Therefore, look for indicators of such intangible qualities as concern for others, desire to help, urge to give, empathy, and ability to nurture. These may be reflected in the interactions of the potential care provider

with children and family members and the responses to questions about the motivation for the new role. With his focus on family foster care for persons with chronic mental illness, Carling (1984) listed the following among those who are usually screened out as care providers: (a) people who depend on foster care for their principal source of income, (b) people with criminal convictions, (c) current service providers (because of potential conflicts of interest), (d) people with other family members not supportive of family foster care, (e) people with grossly inappropriate or unhelpful beliefs, and (f) people who want to be "therapists." Similarly, look for the adequacy of the physical environment and setup of the place, with an eye to its potential for becoming a home for a stranger.

Social Worker as Trainer of Community Residential Care Providers

Despite their importance, the desire and willingness to take on the role of a caregiver for a vulnerable stranger are not enough for the effective performance of that role to the satisfaction of all concerned. Training becomes an important variable that can make caregiving a satisfying and successful endeavor. As the professional responsible for training of care providers, the social worker should consider the following suggestions:

1. *Make the training a multipurpose activity.* Training can be used as an extension of the recruitment effort for screening potential caregivers. It should be used for creating and maintaining a positive relationship with the care provider. It should be so structured that various–foster care providers are encouraged to get to know one another and to form an informal peer support system. The formal coming together and informal ongoing contacts among care providers thus generated can lead to their organizing themselves as advocates for their needs and for greater recognition of their contribution to the field of health care.

2. *Let the principle of flexibility guide their choice of the "when" and "where" of training sessions.* Make it convenient for care providers to attend as many sessions as possible, and also give them incentives to do so. The incentives may be in the form of assistance with transportation, recognition for their service, and coverage of care during their absence from home (Carling, 1984).

3. *Make the content of the training appropriate for the caregiving role.* Important variables that should be considered include the needs of the residents for whom these care providers are or will be caring, their educational background, their health-related knowledge, and their caregiving experience. It is wise to do a simple needs assessment and make that the basis for topic selection. The topics generally considered essential for such training can be clustered into the following groups:

- *Safety and crisis care:* home hazards and accident prevention, first aid, and emergency assistance
- *Drug management and medical treatment:* administration of medication, effects and side effects of medications, common diseases (e.g., in the elderly), signs of illness, infection control, and medical follow-up
- *Food and nutrition:* basic nutrition and special diets
- *Activities of daily living:* basic personal care, use of adaptive equipment and aids, client independence, and realistic expectations
- *Issues related to chronic illness and aging:* experience of losses (sensory and social), depression, mental confusion, aging process, behavioral aspects of mental illness, and death and dying
- *Caregiving and help seeking:* stresses of caregiving, effects of caring on the family, dealing with stress, problem solving, and using community resources (Carling, 1984; Oktay & Volland, 1981; Sherman & Newman, 1988; Sylvester & Sheppard, 1988)

In the foster care program for the frail elderly developed by Johns Hopkins Hospital, the training lasted a week, and at the end of the training course, "potential caregivers were tested on items such as patient's personal care, diet, common

illnesses, CPR, psychosocial and emotional needs. Those who passed the test were ready to be matched with an appropriate patient" (Lawrence & Volland, 1988, p. 28).

4. *Involve professionals with knowledge and expertise in the areas to be covered in the training.* For hospital-based social workers, it is not likely to be difficult because all professionals are directly or indirectly interested in early and appropriate discharge of patients and will be willing to contribute to the development of new residential care facilities. Social workers not associated with hospitals will need to use their contacts with human services professionals in the community to stretch the resources of their agency for training.

Social Worker as Provider of Support and Monitor of Quality of Care

Provision of ongoing support is a necessity for the success of long-term care. When a family begins taking on this responsibility, the need for support is extensive. Vandivort, Kurren, and Braun (1984) considered the first 3 months crucial. During this period, the caregiver is adjusting to a new role, and the resident is adjusting to a new environment. This support can take the form of (a) the worker's frequent visits (at least once a month), (b) easy availability between visits, (c) help in identifying and articulating the resident's needs, (d) assistance with designing a plan for care, (e) linking the caregiver with other sources of services for the resident, (f) quick and appropriate response to crisis situations, (g) aid in organizing and keeping the minimal record of care expected or required by the state certifying or licensing agency if applicable, (h) arrangements for respite and backup care, and (i) periodic retraining or refresher programs. Here are a few suggestions:

1. *Mix and match the various forms of support to address the specific needs of care providers.* Let the principle of individualization of people,

their needs, and circumstances guide the selection and combination of the various modes of support. The Caregiver Well-Being Scale (Berg-Weger, Rubio, & Tebb, 2000) is a comprehensive instrument that can be used for assessment, intervention, and evaluation of social work support of family caregivers. "The scale addresses caregiver's emotional status, physical needs, spiritual or reflective times, special contacts and supports, and whether she or he is able to maintain a personal living environment on a daily basis" (p. 261). Consider using it as needed.

2. *Handle the crisis situations carefully so that the crisis becomes a source of new insight, strength, and positive change.* View the client, other residents, and the care provider as all in "crisis" during an emergency and conduct a "postincidence" evaluation to identify what could have predicted the crisis and what could be alternative responses (Carling, 1984).

3. *Remember that quality of support is often more meaningful and helpful than its quantity.* Try to convey the message that staff are there to strengthen the care provider's commitment and ability to care and that the caregiver, the resident, and the worker are a team bent on deriving the best results from the joint effort.

4. *The quality of care will depend on the combined effect of training, support, and other factors,* such as matching of residents and caregivers and continuous monitoring of the care arrangement. Matching is a difficult task, particularly in the beginning, when there is no good intuitive feeling for the care provider and his or her home. Until the social worker gets to the stage in the relationship with the care provider when she or he knows what type of resident would fit into that provider's home, it will be helpful to (a) solicit from the care provider information about what type of resident would be ideally desirable; (b) share with the care provider as much information about the prospective resident as possible, while protecting the need for privacy and confidentiality; (c) give the prospective resident a clear picture of the foster home; (d) arrange for the care provider to meet the

client/patient in the hospital; (e) arrange, whenever possible, for a visit of the prospective resident to the caregiver's home to give both a chance to decide whether the arrangement is suitable (Sherman & Newman, 1988); and (f) consider as many of the following prospective resident's characteristics and preferences as possible:

Personality characteristics

Social interests

Personal habits

Gender

Race

Religion

Cultural factors

Smoking

Pets

Children

Location

Medical needs

Mental health needs

Rehabilitation needs

Support service needs

Alcohol/drug problems

Wheelchair accessibility (Carling, 1984)

Assurance of quality of care in a safe and healthy environment will result from several efforts. Use follow-up visits to the foster home to provide support and give necessary direction and supervision to the caregiver. In one study, Sherman and Newman (1988) found that about two thirds of care providers considered personal follow-ups beneficial to both residents and providers. The visits should be scheduled as well as unscheduled.

Review the resident's progress and care plan periodically, and modify it in view of his or her changing condition and needs, if needed.

Get to know the residents well enough for them to talk candidly. They can add to the validity of impressions about the quality of care and the success of placement.

Most residents are likely to have health care needs requiring the services and involvement of several agencies and professionals. Act as the case manager and use the opportunities provided by that role to monitor the effectiveness and efficiency of the foster home as part of the total package of care.

5. Because adult foster care has no uniform licensing standards (Oktay, 1987), *push for the certification of family foster care in the state if it does not license or certify this type of care.* Most presenters at a workshop on family foster care favored "a 'certification' approach in which states or local agencies had flexibility in decertifying providers, viewing the certification as a privilege, rather than a right" (Carling, 1984, p. 15).

6. *Encourage the caregiver to join a professional group,* such as the National Association of Residential Care Facilities. Membership in an organized group can be a source of heightened morale, pride and professionalism, support and strength, and training. Professionalism provides a self-propelling force for commitment to providing high-quality care.

Social Worker as Contributor to the Agency's Continuous Quality Improvement

Before we discuss the knowledge and skills necessary for social workers to assume this contributor role, let us briefly look at the concept of "continuous quality improvement" (CQI) and its methodology. This concept was developed in the 1930s by W. Edwards Deming and Joseph M. Juran and was originally implemented in manufacturing. In the late 1980s, its relevance to the health care industry began to be realized (Balinsky, 1994), and as O'Leary (1991a) explained,

American industry is *a,* if not *the,* major purchaser of health care. And like any good American group,

they are quickly deciding that what is good for them is good for you as well. In this case, I would suggest that they are right. (p. 72)

Quality assurance (QA), the approach to quality in health care until then, was punitive in its mind-set, outlier oriented, inefficient, and frustrating. In contrast with QA as a "blame-fixing" activity, CQI is seen as an organization-wide way of life (O'Leary, 1991b). QA separated *production* (the service-providing unit) from *inspection* (the QA department), and *responsibility* for quality (the QA committee) from *authority* (the service). This separation (a) undermined teamwork, (b) delayed feedback, (c) increased cost of data collection, and (d) communicated a less than total organizational commitment to quality (Eskildson & Yates, 1991).

Quality in health care is a multifaceted and multidimensional phenomenon. Dimensions include accessibility, appropriateness, effectiveness, continuity, efficacy, and efficiency of care. Quality is also the safety of the care environment, acceptability of care as judged by the patient and family, and the qualitative interactions between patient/family and care providers (Balinsky, 1994; O'Leary, 1991a). It is believed that CQI will positively affect all facets and dimensions of quality. Eskildson and Yates (1991) considered TQM (total quality management) a new paradigm:

Important components of the new paradigm include commitment to an unrelenting focus on customer satisfaction, continuous improvement, employee involvement, "management by fact" (including the use of statistical process control), effective internal and external teamwork, emphasis on prevention (rather than inspection), cycle-time reduction, and widespread staff training in multiple areas affecting quality. (p. 38)

The basic principles of TQM according to Deming (1986) are as follows:

1. Create constancy of purpose for improvement of product and service.

2. Adopt the new philosophy of doing things right the first time.

3. Cease dependency on inspection to achieve quality.

4. End the practice of awarding business on price tag alone.

5. Improve constantly and forever the system of production and service.

6. Institute training on the job.

7. Begin leadership for system improvement.

8. Drive out fear; create trust.

9. Break down barriers between staff areas.

10. Eliminate slogans, exhortations, and targets for the workforce.

11. Eliminate numerical quotas for production; institute methods for improvement.

12. Remove barriers to pride of workmanship.

13. Institute a vigorous program of education and self-improvement for everyone.

14. Put everyone to work to accomplish this transformation.

The technology of CQI involves use of the following:

1. *Teams*—these are of three types: (a) cross-functional improvement teams, (b) quality circles, and (c) process improvement teams (Keys, 1995)

2. *Methods* such as Plan-Do-Check-Act or Plan-Do-Study-Adjust cycle and benchmarking involve identifying the best practices, studying their applications, and applying them (McCabe, 1992)

3. *Supportive infrastructure,* which is created through vertical alignment, horizontal process management, and independent assessment (McCabe, 1992)

4. *Statistical tools* such as a flow chart, cause-and-effect diagram, control chart, and Pareto diagram (Burr, 1990; Sarazan, 1990; Shainin, 1990)

Social workers in home-based and near home-based long-term care agencies should seize the opportunity offered by these agencies' need to move toward CQI and provide leadership to their efforts. They have an edge over professionals from many other disciplines.

Applying their existing skills or building on them will ensure their readiness for the job. Their basic team-building and teamwork approaches can easily be adapted for CQI. The Plan-Do-Check-Act cycle is similar to the problem-solving process they have thoroughly grasped and practiced. Their understanding and skills for organizational work can help their agency become supportive of the CQI philosophy through structural and procedural changes. Methods of vertical alignment and horizontal process management can be incorporated into their organizational skills. Brushing up on their knowledge of statistical data display techniques would enable them to use the appropriate statistical tools for CQI. The following are some helpful suggestions:

1. *Consider the patient in the same way as a customer is considered in industry.* The application of the TQM approach to health care requires this, with regard to quality.

> Quality is a customer determination, not an engineer's determination, not a marketing determination or a general management determination. It is based on the customer's actual experience with the product or service, measured against his or her requirements—stated or unstated, conscious or merely sensed, technically operational or entirely subjective—and always representing a moving target in a competitive market. (Feigenbaum, 1983, p. 7)

2. *View and involve clients as active partners in the quality improvement work.* This task is difficult in health care because, traditionally, quality has been defined by the provider. A distinction is made between the technical and interpersonal aspects of health care to limit the patient's involvement in quality assessment. It is assumed that the patient is unable to understand the technical aspects of care (Lehr & Strosberg, 1991). This situation will gradually change as, on the one hand, clients become better-educated consumers of health care services, more informed of health care techniques and procedures, more demanding of choices and options, and more conscious of their rights, and as, on the other hand, health care providers start acknowledging and appreciating the role that patients, their families, and other

informal helpers play in the recovery and/or management of patients. Social workers should realize the advantage they have over other professionals. They have been trained to treat their clients as equals, and educating and empowering them are the major social work approaches to enabling clients to exercise self-determination, solve their problems, and manage their lives.

3. *Help agencies institute a threefold approach to involving clients in the CQI endeavor:* (a) service protocols that require client input into all aspects of care; (b) continuing education for professional and paraprofessional service providers on techniques of encouragement, involvement, and empowerment of clients; and (c) ongoing supervision and support for service providers in the field. Besides these organization-level contributions, social workers should monitor their clients as part of the quality improvement work of the agency.

4. *Recognize that, for CQI, all parts of the organization—service management as well as maintenance management—are equally important.* The spirit of quality not only should be visible in the clinical and technical services but also should pervade the total organization. Studies by Bowen (1985) found that (a) a strong correlation exists between customer and employee views of service quality and the internal climate for service; (b) when employees view an organization's human resource policies favorably, customers view the quality of service they receive favorably; (c) a positive work climate directly affects customer service for the better; and (d) human resources is an excellent vehicle for satisfying both employee and customer needs.

The concept of "customer" is much broader in TQM philosophy. It applies internally as well as externally. External customers for a home care agency include patients, families, payers, volunteers, and the community. All employees of the agency are its internal customers. All persons and units function as both "producers" and "customers" at every level and in every process of an organization (Re & Krousel-Wood, 1990). Involvement of both external and internal customers is necessary for CQI. Feedback mechanisms

should be developed for different groups of external customers. Constant effort should be made not only to involve the internal customers but also to develop their full potential. This can be facilitated by such enabling principles as (a) setting clear expectations; (b) maintaining skills and providing resources; (c) providing feedback as a learning tool; (d) granting authority to act; and (e) providing encouragement, support, and recognition (McCabe, 1992).

The creation of a culture of quality and a supportive infrastructure is extremely important for CQI. Social workers can contribute to this task as advisers, technical experts, and team players. The following are a few helpful strategies:

• *The agency must develop a definition of quality that is meaningful for and is understood by everyone.* Management must emphasize that quality improvement is an ongoing effort and look for opportunities to demonstrate its full support for quality (Sahney & Warden, 1991). Although TQM is a participatory and decentralized approach to quality, the involvement of management must be intense and in detail in top-down priority setting and modeling (Eskildson & Yates, 1991; Kaluzny & McLaughlin, 1992).

• *Identification of problems should be considered an opportunity for improvement and not a means for laying blame.* "Long-range thinking and planning should replace the focus on short-term results" (Sahney & Warden, 1991, p. 9).

• *Vertical alignment will aid in the creation of a supportive infrastructure for quality.* Vertical alignment means that everyone in the agency from top to bottom understands what the agency is trying to accomplish and how he or she fits into the big picture. This shared understanding becomes possible through the linking of goals, plans, and responsibilities from the top through all departments to each individual (McCabe, 1992). All goals, plans, policies, and procedures should aim at supporting the agency's mission. Constant efforts should be made for improving communication throughout all levels of the organization and increasing opportunities for meaningful involvement of all employees.

• *It is better to focus on important processes involved in the agency's work than on the people in those processes.* Horizontal process management is aimed at improving the processes. As processes cut across departmental boundaries, this is best accomplished by a team of process implementers. "The team must be given the responsibility and authority to define and control its processes, to assess performance of the processes, and to modify the processes based on assessment findings" (McCabe, 1992, p. 137). This strategy has been presented as a nine-step methodology:

1. Find a process to improve.

2. Organize a team that knows the process.

3. Clarify current knowledge of the process.

4. Understand source of process variation.

5. Select the process improvement.

6. Plan a change or test.

7. Carry out the change.

8. Check and observe the effects of the change.

9. Accept, adopt, or modify the plan (James, 1989).

• *Keep abreast of the literature on the implementation of CQI in the health care field.* Many hospitals and other health care organizations are making impressive efforts in this regard (e.g., Dimant, 1991; Graves & MacDowell, 1994–1995; Re & Krousel-Wood, 1990; Sahney & Warden, 1991). It would be wise to learn from their experience.

Social Worker as Case Manager and Service Coordinator

Case management is likely to continue to expand in a variety of delivery systems. Social workers should seek jobs in home-based care agencies, as well as in near home-based service agencies. In the former, they will be able to take on case management responsibilities; in the latter,

they should apply their case management skills to such jobs as agency director, program planner, and direct service provider. They should keep themselves abreast of the emerging literature on the "what," "why," and "how" of long-term care case management. Gerson and Chassler (1995) described a 15-month project to develop case management practice guidelines. A national advisory committee was created that formulated several basic principles of case management [3]. Hyduk (2002) described the essentials of 11 community-based long-term care case management models for older adults and compared those models on a number of criteria. The models included in her analysis are (1) the National Long-Term Care Channeling Demonstration, (2) PACE (Program of All-Inclusive Care for the Elderly), (3) Social HMO, (4) Project CARE (Community Action to Reach the Elderly), (5) HMO case management, (6) CBLTC (Community-Based Long-Term Care), (7) modified CBLTC, (8) GEM (geriatric evaluation and management), (9) GEM–VA (geriatric evaluation and management–Veterans Affairs), (10) postacute case management, and (11) Physician Practice Case Management. Her analysis revealed great variation in the definition of frail older adults; that the majority of the models did not include important psychosocial variables; that many did not discuss the extent to which older adults and their caregivers are involved in decisions regarding the care process; and that most did not discuss minority status—ethnicity and other attributes of the minority elders. She urged gerontological social workers to recognize the strengths that they bring to the case management role and to embrace that role.

Some case management strategies were presented in Chapter 5. Here, we discuss more ideas regarding case management that are likely to be helpful.

Despite its popularity, case management lacks precise definition. There is no consensus on its exact nature and purpose. It can be viewed narrowly or widely. "It can be a gatekeeping mechanism to control costs and access; it can be an advocacy function to increase access to services and navigate a confusing array of services; or it can serve a diagnostic and prescriptive function" (Williams, 1993, p. 7).

Starting with the assumption that the underlying structure of a program's financing has a fundamental impact on its services, Applebaum and Austin (1990) identified three models of case management: (a) the broker model, (b) the service management model, and (c) the managed care model. Case managers under the *broker model* do not have service dollars to spend on behalf of their clients. They develop care plans and make referrals for services from the existing service system. Under the *service management model,* case managers have access to funds, develop care plans, and authorize services within the predetermined cost caps. The *managed care model* is based on prospective financing that creates "provider risk." Financial responsibility and liability for expenditures are shifted to provider agencies. This puts pressure on the care planning process, creating incentives for the provider to control cost. Social workers should make their understanding of these models of case management serve their agency's mission and program objectives. We discuss social work's role in managed care in Chapter 8. Here, we focus on the broker model of case management.

The most generally accepted components of case management are (a) eligibility determination—financial, medical, and other; (b) level of care determination; (c) assessment of needs, including medical, physical, functional, and psychosocial; (d) place of care determination; (e) care plan development; (f) service prescription or arrangement; (g) coordination of services from multiple providers; (h) budget planning for service units, time periods, or episodes; (i) reassessment of needs; (j) monitoring of delivery and quality of service; and (k) support to family (Williams, 1993). Not all programs incorporate all these functions. In home care programs, for example, the typically covered functions are assessment of needs, planning of appropriate services, ordering or provision of services, monitoring and evaluation of services, and reassessment of the need situation.

Home care programs are offered by many agencies—home health agencies, multiple-service health care providers, free-standing case management agencies, and Area Agencies on Aging. Home health agencies provide nursing and other skilled services, such as physical, occupational, and speech therapy, and home-health aide services. On the one hand, they have historically used a community health nursing model, in which the nurse goes into the home and family setting and performs the assessment, care planning, advocacy, and other roles. On the other hand, Area Agencies on Aging have traditionally focused on social services, meals on wheels, senior activities, and advocacy to the exclusion of health services (Williams, 1993). Social workers should recognize the inherent deficiencies of these models. They should make concerted efforts to move toward a model that combines and coordinates a wide array of health and social services. The integrated health/ social service model (Brody, 1977) can be a good guide. That model includes the following services:

- *Maintenance services* include income maintenance and personal maintenance. Income maintenance is secured through such programs as Supplemental Security Income, Social Security, veterans' benefits, workers' compensation, and food stamps. Homemaker services, home-delivered and congregate meals, and chore services constitute the personal maintenance services.
- *Personal care* is provided through the services of home-health aides representing many public and private health care agencies.
- *Supportive medical services* include nursing; physical, occupational, and speech therapy services, generally provided by hospitals; health clinics; public health departments; and visiting nurse organizations.
- *Personal planning* includes counseling, advocacy, community resources mobilization, and protection services provided by social workers through family service agencies, state social services organizations, community mental health centers, and home health care and vocational rehabilitation agencies.
- *Linkages* include such services as information and referral, transportation, outreach, telephone alert, and friendly visiting services.

Even single agencies can offer packages of the needed health and social services. In some areas, the Area Agencies on Aging are capable of running comprehensive long-term care programs, and some home-health agencies have broadened their scope by including services unrelated to health.

Social workers should consider the following principles of case management proposed by Williams (1993):

- *Only certain individuals should be case managed.* This service should be offered only to those who need it. Possible criteria for selection are (a) high risk because of physical and cognitive impairments and lack of family supports; (b) eligibility for nursing home level of care but electing community-based care; (c) complex care needs; (d) short-term posthospital care needs; (e) high-cost care needs; and (f) high risk for repeat hospitalization.
- *Assessment of service needs and case management are related.* Separating assessment from case management functions is likely to create confusion, delays, and duplication.
- *Case management has multidimensional requirements.* An interdisciplinary approach to staffing is needed. At a minimum, medical and social services must be available; other consultant services could be contracted for.
- *Case management is a team effort.* Links with many types of community agencies, including hospitals, housing providers, meal providers, and others, must be forged.
- *Equity assurance is important in case management.* Services must be distributed equitably among similar clients. "A major goal of case management should be to serve the neediest and spread available resources to do so in a judicious way" (p. 27).
- *Cost control is part of case management.* Incentives for controlling costs must be built into the system.
- *Quality assurance is essential.* QA mechanisms should be made an integral part of both case management and services. These may include the use of standardized, specific, and generally understood criteria, supervision, and quality reviews.

The broker models of case management, which emphasize referrals and linkage, generally within one service sector, are most common in long-term care settings. Even these models are often provider driven rather than client driven. Rose and Moore (1995) brought out the differences between the client-driven and provider-driven approaches. Whereas one (client-driven approach) views clients as subjects, the other (provider-driven approach) views them as objects; one looks for strengths to develop, and the other identifies problems and pathology to manage; one seeks active participation, and the other encourages compliance; the goals of the one are positive direction and self-confidence, and those of the other are improved patterns of service consumption and patient role behavior; the needs assessment is derived in one from the client's direction, plan, and goals, and in the other from the service provider's definitions and outputs; resources to be linked are seen in one as the total community with all its formal and informal networks and in the other as existing formal service providers; monitoring in one involves mutual evaluation of process in relation to direction plan and in the other compliance with treatment plan; and evaluation in one emphasizes increasing autonomy, growing self-confidence, and involvement with informal networks, and in the other increased units of service consumed, use of fewer inpatient days, and improved compliance. Because of their philosophical orientation and as a result of their professional training, social workers are most suited to practice client-driven approaches to case management. They should make sure they are seen as the model, as well as a source of formal and informal training, for client-centered and client-driven approaches in the agency.

In Chapter 5, we discussed strategies and techniques of brokering. Here, we reemphasize that social workers should (a) keep an updated directory of all the formal and informal resources in their community, (b) know the agency eligibility criteria for benefits and services from all the formal sources of assistance, (c) keep themselves abreast of legislation and regulations that are likely to affect policies and procedures of major agencies and programs, (d) develop an awareness of such characteristics of major agencies as the degree of flexibility in accommodating client problems (some agencies are extremely formal and rulebound, whereas others are willing to bend the rules), (e) get to know the contact persons in as many resource agencies as possible, and (f) become involved in the community.

> Join a service club, participate in community meetings, sit in on city council meetings, or attend major community events (pancake day, fireman's chicken dinner, Fourth of July celebration, etc.). These activities will increase your knowledge of community resources and enlarge the circle of people you can call upon in times of need. (Kirst-Ashman & Hull, 1993, p. 497)

Although the case manager's role involves brokering, case management is more than brokering. The client's needs may require more services than are brokered for. The case manager must ensure that those needs are met effectively and efficiently. A commitment to the following principles articulated by Gerhart (1990) would be helpful:

- *Individualization of services* requires that services be developed or designed specifically to meet the identified needs.
- *Comprehensiveness of services* means that the services address needs in all areas of the client's life.
- *Parsimonious services* means that services are well-coordinated, unduplicated, and cost-effective.
- *Fostering autonomy* requires that services and the way they are provided encourage maximum client self-determination.
- *Continuity of care* demands that case management services monitor the client's needs as he or she moves through different settings of care—institutional and community.

Social workers as case managers should give credit to family and other informal caregivers for their work with the elderly and the disabled and "the imaginative way ordinary people invent solutions to problems that disability creates in everyday lives" (Kane, 2001, p. 294). They should also show special sensitivity to the needs and situations of those families. Family caregivers live 24 hours a day, 7 days a week with their caregiving responsibilities, struggling to balance their own needs and those of the ones they care for. Caring for a chronically ill person takes its toll in the form of such problems as family disruptions, psychological stress, physical fatigue, social isolation, financial and at times legal difficulties (Dhooper, 1991), and intrafamilial conflict. With her focus on the effects of Alzheimer's disease, Gwyther (1995) described four types of family caregiving conflicts: (a) normative conflicts around the limits of family solidarity, (b) conflicts arising from family members' disapproval of other members' actions or attitudes toward the patient, (c) conflicts from disagreement over the nature and seriousness of the patient's impairment and the most appropriate care, and (d) conflicts from perceptions that less involved family members either do not appreciate the extent of demands on the primary caregiver or disapprove of the quality of care being given. They should assess the total familial situation and appropriately address the conflicts, problems, and stresses that a family may experience.

Social Worker as Contributor to Improving Hospice Access to People Living in Rural Areas

As pointed out in Chapter 3, terminally ill living in rural areas are less likely to be served by hospice than are their urban counterparts. A review of relevant literature revealed a number of reasons why that is so. We group these reasons into three categories: (1) environment-related, (2) people-related, and (3) hospice-related reasons. A brief listing of these precedes our discussion of social work's role in helping hospice improve its access to people living in rural areas. Most of the material is drawn from Burg et al., 2010; Casey, Moscovice, Virnig, and Durham, 2005; Community-State Partnerships to Improve End-of-Life Care, 2001, 2002, and 2003; Dunham, Bolden, and Kvale, 2003; Gage et al., 2000; and Haxton and Boelk, 2010.

Environment-related barriers:

1. Rural communities have higher rates of poverty and more uninsured individuals (National Advisory Committee on Rural Health and Human Services, 2008), which result in families having fewer resources for end-of-life care of their members.

2. Distance from specialized medical care denies rural dwellers easy access to diagnosis and treatment of life-threatening and terminal illnesses.

3. There is a general lack of community resources, including health and human services, in rural areas and a lack of easy access to the available resources.

4. Long distances between the hospice base location and the rural patient's home (combined with severe winter weather and/or seasonal flooding in many parts of the country) make travel difficult, time-consuming, expensive, and risky, particularly in remote areas.

5. Nonavailability or high cost of medications and medical supplies at local pharmacies puts extra strain on the financial resources of hospice.

6. Local area hospitals, nursing homes, and home health care agencies tend to view hospice as competing with them for patients as well as for locally available health care professionals.

People-related barriers:

1. Most rural folk are independent, self-sufficient, and private.

2. They are used to not having services.

3. They tend to distrust outsiders and formal programs or do not want to abuse the "system."

4. Most of them do not know of hospice and hospice services.

5. They believe that local physicians caring for them should meet all their needs.

6. Local physicians are less inclined to refer their terminally ill patients to hospice, either because they do not know about hospice or do not want to lose control over their patients' care.

Hospice-related barriers:

1. Most rural hospices have low patient volume that makes it hard for them to fund full-time staff positions. They also have difficulty hiring staff willing to travel long distances in remote areas.

2. They have difficulty retaining staff because most home-based care is labor-intensive and puts staff at risk for burnout and compassion fatigue. Staff members who belong to local communities have the extra burden of providing end-of-life care to their neighbors and friends.

3. Providing hospice care in rural areas is financially straining. Medicare pays hospices a capitated per diem for delivering almost all the services needed in a day to treat a patient's terminal illness. Furthermore, Medicare per diem rates are lower for rural hospices.

4. Financial problems also arise because rural hospices have fewer patients to spread fixed costs, and they cannot benefit from economies of scale in purchasing medications and medical supplies.

5. Late referrals to rural hospices result in shorter lengths of stay in the program, and that also causes extra financial strain because first and last days of service are most costly.

6. Long distances and other logistics problems make it difficult for rural hospices to coordinate care.

The above categorization of barriers into environment-related, people-related, and hospice-related reasons makes understanding these barriers easier, but in reality, all these intermingle and overlap to make it hard for hospice organizations to provide high-quality services in effective and efficient ways. The following observations and three sets of suggestions for social work contributions deal with all these barriers.

Two of the barriers—many rural dwellers lacking health insurance and nonavailability of health care services in rural areas because of long distances from medical diagnostic and treatment centers—are likely to become less formidable in the future. As the various provisions of the Patient Protection and Affordable Care Act take effect, most poor in rural areas will become eligible for Medicaid and the spread of new health centers will bring health care closer. It is expected that wellness, illness prevention, early detection, and coordination of care among various settings of medical services will be the hallmark of those health care centers. Hospice social workers should include in their roles educating rural folk about their rights to health care under the new law.

Similarly, as responsible human service professionals working in an area, social workers can contribute to reducing another barrier—that is, lack of community resources or lack of access to available community-based resources. A study by Haxton and Boelk (2010) involving 339 hospice social workers from 34 states found that more than 70% viewed accessing community-based services (adult day care, mental health counseling, etc.) as very much or quite a bit of a challenge for providing social work services to rural hospice patients and families. Similarly, 60% of them considered accessing in-home services (home-delivered meals, supportive home care, etc.) very much or quite a bit of a challenge. Dealing with such challenges becomes a professional responsibility. In this study, responses to the question, "What approaches do you take to overcome challenges you face?" generated several themes.

> Building relationships with other programs and professionals was perceived as even more important in rural areas, where resources are slim and fewer programs, services, and providers exist. Respondents believed that serving hospice patients and families in rural areas has to be more of a collective process involving others outside of the hospice program. (p. 542)

Establishing and maintaining regular contacts with professionals running the various health and human services programs in the area and creating a joint commitment to generating resources and improving the delivery system can go a long way to identifying needs, discussing problems, brainstorming solutions, and creating and coordinating resources.

All other barriers can be clustered according to three themes: (1) recruiting, retaining, and keeping hospice staff energized; (2) making and keeping hospices financially viable; and (3) educating rural families and physicians about hospice. Social workers will find the following suggestions helpful in dealing with each of these.

Recruiting, Retaining, and Keeping Hospice Staff Energized

Acknowledge the reality that the volume of work in rural hospices is not large enough to require a fleet of full-time staff. Therefore, look for potential part-time staff—individuals who have retired, are semiretired, or whose family responsibilities dictate that they work part-time. The need for and purpose of hospice is intuitively attractive to many professionals and volunteers. These can be used to appeal to the service ideal of potential employees.

If the hospice is a part of another organization such as a hospital, home-health agency, or public health department, explore the possibility of (1) employing staff from the parent agency, (2) sharing staff across programs, and (3) training staff to perform multiple roles. The first strategy will ensure that the hospice employees receive salaries and benefits comparable to similar positions in the larger organization. The second strategy is a viable solution for the fluctuations in hospice census. The third can be an adequate response to the problems of inadequate on-call coverage, travel-related expenses, etc. The Haxton and Boelk (2010) study found that the majority of social workers (57.4%) also functioned as bereavement counselors, intake coordinators, outreach coordinators, volunteer coordinators, and administrators. They can easily be role models for others in this regard.

Two dimensions of travel-related problems (i.e., long-distance travels putting physical strain on the hospice staff and economic strain on the hospice organization) can be significantly eased by (1) opening satellite offices in remote areas, (2) planning and coordinating travel to remote areas that combines staff visits so that staff members travel together and the number of cars traveling is reduced, (3) scheduling all visits in one location on the same day, (4) deploying staff members living in communities closest to the patient and family, and (5) using telephone and other technologies (e.g., Internet) creatively to enhance the impact of in-person staff visits with patients and their families.

Retaining and keeping hospice staff energized can be done through (1) setting up a mentoring system for new employees (e.g., matching new nurses with more experienced ones); (2) maximizing communication among staff members through various means, formal and informal as well as in-person and electronic; (3) providing staff members the necessary instrumental support; (4) ensuring that all staff members get much-needed emotional support; and (5) acknowledging and reducing the risk of burnout and compassion fatigue in employees. Familiarize yourself with the growing literature on burnout, compassion fatigue, and compassion satisfaction, and draw practical ideas that can be implemented within your organization.

Making and Keeping Hospices Financially Viable

A threefold approach is needed that aims at (1) improving Medicare reimbursement for hospice services, (2) opening new streams of payment for hospice care, and (3) improving the efficiency of the existing financial resources of hospices.

1. *Improving Medicare reimbursement for hospice services*:

- Know the following facts:
  a. Hospice is widely considered the first and a very successful managed care program in the country, and studies have shown that it is a more cost-effective care option than hospitals and skilled nursing homes. Buck (2006) compared hospital, skilled nursing facility, and hospice Medicare per-day charges for 1998 to

2005. Not only were the hospice charges impressively low—$131 compared with $521 for a skilled nursing facility and $4,787 for a hospital—but the growth in the cost of its care was negligible. It rose by only $18 over a 7-year period. Such cost-effectiveness of hospice has not been appropriately rewarded.

  b. The Medicare payment system for hospice care has remained largely unchanged over the years even though the gap between the actual cost of care and Medicare reimbursement for that care has been growing. Community-State Partnerships to Improve End-of-Life Care (2002) illustrated this gap with the example of the cost of drugs. Whereas per-patient-per-day cost was $15.00, the daily medication allowance was only $2.48.

  c. The average length of Medicare hospice patients' stays in the program has been decreasing. The median length of stay in 2009 was 21.1 days, and 34.4% of patients died in 7 days or less that year (NHPCO, 2010).

  d. It costs rural hospices more to serve their clients than it costs their urban counterparts to serve theirs. Despite that, Medicare reimbursement to rural hospices is lower.

- Generate and gather documented evidence.
  a. Make sure your organization maintains documentation of the actual cost of effective and efficient care (i.e., expenses incurred in serving rural patients and their families).

  b. Undertake and/or seek to participate in systematic research that shows the gap between the cost of care and reimbursement for that care, and proves the inadequacy of Medicare imbursement.

- Join existing coalitions (and/or form a coalition) and actively participate in their work for educating and lobbying members of the U.S. Congress for changes in the Medicare payment for hospice care system.
  a. There are several relevant organizations, such as American Hospice Foundation

(www.americanhospice.org/), Hospice Association of America (www.hospice-america.org/), Hospice Foundation of America (www.hospicefoundation.org/), National Association for Home Care and Hospice (www.nahc.org/), National Hospice and Palliative Care Organization (www.nhpco.org/), Hospice and Palliative Nurses Association (www.hpna.org), Medicare Rights Center (www.medicare rights.org/), and National Family Care-givers Association (www.nfcacares.org/). Find out what the priorities and agendas of these organizations are and how your organization can join forces with them. For creating a coalition, ideas and sug-gestions given elsewhere in this book will be helpful. Community-State Partner-ships to Improve End-of-Life Care (2003) described the successes of coalitions in 21 states that brought about public policy reform, as well as implementing projects to educate and empower patients, fami-lies, and communities to advocate better end-of-life care; building clinical capac-ity among various professionals; and establishing mechanisms for quality improvement in hospitals and nursing homes. There are also examples of how to proceed. Haxton and Boelk (2010) suggested forming coalitions around end-of-life care similarly to the way Area Agencies on Aging were encouraged and funded through legislation to address pervasive social problems of the aging population.

b. In educating and lobbying members of Congress and their staff, the following positives about hospice and hospice care can be highlighted:

o The need of appropriate and adequate end-of-life care is universally recog-nized, and there is no political down-side to this issue.
o The success of hospice as a managed care program is generally accepted and applauded.
o Hospice is a fully integrated system that provides highly skilled palliative care along with emotional, spiritual, and supportive care. It can be a model for a "best-practice" approach to other sectors of health care.
o Hospice represents a mere 1% of the Medicare budget (NHPCO, 2010).

c. The Medicare reimbursement system improvement can be done through sev-eral specific approaches or combinations thereof. These include

o raising per diem rates for hospice care;
o allowing for adjustments for case mix, urban/rural location, costly outliers, etc.;
o paying higher rates for care at the beginning and end of hospice stays; and
o paying different rates for the care of patients with cancer and noncancer diagnoses.

2. *Opening new streams of payment for hos-pice care*: This can be done through identifying and removing hurdles in the way of other sources of reimbursement for hospice care, such as state Medicaid programs and private health insurance, as well as increasing the sources and amounts of donations for hospices.

Most state Medicaid programs include hospice benefit for low-income residents under age 65. Some states do not provide Medicaid hospice benefit. Similarly, not all private insurance poli-cies provide for hospice care. If so, state policy-makers and government officials and/or insurance companies doing business in the state can be tar-geted for lobbying and education. They may yield to pressure and expand their coverage to include hospice care. The work of a coalition in Maine led to the passage of a law that (1) increased Medicaid hospice per diem from $106 to $130 per day for the last 6 months of life (Medicare plus 23%); (2) mandated comprehensive hospice coverage for the last 12 months of life in private insurance policies; (3) provided appropriation of $50,000 in each biennial budget to be divided among Maine's voluntary hospices; and (4) man-dated the creation of the Maine Center for End-of-Life Care (Community-State Partnerships to Improve End-of-Life Care, 2003).

Medicaid pays for care for about 8% of hos-pice patients, but many inconsistencies are built into this benefit. Many elderly dying patients in nursing homes do not benefit from hospice care because of those inconsistencies. Situations differ when a patient is eligible for both Medicare and Medicaid programs and when he or she is eligible for Medicare only. When such a patient who is eligible for both Medicare and Medicaid is referred to hospice, Medicaid considers the hospice the primary caregiver and the nursing home the supplier of room and board. Medicare pays for the hospice care, and Medicaid pays the hospice 95% of the nursing home's room-and-board rate. In such a situation, hospice must pay the remaining 5% of the nursing home's room-and-board charge. When a patient is eligible for Medicare only and is in a skilled nursing facility, the skilled nursing facility benefit pays for the first 21 days and for the next 22 to 100 days the patient is responsible for copayment until the patient spends down his or her assets and becomes eligible for Medicaid. For a dying patient in a skilled nursing home who is eligible for Medicare only, hospice care would cost a whole lot, as he or she would be responsible for the total cost of room and board. Moreover, because Medicaid payment for nursing home care is much lower than payment under Medicare, nursing homes benefit if a new cycle of skilled nursing facility benefit begins. This often works against a referral to hospice for the patient on Medicare who had become eligible for Medicaid (because of spend-down). Instead of being referred to hospice, the patient ends up in a hospital (Community-State Partnerships to Improve End-of-Life Care, 2002).

The nature and quality of hospice care speak for it. The recipients of hospice care—patients, families, and others—are positively impressed and become the sources of or catalysts for donations to hospice organizations. Social workers should encourage their hospice to recognize, appreciate, and encourage that tendency in potential donors or helpers. They will find the suggestions for fundraising given in Chapter 6 equally beneficial in undertaking this work for their hospice organization.

3. *Improving the efficiency of the existing financial resources of hospices*: Social workers should explore or become instrumental in exploring all means of reducing the financial impact of operating in rural areas. The following are a couple of the possibilities:

- Use the pharmacy of the parent organization, such as a hospital or public health department, to buy medications or join a network of pharmacies (rather than the hospice maintaining its own); group purchasing reduces the cost of drugs and medical supplies.
- Institute the travel-related changes we discussed earlier. This will reduce the cost of travel to the homes of patients in remote rural areas.

Educating Rural Families and Physicians About Hospice

This can be done by the rural hospices directly as well as through others such as Medicare and local health and human services organizations. There is a general lack of knowledge and understanding of hospice, and this is probably truer of people living in rural areas than of those in urban areas. Almost half (45%) of the respondents in the Haxton and Boelk (2010) study believed that rural communities know little to nothing about hospice as a resource available to them. More than 80% of people eligible for Medicare do not know that Medicare offers a hospice benefit (Community-State Partnerships to Improve End-of-Life Care, 2002). It is safe to assume that the percentage of rural elderly in this group is even higher. Almost a quarter (22.7%) of the social workers in the Haxton and Boelk study reported that they were very much or quite a bit involved in outreach and education efforts. The foci of their involvement included patients, families, other professionals, and the broader community. They talked to friends and others (hoping that the word of mouth would travel farther) and participated in formal speaking engagements at local churches, human service organizations, and business establishments. Public education is too important for the success of rural hospices and the viability of the social work role therein to remain the concern of less than 25% of social workers. All rural hospice social workers should consider this a part of their job responsibilities. Of all the hospice professionals, they are the most suited for this work because of their education and skills. They can easily learn and/or polish the appropriate techniques. We provided in Chapter 6 many suggestions for social workers' educator role, which are relevant for public education about hospice as well. The following are a few hospice-specific suggestions drawn from the study by Hiatt, Stelle, Mulsow, and Scott (2007).

- Emphasize and build on the strengths of hospice, such as the philosophy, availability, and quality of its care.
- Correct the public information or impression about the weaknesses of hospice, such as the stigma of hospice care being the "end of the road" and its association with death. This can be countered by concepts such as "care at the end of life" and "dignified death."
- Target specific audiences such as the general public, civil groups, etc.
- Use multiple means of communication.
- Reach out to minority groups and communities with culturally sensitive approaches.
- While making presentations to groups, involve bereaved family members of hospice patients who can describe the quality and benefits of hospice care.
- Work out an arrangement with the local nursing homes whereby information about hospice care is provided to residents (and their families) when they are admitted to the nursing home.

Education of local physicians about hospice requires a different approach because there are many reasons why physicians do not refer their terminally ill patients for hospice care or refer them late in the illness. Some do not know of hospice care and/or its availability in their area. Others do not refer their patients because of the difficulty in accepting death, difficulty in predicting the length of time a terminally ill patient is likely to live, reluctance to stop aggressive curative treatment, and concern at "abandoning" the care of the patient at such an important time. For some, the prognosis of 6 months or less leads to fear of indictment for Medicare fraud if the patient survives beyond the 6-month limit (Crawley, 2007).

Hospice admission by regulation must require the physician to certify that a patient is likely to die within 6 months. This is medically very difficult or even impossible with most patients and most diagnoses. In addition, a hospice referral requires a discussion between physician and patient regarding the imminence of death, for the patient will be required to relinquish his or her right to curative benefits under hospice. (Simmons, 2004, p. 819)

A study by Cherlin and her colleagues (2005) examined 218 family caregiver reports of physician communication about incurable illness, life expectancy, and hospice; the timings of these discussions; and subsequent family understanding of these issues. Many family caregivers reported that the physician never told them the patient's illness could not be cured (20.8%), never provided life expectancy (40% of those reportedly told that illness was incurable), and never discussed using hospice (32.2%). The first discussion of the illness being incurable and of hospice as a possibility occurred within 1 month of the patient's death in many cases (23.5% and 41.1%, respectively).

Education of local physicians can be handled in two ways:

1. The medical director of hospice should reach out and meet the local physicians periodically or as often as necessary to educate them about hospice care and the "how" and "why" of the referral process. Evans, Stone, and Elwyn (2004) did a literature review of 26 studies that examined the organization of rural palliative care and the views of professionals involved in that care. Education and strategic issues were dominant research questions. The role of primary care emerged as an important theme, and primary care professionals reported problems in symptom control and management of emotional issues. They also reported difficulty in obtaining education and training. If the hospice is a part of a chain or a member of a group of hospices, the medical director should explore the possibility of using their combined resources to offer local physicians continuing education in palliative care.

Kaufman and Forman (2005) described an educational program organized by the local hospice for nurses and physicians in a rural county of New Mexico. Of about 150 nurses and 20 physicians, 27 nurses and 5 physicians attended the program. Nurses attended a half-day conference, and physicians attended a grand-round presentation by the medical director of the hospice. The number of patients enrolled in hospice nearly doubled in the year following the educational intervention. The hospice medical director can also work with the coalition (discussed earlier) in approaching Medicare to fund educational seminars and continuing education courses for physicians on palliative and hospice care.

2. The social worker and other hospice team members should join and mobilize the area health care providers to work toward enhancing access to health care services and improving collaboration among care providers.

> Educating, empowering, and assisting health professionals to refer people to hospice, and involving them in planning and care, may serve to benefit all parties involved. Additionally, a hospice and palliative care resource directory specific to each local community may be helpful to professionals as well as families in rural settings. (Haxton & Boelk, 2010, p. 546)

Social workers, whose professional socialization emphasizes consensus building, mediation, and negotiation, can help motivate people, create conditions for exchange of ideas and collaboration, and work for policy changes at various levels.

Social Worker as Helper in Reducing Barriers to Hospice Services for Minority Patients

In order to perform this role, social workers should use a threefold approach: (1) knowing more about why various minority groups do not use hospice services, (2) reaching out to those groups and responding to their concerns, and (3) helping make hospice and its services the minority community's own. The following are some helpful suggestions.

1. *Knowing about minority groups' resistance to hospice services.* Keep abreast of the research-based literature that throws new light on the "why" of minority groups' hesitance to use the available services and how to reduce that resistance. If and when possible, use your research skills and undertake simple surveys on topics of interest to the hospice organization regarding a particular minority community or group. Subjects of such surveys can be members of that community or group, their easily identifiable leaders or spokespersons, and human service providers in that community. Encourage and enthuse the organization for such research work. In the age of the Internet, this can be done with limited funds. The potential benefit of such efforts can be tremendous. If there is a college or university in the area the hospice serves, find out about teaching or research faculty who are or can be interested in researching the kinds of questions for which you are seeking answers.

Reese, Ahern, Nair, O'Faire, and Warren (1999) explored hospice access and use by African Americans and found several cultural and institutional barriers. Culturally, there seems to be a difference between the philosophy of life of most African Americans and the philosophy that underlies the hospice approach. Africans Americans often prefer not to plan for death and are opposed to accepting terminality; therefore, they prefer life-sustaining treatment to palliative care. In the absence of such treatment, they will use home remedies. If nothing is working, they will pray for a miracle because they believe that God determines whether a sick person lives or dies. Accepting terminality while everyone around the patient is praying for a miracle would be seen as a lack of faith. Moreover, their cultural values insist that one's own people—family and church members—and not strangers should provide care in terminal illness. The institutional barriers that the study discovered included (1) the unfamiliarity of most African Americans with hospice, (2) a general lack of trust in the health care system and its newer approaches (lest they "end up being a guinea pig in one of their experiments"), and (3) an absence of African

Americans among health care providers. Washington, Bickel-Swenson, and Stephens (2008) did a review of the literature pertaining to the under-use of hospice services by African Americans and found similar factors as discovered by Reese and her associates (1999). Cultural, institutional, and other barriers also stand between hospice services and other minority groups. Randall and Csikai (2003) studied 110 rural Hispanics and found that most (88%) were not familiar with hospice but were willing to accept hospice care in their homes. Among the barriers were language, poverty, low level of education, and lack of health insurance.

2. *Reaching out to minority groups and responding to their concerns.* Acknowledge the reality of the barriers between hospice services and minority groups and plan to break or reduce them. That can involve several activities:

• *Reaching out to groups on the other side of the barriers.* The reaching out should be marked by (a) a genuine interest in the people of the group; (b) respect for their worldview and perspective on life and death; (c) empathy and a desire to serve; and (d) conscious, constant, and sincere efforts. Reaching out can be achieved directly as well as through their leaders and institutions. For example, for African Americans, these would be ministers and churches.

• *Always keeping in mind that trust building with the group or community is extremely important.* Trust building is hard because of the mistrust in many of these groups of the mainstream culture and society at large. For example, many African Americans often view white helpers as an extension of white supremacy and racism. On the other hand, to varying degrees, negative attitudes and beliefs about people in these groups abound in the larger society. Nevertheless, self-awareness in terms of social workers acknowledging their own biases, prejudices, and concepts of what is normal and healthy; ability to accept the validity of others' perspectives on their lives and situations; willingness to consider others as culturally equal to them; and

communication of genuineness, sincerity, and warmth will go a long way to build trust.

• *Recognizing that within a group or community, there is diversity across all spheres of life, including religion and theology, family functioning, socioeconomic situation, acculturation, and political involvement.* The following paragraphs will give an idea of this diversity:

We all know that Native Americans belong to more than 500 different tribes and there are differences among them based on tribal affiliation. There are also differences between those who live on reservations and those off reservations, as well as between those who live in rural areas and those in urban areas. Hence, there are differences based on the level of acculturation. Some have totally assimilated into the mainstream, while others have retained their native language, beliefs, ceremonial practices, values, and customs. Furthermore, there is no universally accepted definition of who a Native American is and what it means to be one. Of course, there are also differences based on socioeconomic status.

Asian Americans represent about 30 countries of Asia and almost as many islands in the Pacific. There are vast differences among them based on national-ethnic variations. Even those from the same country may speak different languages, profess different religions, dress differently, eat different foods, observe different customs, and have different worldviews. There are differences based on immigration status, level of acculturation, and socioeconomic status and situations.

The same is true of Hispanic or Latino Americans. There are differences among them based on the countries they came from or trace their ancestry to. Their major groups are Mexican Americans, Puerto Ricans, Cuban Americans, Central and South Americans, and Caribbeans. Although most Latinos are Catholic, more and more are turning to churches of other Christian denominations. Many Puerto Ricans are also adherents of spiritism, and many Cubans are adherents of Santeria. Sociodemographic factors also divide Latino Americans.

Even among African Americans, there are differences based on when they came to the United States. There are those who are the descendants of slaves, those who came from Caribbean islands, and those who came as immigrants from various African countries. There are differences on the basis of religion, levels of acculturation, socioeconomic status, and sociopolitical experiences (Dhooper & Moore, 2001).

However, there are some commonalities among all these groups, such as the importance of family, extended family ties, religious faith, experience of racism as Americans, and a general sense of powerlessness. Most of them also hold on to different theories of illness and suffering and approaches to healing and help.

• *Looking for commonalities between program ideals, ideas, approaches, and activities, and the views and needs of potential clients.* In any situation, there are always universal as well as unique elements. Looking for the universal and building on those creates the commonality and opens a window for understanding and intervention. Reese et al. (1999) gave an example of how the beliefs of African Americans about illness, death, treatment, and care can be seen as compatible with the hospice philosophy and approach. Their stoicism in the face of death and reliance on God's will as resignation can be interpreted as an ability to accept one's death without fear.

> Some African Americans may feel that since God is in charge, life-sustaining treatment may not determine whether one lives or dies. These views are consistent with the hospice philosophy of acceptance of death without great fear and of preference for palliative rather than curative care. (p. 557)

Furthermore, the large familial network can be the source of family support needed for hospice care in the patient's home.

• *Encouraging the organization to conduct public education campaigns through television ads, newsletters, booths at community festivals, and presentations at local places of worship.* Educational efforts should provide facts about life-sustaining

treatments for terminally ill persons, quality and lower cost of hospice care, etc. They should also show hospice as compatible with the community's overall views about death and the dying. In the case of the African American community, for example, that compatibility can be reflected in such ideas as "caring for one's own," "death as homecoming," and "fulfillment of God's will."

3. *Giving minority communities some ownership of hospice and its services.* The reaching out to minority groups and communities that we suggested above will help break the cultural barriers between them and the hospice organization. The goal should be not only to make hospice services acceptable to minority groups and communities but also to make hospice and its services the minority community's own. That will require breaking down institutional barriers through policy changes at the organizational level. Hospice should consider approaching and recruiting prominent members of the minority communities as members of the hospice board (of trustees, directors, advisors, etc.); hiring minority staff members as hospice care providers, both professional and volunteer; providing translation services; and offering culturally diverse spiritual services. With their focus on the African American community, Reese and associates (1999) made the following recommendations:

- Use churches as referral sources.
- Train African American pastors to serve as community representatives.
- Involve African American pastors on boards of directors of hospices.
- Actively recruit African Americans for full-time positions as hospice chaplains and other staff.
- Develop programs to follow patients from active treatment to palliative care.
- Provide hospice care to African Americans in nursing homes.

RELEVANT ETHICAL CONSIDERATIONS

Since most of the current and likely future recipients of social work services in long-term settings are the elderly and since, with 80% of all deaths occurring in individuals over age 65, death has become the province of the elderly (Kearl, as quoted in Luptak, 2004), we devote this section to issues associated with the end-of-life care and dying of the elderly. A brief description of the historical changes in the "how" and "where" of death and evolution of end-of-life care is provided as the context for our discussion.

In ancient days, people viewed death as a process that could not be helped and sought to find the meaning of death and ways to make the movement from life to death as comfortable as possible in the presence of family and friends. The struggle against death began in the 16th and 17th centuries, but even then, people died at home being cared for by their families and in the midst of their loved ones. Two centuries later, as the causes of disease were discovered, hospitals became the institutions for the study and treatment of the sick, and the process of dying became "medicalized" (Luptak, 2004). Today, most deaths in the United States take place in institutions—hospitals and nursing homes.

The elderly did not dominate the death scene in the olden days. Most people did not live long enough to be old; they died young, and childhood deaths were also common. Throughout the 20th century, increased longevity, changes in family structure, rapid urbanization, and advances in medical technology influenced American attitudes toward the elderly and policies about end-of-life care (Kaplan, 1995). Myths about aging (e.g., old people are resistant to change, unproductive, and senile) developed. In the public mind, the litany of "D" characterized the elderly: decline, disease, disability, dementia, depression, dependency, disengagement, and death. Now, the popular attitudes are slowly turning positive. Society has gradually responded to the needs of the elderly—through Social Security, Medicare, and other programs—and their end-of-life needs are being recognized.

In the first half of the 20th century, the number of older people quadrupled because of lower birth rate, lower mortality, and lessened immigration. Sophisticated interventions became available to cure illnesses and prolong life, and

medical decisions became more complicated and responsibility for decision making began to shift from individuals and families to professionals. Death denial became the prevailing orientation as dramatic shifts occurred in who died, how they died, and when they died. (Luptak, 2004, p. 8)

Thus, "the presence of physicians and hospitals at the end of people's lives has also led to the intrusion of medical professionals and health care systems into the natural process of dying" (Mackelprang & Mackelprang, 2005, p. 315).

Another set of forces was also at work. The consumerism movement of the 1960s and 1970s affected the issues of aging also. Decision making started shifting from a model that fostered medical paternalism to one that emphasized patients' right to self-determination, and the end-of-life care movement started. End-of-life care has become institutionalized, but the treatment choices have also expanded, which has complicated decision making. Mackelprang and Mackelprang (2005) conceptualized end-of-life care on a four-level continuum: (1) care that is palliative—alleviates pain and provides comfort but does not prolong life; (2) care that involves noninvasive efforts to preserve or prolong life and may involve oral antibiotics; (3) care that involves intravenous medications and artificial hydration and nutrition; and (4) care that involves invasive treatments such as artificial ventilation and cardiopulmonary resuscitation. Terminally ill persons have to decide the level of care they want. When they are incapable of deciding and did not make their wishes known beforehand, surrogates decide for them.

There are also interventions that hasten death, which equally require a decision by terminally ill persons or their surrogates. Mackelprang and Mackelprang (2005) put those interventions into four categories: (1) declining curative or restorative treatment, such as surgery, chemotherapy, and radiation for a cancer patient, so that death can take its natural course; (2) allowing the withholding or withdrawal of life-extending measures such as intravenous medications, feeding tubes, and ventilators; (3) allowing treatment such as the use of high levels of morphine that results in depressed respiration and cardiac functioning; and (4) seeking assisted suicide and euthanasia. Oregon is the only state in the United States that gives people the right to die and allows physician-assisted suicides. Decisions about these options have become public, resulting in the involvement of the courts. Besides the court judgments, society has responded with such measures as the Patient Self-Determination Act of 1991, advanced directives, and do-not-resuscitate orders.

The Patient Self-Determination Act (P.L. 101-508) is the first federal law that reinforces the right of adults to refuse life-sustaining treatment. It requires all health care organizations that receive Medicare and Medicaid payments (hospitals, nursing homes, and in-home care providers) to provide adult patients information about state laws regarding advanced directives. At the time of admission, patients are asked if they have an advanced directive or desire one. If one is created, it is placed in the patient's chart. The law also directed the Department of Health and Human Services to conduct a national campaign to inform the public about advanced directives.

Advanced directives allow competent adults to make a written statement about how they wish to be treated at the end of life, including medical care preferences. These directives include the durable power of attorney for health care and living will (also known as directive to physician) documents (NASW, 2006). The durable power of attorney for health care, or health care proxy or agent, is an individual appointed by a patient to make health care decisions if the patient becomes incompetent. A living will is written by a competent adult to control health care decisions in the event of that person's incompetency. Every state has created legislation and a set of regulations for advanced directives. They provide that (1) patients can maintain control over what happens to them when they become physically or mentally incapable to participate in decision making; (2) guidance is given to decision makers regarding life-sustaining treatments; and (3) immunity is available to health care providers from civil or criminal liability when they honor advanced directives in the face of objections by family or surrogates (O'Donnell, 2004).

Do-not-resuscitate orders (DNRs) can be a part of an advanced directive along with a durable power of attorney, living will, and health care proxy. A DNR is an order written by a physician indicating that no cardiopulmonary resuscitation is to be performed if the patient's heartbeat and breathing stop. This order is in response to a decision by the patient, his or her health care agent, or a family member.

Ethical Challenges. The decisions about terminally ill persons' levels of care and interventions that hasten death, and even the societal prescriptions about the "who" and "how" of those decisions, are fraught with ethical challenges.

The issues related to end-of-life care revolve around the concept of a "good" death. However, there is no universally accepted definition of a good death. The quality of life—determined as it is by a host of socioeconomic factors, including health care—and cultural beliefs decide how individuals view death and dying. Crawley (2007) captured this reality in his question,

> How does one define a "good death" for the person whose life has been constrained by disadvantage, or whose imminent death may result, in whole or in part, from societal factors responsible for socioeconomic inequalities or racial or ethnic-based inequalities? (p. 223)

In general, it is difficult for most people to discuss death and dying, partly because of death anxiety, which can include fears about the process of dying, death itself, and what happens thereafter. "Nowhere is death anxiety seen more clearly than in patients suffering from terminal or potentially terminal conditions. Facing one's own mortality is a frightening experience that one cannot totally prepare for" (Zilberfein & Hurwitz, 2004, p. 298).

As stated earlier, the process of death has been medicalized. Advances in medical technology have transformed previously fatal illnesses into chronic illnesses that can be treated (Callahan, 2000). Thus, death is viewed as something that should be controlled, and it continues to be seen as a medical failure (Silverman, 2004). Cure-oriented treatment to extend life is preferred over end-of-life care, and there is a reluctance to withdraw treatment (on moral or legal grounds) even when it is not working. At the same time, decisions about the use of medical technologies raise ethical questions about the equitable allocation of expensive and limited resources. The concept of medical futility—defined as treatment that will not alter the natural course of disease but may add physical, social, and emotional burdens to the patient (Schneiderman, Jecker, & Jonsen, 1990)—is gaining ground. However, there is no agreement on what the criteria for futile treatment should be and who should determine futility.

The proportion of those who have executed advanced directives continues to be low—only 1 in 4 patients has done it (Gerbino & Henderson, 2004). In the absence of these directives, as the decision-making capacity of patients diminishes, the likelihood of their wishes being ignored becomes high. This is true not only of patients being treated in hospitals but also of those receiving palliative care. Other factors become reasons for raising questions about patients' decisional capacity and often deprive them of autonomous decision making. It is also likely that families and/or care providers will decide for those who have limited command over the English language (and must rely on others to translate and interpret their wishes), persons with psychiatric disorders, those with cognitive impairments such as dementia, ones with histories of substance abuse, and those who are incarcerated or in foster care. Csikai (2004) talked about the dilemma caused by attempts to balance the rights of self-determination of patients and their families in end-of-life care. Reese (2000) studied hospice care patients and found that caregiver denial often resulted in inpatient hospice stays for patients who had desired to die at home.

The United States is increasingly becoming a multicultural society, but in the eyes of most health care professionals, the "ideal" patient is one who shares the Western ethical precepts of truth telling and respect for patient autonomy (Davis, 2000). Patients whose cultures emphasize different values become difficult to deal with. The Patient Self-Determination Act, which is underpinned by the principle of autonomy, reflects the belief that all patients have the same belief system and that cultural differences are not important. In reality, in many cultural groups, families or elders make all vital decisions affecting a family member, may prefer that the member not be told the truth about his or her diagnosis/prognosis, and may believe that discussing death will somehow bring death on the patient. However, acculturation is another reality, and there are variations in the observation of cultural values by individuals and families. Working with such patients and their families is ethically challenging.

Social workers will find the following suggestions helpful in dealing with ethically challenging situations:

1. Strive constantly to strengthen your knowledge base of policy and practice issues pertaining to aging, death and dying, and end-of-life care. Improve and refine your assessment and intervention skills for work with clients of varied socioeconomic and cultural backgrounds. This improvement may also involve confronting your own mortality and/or unresolved grief from a personal loss (Crawley, 2007).

2. Let the NASW (2004) Policy Statement on Client Self-Determination and End-of-Life Decisions guide your professional roles and behaviors. This statement defines end-of-life decisions as choices made by a terminally ill person regarding his or her continuing care or treatment. It emphasizes the *right* of individuals to choose among all available care options and social workers' *responsibility* to ensure that all options are presented to patients and families and that they are assisted in understanding the meaning and possible outcomes of treatments as they affect quality of life. It provides specific action steps for both worker-client–level activity and cause-related advocacy.

3. Know that despite the difficulty of defining a "good" death, consensus is emerging about the attributes of such a death. These include the following factors: (1) It happens at a very old age; (2) it is not a prolonged process (as in a coma); (3) it does not involve uncontrolled pain and suffering; (4) the dying person's physical and emotional capacities are intact; (5) there is no loss of control or personal dignity; (6) it happens in the midst of one's loved ones (not in isolation); (7) all family conflicts are resolved; (8) it does not cause undue burden (financial or emotional) to the family; and (9) there is meaning in the person's death—the death matters to others (American Medical Association, 1999; Callahan, 2000; Zilberfein & Hurwitz, 2004). Deal with factors (e.g., professional attitudes and institutional policies) that make it difficult for many terminally ill persons to experience good deaths.

4. In many acute care settings, it is not uncommon to be confronted with a situation where a patient has not made his or her wishes regarding end-of-life care known and can no longer do so. In such cases, use your advocacy skills to ensure "that persons who do not explicitly state their wishes still get treatment that is close to what most people would want" (Lynn et al., 2000, p. S221).

5. In many acute care settings, palliative care is not an option in the treatment of terminally ill patients. Advocate for incorporating the palliative care perspective. That will enable caregiving professionals to remain focused on and provide for the total care needs of the patient (O'Donnell, 2004).

6. Know that sometimes the reluctance to withhold and withdraw treatment is based on moral or legal myths. "Many believe that withdrawal of life support is equated with murder and suicide. Others believe that once a treatment is initiated, it cannot be discontinued" (O'Donnell, 2004, p. 177). Understand the legal and moral contexts of withholding and withdrawing treatment, and participate in the education of all involved in such situations. "In some cases, dying patients who have lacked access to health care may view discussion of withdrawal or withholding of care as yet a further example of social injustice" (Crawley, 2007, p. 227). Make sure that ethical principles of justice and equity inform decision making in all such cases.

7. Actively participate in the education of patients and their families about the legal and moral rights of patients to decide what treatment they want or do not want. Give them clear information about all the available options, and support them in their choice. Cagle and Kovacs (2009) urged that education be recognized as an essential component of professional practice. They provided a theory-based approach to education.

8. Remember that in palliative care, social workers are not as focused on individual treatment as are other members of the care team and, therefore, can focus on the overall goals of care as desired by the patient and family. Furthermore, they have a bridge role in explaining the context of care to patients and their families and explaining concerns of patients and families to staff members (O'Donnell, 2004).

9. Recognize that the principles of palliative care are reflective of the core social work values. "Viewing the individual in a holistic way, considering the family as the 'unit of care,' examining the client's experience across the continuum of care, and building on the strengths of the family system are inherent to social work practice" (Blacker, 2004, p. 419).

10. Be actively involved in the ethics committee of your institution in resolving ethically challenging situations. In many such committees, social workers are playing leadership roles. Wherever an ethics committee is not available, as in the case of many hospices, participate in the meetings of the interdisciplinary group discussing ethical issues and enrich its deliberations with social work's ethical perspective, along with case-specific information. You should suggest and participate in the development of policies

that address common ethical issues and in the education of the hospice staff. You can make this contribution by using your communication skills, by promoting your profession's central values of self-determination and respect for individual worth and dignity, and by helping others recognize the interplay of people and their environments (Csikai, 2004).

11. In Chapter 6, we presented a model of culturally proficient and ethical practice. Skills discussed there are relevant in the end-of-life care situations of culturally diverse patients and their families as well. Koenig (1997) suggested the following questions to enhance the cultural sensitivity of social work assessment:

- Is information about diagnosis/prognosis openly discussed in this culture? If not, how is information managed?
- Is death an appropriate topic for discussion?
- Is maintaining hope considered essential?
- How is the decision making done? Is it shared with patient/family or delegated by patient to someone else?
- How is quality of life versus quantity of life weighed?
- Does the patient/family trust that the health care providers will act in their best interest? (p. 373)

12. Reflect on how answers to the above questions will affect your intervention approach and strategies. Keep abreast of the various theories and approaches of bioethics and see how those can enrich your repertoire of knowledge and skills. Generally, added sensitivity, some creativity, extra efforts to build and retain trust, discussion with colleagues, or assistance from an ethics committee would suffice in dealing with difficult situations (e.g., telling the truth without doing undue harm) and dealing with questions of diversity and justice.

13. Csikai (2004) surveyed 110 hospice social workers in six states regarding ethical issues in hospice care. These social workers had no access to an ethics committee. The issues of assisted suicide and euthanasia were the least discussed

among ethically challenging situations listed by the participants in this survey. However, 32% of them indicated that they had received a request from a patient to discuss assisted suicide and 17% had received a similar request from a family member. How should social workers respond to such requests? The NASW (2004) Policy Statement on Client Self-Determination and End-of-Life Decisions provides the following guidance.

- Facilitate client and family understanding of all aspects and options in end-of-life care.
- Assess mental health functioning to include assisting in decisional capacity determinations, depression, anxiety, suicidal ideation, and facilitate or provide intervention or referrals for care.
- Be knowledgeable about state-specific policies on end-of-life care.
- Be present (if the social worker is comfortable with being present) with a client or family in assisted-suicide situations in states where this practice is legal and requested by the client. (NASW, 2006, pp. 133–34)

Critical Thinking Questions

1. We have discussed the evolution of the societal response to death and dying. Changes in society, family, and medical science and technology have led to the medicalization of death. Medical and health care personnel and establishments are deciding when, where, and how death takes place. Assuming that the anticipated changes in the various dimensions of life (projected in Chapter 1) come true, what is likely to be the next stage in this evolutionary process and what will be the major features of that stage?

2. Study the concepts of "good death" and "medical futility" and how these are operationalized in the health care setting with which you are associated. Do the "dos" resulting from that operationalization allow for significant options for patients and their families in view of the "dos" drawn from the NASW Policy Statement on Client Self-Determination and End-of-Life Decisions? How can you increase the options and/or improve the substance of those options?

NOTES

1. As per the federal regulations, a qualified social worker is an individual with (i) a bachelor's degree in social work or a bachelors' degree in a human services field, including but not limited to sociology, special education, rehabilitation counseling, and psychology, and (ii) 1 year of supervised social work experience in a health care setting working directly with individuals (Bern-Klug, 2008, p. 383).

2. The goal of palliative care is similar to that of hospice care—that is, the treatment of the whole person. That involves meeting all the patient's medical, physical, psychological, social, and spiritual needs. However, palliative care is not necessarily for those who are terminally ill. Many who receive palliative care will improve and do well, whereas the recipients of hospice care are dealing with the reality of imminent death.

3. The National Advisory Committee identified the following principles:

o Case management is a consumer-centered service that respects consumers' rights, values, and preferences.

o Case management coordinates all and any type of assistance to meet identified consumer needs.

o Case management requires clinical skills and competencies.

o Case management promotes the quality of services provided.

o Case management strives to use resources efficiently (Gerson & Chassler, 1995).

8

THRIVING IN HEALTH CARE

In this chapter, we present strategies, based on an extensive review of the literature, that are helpful in enhancing social worker effectiveness and efficiency. Most social workers can easily acquire and refine these strategies. As in any host setting, social work in health care is strenuous. It involves not only providing social work services to clients but also constantly educating others and demonstrating how social work contributes to the setting's overall function, helps fill the gaps in its services, and enriches the quality of those services.

> Whether the practice domain be a hospital, a clinic, the legislative or public health district, an HMO [health maintenance organization] or a shelter, the health social worker is constantly moving on a moment's notice between potentially conflicting roles, statuses, functions, and contexts. (Dillon, 1990, p. 91)

The strategies for thriving in health care have been clustered into two groups: worker-focused strategies and other strategies. Table 8-A shows a list of those strategies.

WORKER-FOCUSED STRATEGIES

Stress Management

Stress has been the subject of a lot of theorizing and research over a long period of time.

Table 8-A Strategies for Thriving in Health Care

Worker-Focused Strategies

- Stress management
- Time management
- Self-empowerment
- Using research skills

Other Strategies

- Conflict resolution
- Coalition building
- Community work
- Culturally sensitive practice

Cooper and Dewe (2004) wrote a book on the history of stress. They traced the use of the term *stress* back to the 17th century and discussed the work of Robert Hooke, Walter Cannon, Hans Selye, Harold Wolff, Richard Lazarus, and others, as well as the ideational and societal contexts in which the concept of stress developed. A lot of attention also has been devoted to coping with stress through various approaches to and models of stress management. There is no agreement among scholars about the precise meaning of the term *stress*.

Nevertheless, evidence continues to accumulate and be reported in terms of the millions of dollars lost each year in production, sickness absence, premature death, and retirements, escalating health insurance costs, the increasing use of stress management interventions, and the wide range of health and well-being issues reported under the banner of stress. (Cooper & Dewe, 2004, p. 117)

The stressfulness of social work in health care settings is a major reality that must be acknowledged and dealt with. Otherwise, this stress tends to result in burnout.

Stress is influenced by a host of factors, including genes, events, lifestyle, attitudes, and thoughts. Whereas we may not have much control over the genetic factors, we can alter our lifestyles, attitudes, and thoughts, and can change the stressful events and/or modify our perception of them. Various models for understanding and management of stress have been proposed. For example, Meichenbaum and Jaremko (1983) hold that stress lies neither in the individual nor in the situation but, rather, depends on the transaction of the individual in the situation. The transactional model of stress views stress as resulting from an imbalance between demands and resources—that is, when the demands of the situation exceed the individual's resources for dealing with it or when pressure exceeds one's perceived ability to cope (Lazarus & Folkman, 1984). On the other hand, the health realization/innate health (HR/IH) model views stress as resulting from appraising oneself and one's situation through a mental filter of insecurity and negativity. "HR/IH proposes that 'stressors' are the moment-to-moment perceptions of a mind innocently caught up in negative, upsetting thinking without recognition and understanding of the process that is driving the experience" (Sedgeman, 2005, p. HY49). It does not question the existence of external, unpleasant, and sometimes tragic circumstances but emphasizes an internal mediating factor between external circumstances and one's experience of them and that each person has the power to determine how those circumstances will affect him or her.

A manifold approach to stress management would yield the best results. It should include an assessment of the stressful situation, one's reaction, and resources, and should aim at developing skills

appropriate for preventing, preparing for, and responding to stress. Drawn from various sources, the following are a few helpful suggestions for social workers to follow.

- *Take an inventory of their attitudes and consciously work on modifying the ones that are unhealthy, unhelpful, and dysfunctional.*
- *Look at their lifestyle critically and incorporate into it on a regular basis (a) some exercise, (b) some recreation, (c) some relaxation, and (d) an appropriate, nutritious diet.* These strategies have significant preventive and preparatory stress management relevance. The literature—both popular and professional—on the "how" of these strategies is enormous and rich. Techniques abound. For example, relaxation techniques include deep breathing, progressive muscle relaxation, imagery, meditation, self-hypnosis, and biofeedback.
- *Leave their work at the office and not let work-related stuff clutter their personal lives.* At the same time, they should attend to the potential or present stresses in their personal lives because these tend to deplete their energy and adversely affect their ability to deal with work-related stress. Improving interpersonal communication, problem solving, using social skills, and seeking professional help, if needed, are appropriate measures.
- *Identify major situational factors that cause stress and devise appropriate strategies to deal with them.* Dillon (1990) listed several of these, including (a) existential stressors, (b) team stressors, (c) sex role stressors, (d) membership stressors, (c) family influences as stressors, and (f) vulnerability (because of the relative unimportance of psychosocial functions) as a stressor. Some of these require renewed commitment to the social work mission and values, others improved professional skills, others the creation or strengthening of formal and informal support systems, and still others organizational work aimed at improving the status of the social work department or unit.
- *Build a support group of colleagues or friends who can understand and relate to their frustrations.* Without support, a stressful situation becomes harder to deal with. Mix some enjoyable activity with the sharing, ventilation, and problem solving within the group.

• *Consciously try to recognize how they respond to stress.* The beliefs people hold about themselves and the world around them also affect their responses to stress. De-emphasize beliefs that are unrealistic and have the potential to create or add to stress. Klarreich (quoted in DiNitto & McNeece, 1990) identified 13 such beliefs, including (a) something terrible will happen if I make a mistake, (b) it is awful to be criticized, (c) people in authority should not be challenged, (d) life must be fair and just, (e) I must be in control all the time, (f) I must anticipate everything, (g) I must feel perfect all the time, and (h) I was promised a rose garden.

• *Convince themselves that positive thinking provides a positive view of people, problems, and possibilities, and generates hope and optimism.* Positive thinking is likely to lead to positive actions with desirable consequences. Social workers should form the habit of thinking positively and thereby looking for the positive side of things. They should remember that they have the ability to create a new experience via thinking. The following observation of Sedgeman (2005) about clients applies to others as well:

When they begin to see the nature of thought, they are able to use distress as a warning sign to stop ruminating. Then their natural, resilient flow of thinking can resume. Upsetting thoughts lose their power; they are no more real, and just as real, as any other thoughts. (p. HY50)

• *Recognize that most work-related tasks do not require perfection*; even with the best of intentions, planning, and problem-solving skills, mistakes are likely to be made. Social workers should think of their previous accomplishments, put the situation in the proper perspective, and try to recover from their mistakes.

• *Try not to be immobilized by fears, whether real or imagined.*

As a technique for handling your fears, try exaggerating them all out of proportion. For example, if you fear being embarrassed, visualize yourself blushing to the point of turning beet red, sweating buckets, and shaking so hard your watch vibrates off your wrist. Exaggerating your fears to the point of being ludicrous may help you laugh at yourself and put your fear into perspective. (Sheafor, Horejsi, & Horejsi, 1988, p. 174)

• *Develop and maintain a sense of humor.* Humor helps diffuse potentially unpleasant situations, put things in perspective, reduce negative feelings, and relax us. Social workers may find "Saving Face in the Status Race" by Winkler (1980) humorous.

Time Management

Lack of time management can add to the loss of control over one's situation and to a sense of being overwhelmed. In busy health care settings, time is always a scarce resource. Some research has been done on time's place in medical settings (e.g., see Finley, Mutran, Zeitler, & Randall, 1990; Frankenberg, 1992; Yoel & Clair, 1994). Yoel and Clair (1994) studied how medical residents learned to manage time over the course of their residencies and found that controlling time was an ongoing concern and a central dimension of their subculture. This controlling is influenced by the structural constraints of the residency program, such as the year of residency; patient care loads; and time management strategies. The latter included learning to work quickly, focusing on only bodily symptoms (to the neglect of the psychosocial realm), making themselves scarce (by not being visible, not wearing lab coats so that patients would not remember the resident's name), manipulating the appointment schedule, deflecting time complaints onto nurses, and using other residents for shortcuts (e.g., asking others for advice rather than reading journal articles).

Lack of adequate time to do a job well has the potential to force one to let the quality of one's work suffer, to experience burnout, or both. Hence, to guard against damage of the quality of their work and/or burnout, social workers should master time management strategies. They have some advantages over many other health care professionals. Their work is not unidimensional; it has much variety, involving as it does interventions with individual clients and their families, interventions on behalf of those clients within the agency and outside, work with other professionals, and organization- and community-level activities. Most social workers are female, and most females with outside-the-home jobs are used to accommodating work-related and household demands. Hessing (1994) studied how women employed in clerical and related office positions managed their time and coordinated their work and household responsibilities. She found that time use was not simply dictated by external demands but, rather, was mediated through an innovative time management process. The methods they used included conformity to and prioritization of the office schedule, manipulation of time use (especially in household schedules), routinization of activities (both in the office and at home), synchronization of events, and preparation for any contingency. These methods highlight the importance of thorough assessment and planning as the basis of time management. Social workers can use the following helpful time management strategies:

- *Understand their job requirements and become clear about their responsibilities.* Analyze the different dimensions of the job either by roles or by major activities. Learn about the priorities of the agency and the order of those priorities and examine how their roles or activities relate to those priorities.
- *Work for a convergence of the agency's goals and objectives and their roles and responsibilities.* Have a clear understanding of how their roles and responsibilities fit into the larger picture. Negotiate, if necessary, with their supervisor or the agency boss to reach that understanding and clarity.
- *Convince themselves that planning their work and setting priorities are absolute necessities.* "Don't hide behind the claim that you are too busy to get organized" (Sheafor et al., 1988, p. 123).
- *Spend a few minutes at the end of each workday to plan for the next day.* List all the tasks to be accomplished and prioritize the list. Setting priorities has several approaches. Lakein (1973) suggested a simple priority system. In his ABC priority system, one assigns an A to all those tasks that are the most important, a B to those tasks that are less important, and a C to those that are the least important. Next, one looks at the tasks within each of these groups and prioritizes

them according to their importance or urgency. The result will be a list of tasks that have been labeled A-1, A-2, A-3; B-1, B-2, B-3; C-l, C-2, C-3; and so on. Another approach is to divide the work into such categories as (a) routine work, (b) regular job duties, (c) special assignments, and (d) creative work, and to assign importance and allot time to the tasks in each category. Still another approach is to create a list of "things to do" for each day, with an estimate of time required to do each thing. One can divide a things-to-do list not only by priority but also by persons involved so that one over-the-telephone or in-person contact can cover several items of business (Sheridan, 1988).

- *Let the priority list or the list of things to do guide their task performance each day, starting with the most important task.* Make sure that the date book containing the priority lists is in a format that best suits their life. Although unforeseen situations and crises will, at times, claim immediate attention and accommodation on the priority list or push a low priority task up into a high-priority position, these do not minimize the importance of establishing priorities as an approach to controlling and managing time.
- *Allow time for emergencies.* Social workers should look for a pattern in emergencies, however, and plan accordingly. If uncovered areas or hours of service generate emergencies, improved coverage may be the answer. Similarly, they should analyze why and when situations tend to escalate into crises. Answers to the following questions will help prevent emergencies: Who is truly experiencing the crisis—the patient, another staff member, or the social worker? Could the crisis have been prevented, as by more thorough work ahead of time? Does an individual emergency actually represent a chronic problem? Procrastination causes matters to become more urgent priorities and usually generates far more anxiety than relief (Sheridan, 1988. p. 98).
- *In noncrisis situations, attend to more difficult and more time-consuming tasks first.*

It is usually best to tackle lengthy tasks before those that can be done in a short period of time. It is also best to schedule work on the most difficult tasks when your energy level is highest (e.g., first thing in the morning). (Sheafor et al., 1988, p. 124)

- *Have a large month-to-month wall calendar hanging in the office.* It will help them keep long-range projects and plans in perspective (Rogak, 1999).
- *Keep handy an updated information file on the "who," "what," and "how" of frequently used resources.* This will prevent the wasting of precious time in locating resources. Similarly, keep the needed forms, handouts, and telephone numbers within easy reach. It will save time.
- *Look for ways of saving time while making referrals to outside resources.* "Community inquiries and referrals can be made in the presence of the patient concerned so that needed information can be exchanged on the spot and the sometimes lengthy process of reporting back is eliminated" (Sheridan, 1988, p. 97).
- *As much as possible, try to do one thing at a time.* Tackling several things at once is often at the cost of both efficiency and quality. Social workers should look around their workplaces and creatively work out ways of reducing interruptions. It may be as simple as closing the door when they are working in the office or gracefully saying no to avoidable demands on their time. It is best to give an unqualified "no," lest the requester interpret it as a conditional refusal (Gillies, 1989).
- *Wherever possible, delegate to others those tasks that do not require professional decision-making skills.* Spending less time performing low-priority items allows more time for important tasks (Pagana, 1995).
- *Master the use of computers.* The use of computers for communication and documentation is already commonplace. However, there is room for individual discretion in the use of computers, from the minimal required to the maximum possible. Social workers should go for the maximum, master the various software, and use the computer as a powerful timesaving and management aid.
- *Use other wonders of technology that can help in time management.* These can include electronic organizers as well as scanners and voice recognition software that can streamline their work and reduce the time spent at the computer (Kogak, 1999).
- *Use the telephone judiciously.*

The problem arises because many people perceive a ringing phone as an urgent signal that has to be answered immediately. They believe that if they're sitting there, they should interrupt whatever they're working on and pick up the receiver instead of letting the answering machine or voice mail handle it. (Kogak, 1999, p. 93)

- *Get the most of their phone time.* Set aside a particular time for making outgoing calls and stick to it. It can be the first thing in the morning or in the mid- to late afternoon. When leaving a voice mail message, let the recipient of the message know when they will be answering the phone. "It's also a good idea on your outgoing voice mail message to let people know the specific times that you do pick up the phone" (Kogak, 1999, p. 93).
- *Limit time spent in meetings.* Meetings are often the source of time loss. For limiting the time spent in meetings, Sheafor et al. (1988) provided the following helpful recommendations:

Consider alternatives to a meeting, such as telephone calls.

Choose the location and time for the meeting that would ensure the most efficient use of time

Attend the meeting for the time needed for one's contribution.

Define the purpose of the meeting clearly so that everyone comes prepared.

Prepare an agenda and follow it.

Stay on the task.

Start on time and end on time.

Control interruptions.

Evaluate the success of the meeting and make that the basis for improvements in the future.

- *From time to time, analyze how they spend their time on different dimensions of the work, the degree of control they have over their time, and the time management strategies they use.* Let that analysis help them discover their mistakes and guide their future planning and organizing. A comparison of time actually spent with time estimated for specific tasks can be particularly helpful. Social workers can identify their most productive hours for high-priority tasks or activities requiring high concentration (Sheridan, 1988).

Self-Empowerment

Working in host settings dominated by high-power professionals who may not fully realize the significance of one's professional contributions has the possibility of creating a sense of power-lessness. Although the client's self-determination always has been a basic value of social work practice, during the past three to four decades the profession has emphasized the importance of empowerment as a fundamental practice principle. "Building on empowerment theories of the 1980s and 1990s, social work has moved the concept of empowerment from value and philosophical levels to practice principles, frameworks, and methods" (Parsons, 2008). Empowerment-based practice is strength oriented so that social workers look for strengths in their clients and clients' situations and environments, as well as help them acquire new strengths in the form of problem-solving skills and resources. The same workers, however, have not always used their professional skills for self-empowerment. There has been a perception that power is bad. Now it is being realized that empowerment also involves enhancement of workers' feelings of self-efficacy by identifying and removing conditions that foster powerlessness (Bartle, Couchonnal, Canda, & Staker, 2002). Assuming that a powerless worker cannot be an optimum source of empowerment for others, we discuss below the concepts of "power" and "empowerment" and approaches to self-empowerment.

Power is the ability to carry out one's will. It manifests itself in the form of authority, as well as influence. *Authority* lies in the position and not the occupier of the position, whereas *influence* comes more from the individual than from his or her position (Berger, 1990). Power has several bases. Building on the work of French and Raven (1959), Bisno (1988) identified the following:

Reward power is based on the ability to provide rewards.

Coercive power is based on the ability to punish.

Expert power is contingent on the desired knowledge and skills.

Positional power is derived from filling an "official" position.

Informational power lies in the capacity to control the flow of information.

Exchange power comes from the ability to create an imbalance in exchange relationships (e.g., "calling in" a political IOU).

Mobilizational power is based on the capacity to mobilize other people's support for desired goals.

Moral power lies in the capacity to gain one's objectives by invoking moral commitments from others.

Personal power is contingent on personal characteristics (e.g., attractiveness, persuasiveness, charisma) that enable one to affect the behavior of others.

Positional or legitimate power is based on the formal delegation of rights and responsibilities. This comes from the formal authority designated by the structure of the organization. It is, however, only one of several sources of power. "Individuals in the organization can acquire some degree of power regardless of their location in the hierarchical structure, professional training, or status" (Berger, 1990, p. 80). Power is dynamic and relative. This discussion of self-empowerment emphasizes strategies for increasing one's influence irrespective of one's official position in the organization. The strategies are divided into two groups: one focused on attitudes and the other on skills.

Social workers should consciously develop and cultivate attitudes that reflect a brighter and positive view of the world and their ability to affect it. They will find the following suggestions helpful:

• *Carefully study the situations that seem "impossible" and look for the presence of hope, howsoever feeble. A simple apostrophe has the power to turn Impossible into I'mpossible. Substitute "something" for "nothing"; instead of assuming that nothing can be done about the situation, shift to the stance that "something can be done about the situation." That leads to exploring "what can be done" and moving on to* "this is what can be done" about the situation. This idea of the possible was impressively conveyed by a cartoon accompanying a paper by Lawrence (1980). It showed, on the one end, a man looking at a flying bird and wondering whether he could do likewise and, on the other, a flying jet. Underneath were written the words spoken by an ancient philosopher: "Anything the human mind can conceive it can one day consider; anything the human mind can consider long enough it can one day accept; anything the human mind can accept it can one day believe; and anything the human mind can believe it can act upon."

• *Consciously guard against acquiring a victim mentality.* Settings dominated by more powerful professionals and social workers' identification with weak and powerless clients tend to encourage such a mentality. Although appealing, it is not helpful. Anyone who has choices is not a victim; social workers have choices and the ability to make and increase choices. The notion of choices is applicable to the realm of feelings as well. John Wax, a social worker with the Veterans Affairs medical system for years, advised that to increase their choices, social workers should practice controlling their first response to a stimulus.

Feel your response but do not go with it. Process your experience and multiply your responses, then use the best response. That allows you to ensure that others do not control your emotions and you are able to make it the other party's problem. (Wax, 1982)

• *High self-esteem is a must for self-empowerment.* High self-esteem comes from many sources, some of which one has control over. Social workers can build strong attitudinal views of their capabilities, and "the world largely accepts us at our own estimate of ourselves. There is a good reason: It is because we almost always live up to our own estimate of ourselves" (Lawrence, 1980, p. 19). Programming their thinking positively will help improve their self-image. The programming tool is the subconscious mind. It is always moved by a positive suggestion. It will respond to the direction of the conscious mind, and it will not consider whether the suggestion of the conscious mind is right or wrong. The subconscious simply accepts. If one says, "I am

angry" or "I am afraid," the subconscious mind will accept the dictate of the conscious mind and create the characteristics of fear or anger in the body. It is important to realize that a statement such as "I am not afraid" or "I am not angry" has no impact on the subconscious. The subconscious does not understand the word not. Therefore, the suggestion must be positive: "I am calm" or "I am courageous" (p. 19).

• *Labeling one's experiences determines the meaning one gives to those experiences, and one's ability to give meaning to one's experiences is the most powerful thing going for a person* (Wax, 1982). This ability can be developed and enhanced. Social workers should work on assigning positive labels to stressful and unpleasant experiences. Adverse situations can thus be turned into opportunities for learning and growth.

• *Recognize one's strengths and the relevance of those strengths to the mission and purpose of one's organization.* For example, social work's holistic approach to people and their problems, and workers' comprehensive understanding of clients and their ability to intervene at different levels are some of the unique strengths they bring to their work.

• *Learn to be assertive but not aggressive.* Assertiveness is a learned attribute. Assertive statements start with *I,* whereas aggressive statements start with *You.* Social workers should use their professional and interpersonal communication skills for self-empowerment.

• *Treat one's job as the gateway to power.* Social workers should take responsibility for their job, take it seriously, and do it so well that they acquire a high reputation for their knowledge, skills, wisdom, integrity, and credibility. They should cultivate dependency in others, professionally and otherwise.

• *Remember that the approaches and strategies that are effective with clients are equally effective with other people as well.* The relevant practice principles are as follows: (a) Start where the other person is; (b) recognize his or her needs; (c) affirm his or her strengths; (d) understand his or her point of view or let him or her know that you really want to understand that point of view; (e) respect differences; (f) use all the channels of communication—verbal, extraverbal, and nonverbal; and (g) give credit for his or her situation-related efforts and accomplishments.

- *Use the problem-solving process learned and mastered as social workers.* Every situation lends itself to the use of that process.

- *Wherever possible, use group work skills.* Monitoring and careful handling of the group process can make social workers significant contributors to group problem solving. Fighting in groups is a time-limited phenomenon; people get tired. Keeping out of the conflict, looking for the first sign of the desire for reconciliation, and introducing a new idea or solution will save the situation (Wax, 1982).

- *Put one's understanding of the crisis theory and crisis intervention skills to use in dealing with other professionals and the organization in crisis situations.* In crises, people and organizations are much more open to suggestions and amenable to change.

- *Look for other sources of power and borrow it from those sources.* Building and strengthening coalitions and alliances with others increases one's power base and provides opportunities to influence those in the alliances and others through those alliances.

- *Understand that power can be derived also from structural sources.* Resource control and network centrality are among the major structural sources. Those who secure or control the supply of essential resources for the organization acquire power (Astley & Sachdeva, 1984; Jansson & Simmons, 1984). Similarly, those who are in the center of the network of relationships among the many positions essential for the organization's workflow gain power (Gummer, 1985). Social workers should explore ways of encroaching on both these sources of power individually or as a unit. In earlier chapters, we discussed ideas for social work contributions to creating new resources for organizations. In the words of Berger (1990),

> For example, social work departments are creating fiscally sound plans for the development and management within the hospital home health care programs, revenue producing counseling services, case management for a variety of clinical groups (elderly, maternal-child health, AIDS and transplant patients), and bio-feedback programs within the hospital setting. (p. 88)

- *Realize that making one's activities essential to the organization's workflow will bring one into the network.* The role of a case manager is potentially powerful because all service providers depend on the case manager for the maximum effectiveness of their interventions. With her focus on hospital-based social work, Berger (1990) said, "Social work is often at the central point or node in the network for discharge planning by virtue of its skills in helping individuals in crisis, its counseling skills, as well as its knowledge of community resources" (p. 89).

In short, social workers should be alert to "the potential power opportunities residing in the multiple sources of power that exist in every organization, including both individual and structural sources" (Berger, 1990, p. 91).

Using Research Skills

Social workers should view their knowledge of research methodology and their research-related skills as essential parts of their professional repertoire.

> An important attribute of a profession is the systematic study of its practices, to continually advance its service modalities. Throughout its history, the social work profession has engaged in research and sought to strengthen connections between research and practice. (Tripodi, Lalayants, & Zlotnik, 2008)

Examples of early research work include the study of deserted wives reported by Mary Richmond in 1895 and the 1907 Pittsburgh survey that was an elaborate social investigation of the conditions of that city (Task Force on Social Work Research, 1991). Austin (2003) provided other examples from the early history of research in social work, including links between social work and social sciences. Those include case studies from the Charity Organization Society and the 1909 Russell Sage Foundation-supported survey research "The Standards of Living Among Workingmen's Families in New York City." Those studies led to workers' compensation and child labor laws. Thus, social workers all along have appreciated the importance of systematic research for dealing with social problems and strengthening the scientific base of the profession. The Institute for the Advancement of Social Work Research (2003) defines social work research as addressing psychosocial problems, treatment of acute and chronic conditions, and community, organizational, policy, and administrative issues. Reid (1995) divided social work research literature into four categories:

> studies of (1) behaviors, personality, problems, and other characteristics of individuals, families, and small groups; (2) characteristics, utilization, and outcome of services; (3) attitudes, orientations, and training of social workers, the profession, or interdisciplinary concerns; and (4) organizations, communities, and social policy. (p. 2044)

Social work research initially occurred in social service agencies and was supported by funds from foundations. As social work training moved from agencies to universities, so did researchers with studies supported by public dollars. Over time, tension developed between research and practice. On the one hand, there were concerns about practitioners' lack of demands for and use of empirical research, and on the other, researchers' studies were viewed as not relevant to practitioners (Tripodi et al., 2008). A gap still exists between much of the research conducted on clinical practice and clinical practitioners' usage of that research (Epstein & Blumenfield, 2001). More recently, the evidence-based practice movement has further emphasized the division of labor between academics as knowledge producers and practitioners as knowledge implementers (Gambrill, 2006). A strategy for addressing this gap is for practitioners to design, implement, and use research on their own practice within the agency setting (Vonk, Tripodi, & Epstein, 2006). Such research will help them improve their practice and enhance the effectiveness of their agency in serving its clientele and achieving its mission, as well as make contributions to professional knowledge. In addition, agency-based research accommodates the dynamic context of the organization. There are three primary stakeholder groups who can benefit from research endeavors: administrators and program managers, supervisors, and direct service workers and clinicians (Epstein & Kapp, 2008).

At the level of individual social workers as well as social work agencies and programs, attitudes toward research vary widely. These attitudes reflect varying degrees of commitment to systematically creating and testing practice knowledge and skills, as well as incorporating research-based knowledge into social work practice and programs, with the result that "a hundred years of effort to construct a base of scientific knowledge for the profession has fallen far short of the enthusiastic hope of the pioneers" (Reid, 1995, p. 2041). Here are a few suggestions for ensuring that the future of the profession in this regard will be brighter than its past:

- All social workers should view themselves as practitioners/researchers (Grinnell, 1985) and consciously incorporate elements of research into their everyday professional activities. The practitioner–researcher role highlights the importance of practitioners' systematically gathering and utilizing information about their practice, client attributes, and service outcomes. This task may require their convincing themselves that it is necessary and possible to be a practitioner and a researcher at the same time. Attitudinal barriers are often more difficult than logistical and methodological difficulties. The ability to contribute to the strength and prestige of their profession, improvement in their professional skills and strategies, and enhanced respect from other professionals and society at large are benefits of operating on the practitioner/researcher model. They should keep such benefits in mind.
- Every setting can lend itself to being imbued with the desire for improved service approaches and systematic data collection.

Social workers would do well to seek out opportunities for knowledge building by participating and collaborating in existing efforts, proposing and undertaking new projects themselves, building elements of research into their service activities, and systematically evaluating the effectiveness and efficiency of their programs, roles, and tasks. (Dhooper, 1994b, p. 189)

- In health care settings, the atmosphere is generally much more congenial for research-oriented thinking and practice than in many social work agencies. There are numerous potential research topics that can be explored. Social workers should take advantage of that atmosphere. They should also initiate, encourage, and collaborate in interdisciplinary research endeavors. These endeavors carry more clout, command more resources, are richer in their design, and have greater impact on agency policies, programs, and procedures. They will find physicians willing partners. The nursing profession also urges its members to view research as an important professional activity. Martin (1995) suggested a number of ways for nurses to find time for research.
- With most health care agencies subscribing to the concept of continuous quality improvement in all dimensions of their work, there will be room for innovative approaches to continuous quality improvement and its measurement. Social workers should creatively mix and match the quantitative and qualitative methodologies and the various data collection approaches they have learned as part of their professional training. These include (a) survey approach, (b) interview approach, (c) observational approach, (d) experimental approach, (e) program evaluation approaches, and (f) analyses of secondary data.
- They should keep themselves abreast of the emerging research-related approaches and methodologies. For example, Epstein and colleagues developed an innovative, direct-service, practitioner-friendly approach described as clinical data mining. In this approach, the individual clinician functions as the primary researcher responsible for designing, implementing, and utilizing research. His or her research questions are addressed by collecting and analyzing data directly from the case files (Epstein, 2001; Epstein & Blumenfield, 2001).
- They should also be in the forefront of the growing interest in evidence-based practice across disciplines. Several sections of the National Association of Social Workers (NASW) Code of Ethics point to the moral duty of social workers to provide clients their best-practice efforts. They are expected to understand and use research evidence in defining client problems and in selecting interventions that lead to best outcomes (Proctor, 2003). That involves review of professionally relevant research from basic and applied scientific investigations, research evaluating the outcomes of social work interventions, and studies on the reliability and validity of assessment measures (McNeece & Thyer, 2004). Identifying the "best available evidence" also draws attention to the need for meta-analysis and systematic reviews of high-quality research. They should weave into their practice essentials of evidence-based practice by (1) treating every intervention as "an explicit, systematic, and rational problem-solving process" (Rosen, 2003, p. 201); (2) locating and employing the strongest research-supported interventions; (3) engaging in an "ongoing recursive evaluation of outcome attainment, further adjusting the intervention based on evaluative feedback" (Rosen, 2003, p. 203); and (4) sharing their experience of what has worked with the professional community.

- The availability of computers in health and social service agencies will become universal in the future. Computers will do much more than make client records and agency-generated data easily accessible to professionals. Computers will put within easy reach of professionals the resources of libraries, consultation with research experts, and tools for data processing and analysis. With advances in software and statistical programs, data analysis will become more sophisticated, leading to better understanding of outcomes—for example, relationships between length of stay in care and time of entry for foster children or differential health outcomes related to health disparities (Tripodi et al., 2008).
- Coulton (1985) reviewed the impact of several social work research studies on different aspects of social work practice in health care and saw in the cumulative effects of that research a movement toward what Kane (1984) called "science of health care social work." She also identified general trends about the types of social work research. These included movements toward (a) a greater focus on specialty areas, (b) interdisciplinary research, (c) greater emphasis on analysis and evaluation rather than simple description, and (d) a concern over health care cost. The themes reflected in these trends will continue in importance and

will be joined by others. The concern over health care costs will definitely persist. Social workers should take note of these and contribute to the related efforts.

- Other areas for ongoing research will include quality of care in terms of access, comprehensiveness, and sensitivity to the characteristics and needs of clients and communities, and the impact of quality of care on the quality of life. Social workers should view these as areas of their special knowledge and expertise and take initiative in researching these. Setting-specific areas that can benefit from a research-oriented look abound.
- For disciplinary research, social workers can benefit from the experience of Adler et al. (1993), who, as social work practitioners in a Veterans Affairs medical center, overcame barriers to research and publication activity. They formed themselves into a support group that emphasized "peer involvement, acceptance and trust, combined with a commitment to measurable progress on an ongoing basis" (p. 125). Their efforts resulted in the publication of seven articles and submission for publication of five articles over a period of a few years. Wade and Neuman (2007) provided a number of helpful suggestions.
- Social workers should help their agencies/ departments create a climate supportive of research and research-oriented activities. This can be done in many ways, including (a) encouraging intellectual discussion about practice issues and treatment techniques, participation in case conference presentations and grand rounds, and program evaluation as a means of developing interest in research; (b) providing tangible support such as time for specific research-related activities, access to library resources, consultation regarding methodological issues and statistical data analysis, and clerical assistance; (c) matching those practitioners who are experienced or are better at combining the practitioner and researcher roles with those who are just starting; and (d) providing a "clear understanding between administration and clinical researchers about what research is allowed, how resources are to be allocated, and what avenues of appeal exist when conflict develops" (Adler et al., 1993, p. 125).
- Social workers should understand their profession's stance and approach to consumer involvement in agency-based research. Social work ethical directives focus on consumer empowerment by increasing the role of the consumer in service provision as well as involvement in agency-based research efforts. Strategies have been developed and implemented for including consumers in study design, data collection, report writing, and utilization of agency-based research findings (Linhorst & Eckert, 2002).
- Social workers should also seek the assistance and collaboration of faculties of local or nearby social work education programs. University-based teachers and researchers are always looking for ways to stay connected with the field. Rathbone-McCuan (1995) listed reasons for this linkage, including (a) the need to field test instruments and practice models developed in nonagency settings; (b) the need to reach specific client populations as research subjects; (c) the need to test methodological validity through an agency's database; (d) the need for an agency willing to cooperate in a research project or a grant application; (e) the need to create research opportunities for students in the agency; (f) the need to reconnect with the field to update professional knowledge about practice, programs, and policies; (g) the need to learn the perspectives of different age, ethnic, racial, and socioeconomic groups; and (h) the need to supplement income by providing consultation or doing research on a contractual basis. Joubert (2006) described a mentoring model of practice-research collaboration in Australia that is focused on supporting practitioners in developing rigorous research projects from within their own practice or from available data collected as part of a routine hospital service. Find out if a similar possibility exists or can be created at the local college or university.

OTHER STRATEGIES

Conflict Resolution

Conflict is inevitable; it is a universal part of life. Whatever its causes, conflict appears at various levels—internal, interpersonal, and intergroup. Internally, it represents the mental struggle of two or more mutually exclusive impulses, motives, drives, or social demands; at other levels, it reflects the striving by two or more parties to achieve opposing or mutually exclusive goals (Barker, 2003). People can be in conflict with themselves, their families, peers, other groups, institutions, and communities. Costs of conflict are huge. Conflict, even within a group, uses up energy, wastes time, weakens the group bond, saps the group's morale, lowers the self-esteem of its members and accelerates their burnout, and diverts attention away from the group's purpose (Wax, 1982). Drawing on various sources, Mayer (2008) discussed the nature of social conflict and highlighted its (1) functions, (2) dimensions, and (3) components. Functions may be necessary or nonnecessary. Necessary functions are related to a need/problem that requires a solution, an outcome, or an agreement, whereas nonnecessary functions are related to the need for acknowledgement and "venting" and not for a specific outcome. Its dimensions are behavioral, emotional, and cognitive. Its components are relationships, data, interests, values, and structure. Mayer (1995) pointed out two essential elements of a conflict: (a) the perception of being in conflict and the feelings that accompany it and (b) the objective differences in the expected outcomes of conflict. The first requires attention to the emotions and tensions created by the conflict; the second demands that the issues and interests of the parties be addressed.

Major causes of social conflict are (a) relationship issues, (b) value conflicts, (c) inconsistencies in data, (d) structural problems, and (e) conflicts of interest. Some or all of these elements may be involved in a particular conflict (Moore, 1986). The various possible causes of conflict must be acknowledged and understood for conflict resolution. The different issues involved in a conflict make it harder or easier to resolve it. In general, issues about facts are easier to resolve than those about methods. Conflicts about methods are easier to resolve than those about goals. Conflicts about values are the hardest to resolve.

In their therapeutic roles as case workers, counselors, and case managers, social workers help their clients deal with conflicts in the personal and interpersonal realm, as well as in their relations with human service organizations. In conflict situations at the interpersonal and person-organizational levels, they function as mediators. Mediation as a social work approach to serving clients is particularly useful in marital problems, child custody and divorce disputes, adoption disputes, child protection conflicts, conflicts between adolescents and their families, care of the elderly, victim-offender situations, equal employment opportunity disputes, and conflictual relationships among the various elements of the mental health system (Mayer, 1995). The NASW (1991) has established standards of practice for social work mediators. The negotiation skills that social workers use in dealing with involuntary clients are also helpful in conflict resolution.

Health care organizations are no different from others in breeding conflict. Social workers already have client-related conflict resolution skills involving both mediation and negotiation. They also appreciate the values of constructive conflict resolution, which Deutsch (2006) listed as (1) reciprocity—fairness to and from the other, reflected in the old maxim, "Do unto others as you would have others do unto you"; (2) human equality—implying that all are equally entitled to just and respectful treatment; (3) shared community—mutual recognition that they belong to a broader community whose norms and values they share and wish to preserve; (4) fallibility—acknowledgment that the sources of disagreement between people are manifold and reasonable people understand that their own judgment as well as that of others may be fallible; and (5) nonviolence—implying that coercive tactics are not to be employed by either party to obtain agreement or consent. By building on these values and their therapeutic skills, social workers can become a significant resource for conflict resolution in health care settings. This will add another dimension to their position.

With our focus on conflict resolution within and between organizations, the following are a few helpful suggestions. Social workers should apply to conflict resolution the problem-solving framework in which they are well versed. This can be a simple process. Pickering (2000) suggested a four-step ACES framework: (1) assess the situation, (2) clarify the issue, (3) evaluate alternate approaches, and (4) solve the problem. We propose a three-step process of (1) recognizing the conflict, (2) assessing the conflict, and (3) choosing a strategy and intervening accordingly.

1. *Recognizing the conflict* is not difficult; its existence is generally obvious.

2. *Assessing the conflict* should involve knowing something about

    a. the characteristics of the parties in conflict, such as their values and motivations, beliefs about the conflict, and resources for waging or resolving it;

    b. the prior relationship of those parties to one another, particularly attitudes, beliefs, and expectations;

    c. the nature of the issue giving rise to the conflict in terms of its scope, rigidity, and motivational significance;

    d. the social environment within which the conflict occurs;

    e. the interested audiences to the conflict, their relationships to the parties in the conflict, and their interest in the conflict and its outcomes;

    f. the strategy and tactics employed by the parties in the conflict; and

    g. the consequences of the conflict to each of the participants and to other interested parties (Deutsch, 1973).

They should gather as much information from as many sources as possible about the parties in conflict or their opponent if they are a party in the conflict and are negotiating for themselves.

3. *Choosing and using the appropriate strategy* for intervention should be given careful consideration. This should be done with the following things in mind: (1) an overall philosophy of conflict resolution, (2) a set of general principles, (3) an assessment of the level of the conflict, and (4) a preference for a win-win approach.

    a. *The philosophy of conflict resolution* should remind social workers that

- the relationship must not be sacrificed—the issue will pass, but the relationship must go on;
- the issue must not be personalized;
- they have nothing to gain by undermining the other party—they must not get into win-lose situations;
- the issue must not be defined as "you against me" but, rather, as "we against the problem";
- they must take responsibility for their feelings and behavior; and
- they have the power to give meaning to their experience (Wax, 1982).

    b. *The general principles* they should observe are as follows:

- Maintain fairness and objectivity.
- Do not criticize a participant in front of others.
- Do not be critical of the other relationships of the adversary.
- Do not attack the opponent's motives.
- Do not indicate "concern" or doubts about the adversary's emotional well-being.
- Do not attribute the divergent views of the opponent to personality or personal factors.
- Do not depreciate another participant behind his or her back.
- Reciprocate debts, favors, and compliments.
- Keep confidences.
- Demonstrate a caring concern and be emotionally supportive, even with respect to an adversary.
- Take into account the opponent's desire for recognition and self-esteem and other matters of "face."
- Avoid blatant or subtle manifestation of arrogance (Bisno, 1988, p. 57).

    c. *Understand the level of the conflict.* Levels of conflict include

- survival,
- basic values,
- resources,
- turf,
- priorities,
- communication, and
- semantics (Wax, 1982).

Social workers should try to go up or down the scale to stay in control.

d. *Prefer a win-win approach,* which involves the use of negotiation. Fisher and Ury (1981) urge those negotiating to

- separate the people from the problem,
- focus on interests (needs and concerns) and not positions (demands and desired outcomes),
- look for principles that can frame an agreement, and
- develop one's BATNA (best alternative to negotiated agreement) as a means to promote one's influence in negotiation.

The following are a few helpful guidelines for negotiating:

- Listen carefully to what the other party is saying and where he or she is coming from.
- Allow the other party to be right, too.
- Do not try to prove the other party "wrong."
- Do not move from being right to becoming righteous.
- Stay out of the blame game; it weakens your creativity, initiative, and control.
- Try to know how much authority/power the other party has and what the range of bargaining is.
- Challenge the other party's data and assumptions, if needed, but never attack his or her motives.
- Make a clear statement of your need that the other party can understand.
- Let your total being—your oral and body language—convey the message, "I am entitled to what I am asking."
- Give the other party several options regarding your need.
- Do not make a threat unless absolutely necessary, and even then, make a veiled threat.
- Do not remove the threat from the other party's threat.
- Be prepared to make concessions for what you get (Wax, 1982).

They should also realize the importance of framing and labeling as significant techniques. "One of the subtlest and most powerful ways in which conflict can be exacerbated or reduced is the framing of the conflict itself" (Mayer, 1995, p. 617). For instance, labeling a problem as a communication problem defuses the issue.

Coalition Building

Health problems with profound social dimensions, such as AIDS and alcohol and drug abuse, as well as social problems with powerful health consequences, such as poverty, homelessness, and violence in homes and on the streets, will persist in the future. These problems cross professional and organizational boundaries and require comprehensive, multipronged approaches that demand multiprofessional and multiorganizational involvement. To retain their prominence in the community, health care organizations will feel compelled to go beyond the narrow scope of their traditional involvement and become partners with others in dealing with major social problems. Social workers can be instrumental in helping these organizations take on this added social responsibility. With their professional knowledge and skills, as well as their ongoing relationships within the wider human services community, social workers should be able not only to represent their organizations in the various community efforts but also assume leadership roles in generating those efforts. Coalition building is an important approach to dealing with social issues and problems.

A coalition represents a time-limited organization in which there is a convergence of interests of a number of actors, both individuals and organizations, and interactions around furthering those common interests (Warren, 1977). In the words of Staples (2004), "By 'coalition,' I mean a formal alliance (usually temporary) that creates a structured relationship between two or more organizations" (p. 134). The goals of a coalition may be both political and nonpolitical (Dluhy, 1990). Rosenthal and Mizrahi (2004) view coalitions as the means to achieve specific outcomes and as models of interdependence. They included in specific outcomes (1) service integration and strategic partnerships, (2) asset and capacity building, (3) political action and progressive social change, and (4) movement building. As models of interdependence, coalitions enable their members to appreciate diversity, undergo attitudinal and behavioral change, and experience transformation, a shift from an autonomous to a collective perspective (p. 321). Braithwaite, Taylor, and Austin (2000) gave examples of health coalitions in the black community. Coalitions have a special appeal for organizations. They allow individual organizations to become involved in broader issues without total responsibility for managing those issues.

> Thus, coalitions give organizations greater power and influence over an issue than any single organization would have working alone. They enable the mobilization of a greater number of resources, and they bring a wider variety of effective strategies to bear on an issue. (Dluhy, 1990, p. 12)

For improving their ability to build coalitions on behalf of their organizations, social workers will find the following suggestions helpful.

1. *They should familiarize themselves with the various theoretical explanations of the coalition phenomenon and models of coalition building.* Hill (1973) identified three major theoretical models: (a) the mathematical-normative model, based on game theory, which uses mathematical analysis to discover rational outcomes for conflict situations; (b) the economic or cost-benefit model, which is also related to game theory and seeks to maximize the net payoff (gross payoff minus the cost of making the decision and living with its consequences); and (c) the sociopsychological model, which endeavors to explain "coalition-forming behavior as a result of specific modes of cognitive processing (psychological) or as the result of the interaction of group behaviors and individual cognitions (sociological)" (pp. 13–14).

2. *They should keep themselves abreast of the relevant emerging research- and practice-based knowledge on coalitions.* For example, Dluhy (1990) studied coalitions in terms of such characteristics as selection and recruitment of members, ideology, resources, staff, communications, longevity, issues, and organizational structure. He developed a typology of coalitions that include bread-and-butter, consciousness-raising,

network, preassociation, prefederation, and pre-social movement coalitions. The first three are more short-term, ad hoc coalitions formed around a single issue. The other three have a longer life and tend to move beyond a single issue. Mizrahi and Rosenthal (2001) studied social change coalitions and tested the validity of a conceptual framework for successful coalition building. The components of the framework, "the four Cs," are (1) *conditions*—the right political, economic, and community conditions for a coalition to form; (2) *commitment*—a group of representatives of different organizations with the commitment to achieve the common goal as well as commitment to the coalition model for achieving it; (3) *contributions*—the availability of the necessary contributions (resources, ideology, and power) to the coalition; and (4) *competence*—the coalition's competence to move forward, maintain its leadership core, and sustain its membership base. They found that (1) while political, economic, and community conditions are important, more critical are the issue, the right timing, and the social target; (2) commitment to the coalition's unity and work is as important as the commitment to the issue/cause/goal of the coalition; (3) a variety of member contributions are necessary, and the more resources members give and receive, the more committed they stay; and (4) competent leadership is critical to coalition success.

3. *They should visualize the type of coalition they would like to build.* With their focus on relationship building, Tucker and McNerney (1992) viewed coalition building as an opportunity for organizing a team of opinion leaders to build public trust and supportive behavior. They identified four types of coalitions: (a) representatives of stakeholder groups that are tired of expensive confrontation and need to create consensus on an active issue, (b) representatives of stakeholders who find themselves on the same side of the fence on an issue, (c) multidisciplined groups brought together by their "sensitivity or empathy to a point of view on an emerging issue" (p. 28), and (d) representatives of stakeholders who share

a position on an issue that already enjoys widespread acceptance. Whatever the type of coalition, its purpose, and degree of existing agreement on the issue among the coalition members, success is dependent on the strategy and tactics and the ability to mobilize those members. They suggested a fivefold approach: (a) manage the issue, (b) identify coalition participants, (c) conduct research, (d) organize meeting design, and (e) develop messages and tactics.

4. *They should know that managing the issue is very important.* Coalition building should result from a systematic process of issues management (Tucker & McNerney, 1992). It involves developing a position and creating a strategy to pursue that position. Social workers should help their organization develop its position on the issue around which a coalition should be built. This task will require a thorough analysis of all the forces affecting the issue: those driving the issue, those working for and against it, those likely to be affected by it, and those who may perceive themselves to be affected by it. They should try to ensure that the position developed is beneficial to their organization, as well as to others who are likely to be affected by the issue.

5. *They should look at their analysis of the stakeholders in the issue for help in identifying candidates for participation in the coalition.* Criteria for selecting coalition participants can include credibility with peers and broader audiences, interest in the issue, moderate (vs. extreme) point of view, receptivity to the organizer's position or willingness to seek common ground, ability to work in a group seeking consensus, and availability of avenues to reach out to peers and broader audiences (Tucker & McNerney, 1992, p. 29). They can either approach stakeholder organizations for recommending participants or start with a core group that generates a list of people to be approached for participation. In recruiting (and retaining) members, the key is a shared goal "that does not require members to give up their individual, professional, or organizational or agency goals" (Dluhy, 1990, p. 52).

6. *They should realize the crucial importance of the first meeting of a coalition.* Its goal should be to establish an organizational framework, elect temporary leadership, and plan organizational action (Staples, 1987). The "temporary governance committee," as Dluhy (1990) termed this leadership, should determine the formal process of electing the coalition's leaders and provide a forum for discussing its strategy and tactics. This meeting should also clarify the extent to which

> the coalition should remain narrow or be broadened. Because there may not be a specific answer to this question, making this tentative or approaching the issue as a preliminary discussion may take some of the edge off of disagreement. (p. 52)

Such decisions can always be reviewed.

7. *They should know that coalitions can have many organizational structures, depending on the scope of their work and the geographic area they cover.* The old adage that "structure should follow function" (Staples, 2004) should be remembered as a guiding principle. A coalition can be organized into committees or work groups. Dluhy (1990) proposed an organizational model of a statewide coalition that provides for seven committees: (a) long-range planning, (b) talent and recruitment, (c) communications, (d) special events, (e) monitoring and oversight, (f) medical and public relations, and (g) advocacy strategy. The advocacy strategy committee is at the core of the structure. He recommended that this committee be composed of five to seven people who are able to devote considerable time and effort to the coalition work and can meet regularly. This committee would be responsible for the overall plan of action, coordination of the various activities, and continuous evaluation of the plan of action.

8. *They should recognize the extreme importance of adequate professional staff for the coalition's work and explore all possible avenues for that.* These include (a) the coalition's own fiscal resources that can be used for hiring needed staff, (b) the member organizations that may be

willing either to share the cost of hiring staff or to lend the services of their employees with appropriate skills, (c) people involved with the coalition who have professional qualifications and skills, and (d) student interns from various professional programs of the local educational institutions.

9. *They should remember that continuous, careful attention is needed for maintaining coalitions.* Members' willingness to continue involvement in and remain committed to the coalition depends on several factors. Dluhy (1990) listed principal incentives for participation in a coalition, including (a) ideological or symbolic benefits, (b) tangible benefits for the member's agency or profession, (c) tangible benefits for the person, (d) social benefits for the person, (e) enhancement of agency or professional reputation, (f) improvement of client situation, (g) civic duty or pride, and (h) critical up-to-date information and knowledge about clients, services, or the broader field (pp. 60–61). Let these incentives guide them in the management and maintenance of the coalition.

10. *They should always be open to learning from the work of others.* Rosenthal and Mizrahi (2004) discussed a number of challenges that coalitions are likely to experience. These include (1) dynamic tensions caused by members' mixed loyalties, the phenomenon of unity and diversity, differential amounts of power of member organizations, and the need to balance autonomy and accountability; (2) operational difficulties in terms of the coalition's structure, membership, and struggle for resources; and (3) tacit expectations and risks involved in or because of competing priorities, interdependence, uncertainty, and lack of trust. They also suggested ways to deal with such challenges.

To summarize, for ongoing successful coalition work, social workers should

- remind the members of the benefits of membership from time to time;
- give equal importance to the needs of the members and the tasks of the organization;

- maintain an effective communication network within the coalition and not let the organization become too formal and rigid;
- make sure everyone has a place in the coalition and is matched with the tasks he or she enjoys;
- keep issues in front of the members and highlight even small successes;
- take advantage of external events or crises, whenever possible, to validate the coalition and energize its members;
- stress organizational and professional credibility above all else;
- develop internal decision-making processes that keep members coming together;
- design strategies that require maximum participation and interaction among members;
- use periodic retreats and other self-assessment techniques (Dluhy, 1990; Friesen, 1987; Hasenfeld, 1983); and
- manage and resolve conflict as it emerges (we discussed several approaches to conflict resolution earlier in this chapter).

Community Work

In Chapters 4, 5, and 7, we discussed some community-work-related knowledge and skills relevant for social workers in different health care settings. The purpose of adding more material on social workers' community work on behalf of their agencies is to emphasize the importance of that work as a strategy for thriving in health care. Social workers' skills related to community work will set them apart from many other professionals and not only give them an edge over others but also provide them opportunities for leadership. In our earlier discussion, we presented models of community social work appropriate for the needs of particular health care settings. Here, we present a view of the larger picture, highlighting the basic similarities among the various modes of social work practice—clinical-, organizational-, and community-level work—and offer helpful ideas/suggestions.

The history of community organizing in the United States is closely tied to the development of social work theory and practice (Kahn, 1995). The roots of community practice can be traced to the settlement house and charity organization movements (Mondros & Staples, 2008; Weil & Gamble, 1995). Knowledge of community variables always has been an important part of social workers' professional assets.

> In spite of the influences of the scientific charity movement of the early 20th century and of Freudian psychology and its intrapsychic corollaries, social work never totally removed itself from its early roots in the community. Social work practice, regardless of the context or specialty, requires an understanding of the ties that bind the individual, the family, or the group to larger societal networks. Further, as resources dwindle, social workers increasingly fill the role of mobilizer of community resources to resolve personal problems or address public issues. (Martinez-Brawley, 1995, pp. 545–546)

Social work profession embraces a person-in-environment perspective, and, therefore, every practitioner is expected to be sensitive to and willing to engage in macro practice activities. Furthermore, macro work is also "direct" practice because there are ongoing interactions among people, although it is not always one-on-one (Netting, 2008). However, some social workers trained as specialists in clinical practice might not have acquired adequate skills for effective community-level work. They will find the following material helpful.

On the basis of an extensive review of the community practice literature, Weil and Gamble (1995) identified eight models of community work. These models are (a) neighborhood and community organizing, (b) organizing functional communities, (c) community social and economic development, (d) social planning, (e) program development and community liaison, (f) political and social action, (g) coalitions, and (h) social movements. They discussed these models in terms of the desired outcome, system targeted for change, primary constituency, scope of concern, and social work roles. According to them, the future will witness a resurgence of community practice aimed at supporting various trends.

Ideologies, theories, and practice methods that support these trends will expand, with particular focus on applied democratic development, consumer participation, neopopulist ideology, feminist theory and practice, and theory and practice for sustainable development. The knowledge and research base for community practice will continue to grow and use more-sophisticated quantitative and qualitative methodologies to assess the outcomes of service reforms and planning and development efforts. (p. 591)

With a focus on effective community-based services for vulnerable populations by direct service agencies, Johnson (1998) did an extensive literature review. That review yielded the following six characteristics of community-based services delivery: (1) It is neighborhood based and family focused; (2) it is strength and empowerment oriented; (3) it is culturally sensitive and multiculturally competent; (4) it provides comprehensive services; (5) it provides access to integrated services and supports; and (6) it reflects teamwork and leadership skills. Mondros and Staples (2008) analyzed the contemporary community organizing and forecast the following.

Constituencies and Issues. Populations that will be organizing or will be the foci of community organizations in the future include the elderly, foreign-born Americans (of whom Latinos will be the largest group), racially and ethnically diverse groups, and immigrant workers. The needs of these groups, including their health care needs, will become the compelling issues for community organizational activities. Other issues will be related to environmental justice, environmental racism, and environmental classism—which is reflected in dumping of pollutants and storage of toxic wastes in communities of color and low-income neighborhoods.

Ideas for Organizing. Community organizing is no longer only around geographic communities, as the meaning and scope of the term *community* is changing. Many "communities" are organizing or being organized around a common identity, along such dimensions as race, ethnicity, faith, gender, age, physical or mental disability, and sexual orientation. Others are organized around issues of shared experience, such as being day laborers, homeless, immigrants, prisoners, single parents, students, welfare recipients, and women.

Organizing Approaches. Newer community organization methods and strategies will continue to evolve. Information and communication technology will have a profound effect on those approaches. McNutt (2000) identified six ways technology can help an organizing campaign: (a) coordinating activity and community with stakeholders; (b) gathering tactical and strategic information through online databases and discussion groups; (c) analyzing data with mapping or Geographic Information System programs, community databases, and statistical packages; (d) using webpages for advocacy; (e) fundraising and recruiting volunteers or members through online venues; and (f) automating office and administrative tasks. Schultz and associates (2000) described an Internet-based support system for community work known as the Community Tool Box.

Models of community organization incorporating the above approaches and trends will continue to appear in the future. An example of such work is the community management approach proposed by Smith, Loppnow, and Davis (1995), which blends selected elements of traditional community social work concepts and methods with mainstream modern corporate leadership and management concepts and methods. Similarly, models for integrating social work practice at different levels (micro, mezzo, and macro) are appearing in the literature. One such model was proposed by Frankel (1989) and named the community intervention model of clinical social work. This model presented parallel steps involved in the clinical, community, and agency-organizational work [1]. Social workers in clinical practice positions venturing into community work often must do extensive work within their own agency as a precondition for effective community work. While discussing her approach to integrating micro, mezzo, and macro

practice perspectives, Kirst-Ashman (1994) proposed two process-oriented tools, one with the acronym PREPARE for assessing organizational change potential and the other called IMAGINE for intervention. The steps included in PREPARE are (a) identify *problems* to be addressed, (b) assess one's macro *reality*, (c) *establish* primary goals, (d) identify relevant *people* of influence, (e) *assess* potential costs and benefits to clients and the agency, (f) evaluate professional and personal *risk*, and (g) *evaluate* the potential success. The process represented by IMAGINE includes the following steps: (a) Start with an innovative *idea*, (b) *muster* support, (c) identify *assets*, (d) specify *goals*, (e) *implement* the plan, (f) *neutralize* opposition, and (g) *evaluate* progress.

Below are some suggestions that social workers in health care settings embarking on community organizational projects will find helpful.

1. *Study the various models of community work and determine how mixing and matching elements of those models will help create an approach peculiarly suitable for their purpose.* The actual work in any community will require the combining of different aspects of the various models, depending on the purpose of that work and a host of other factors.

2. *Remain familiar with other emerging practice models that propose newer approaches to community work or ways of integrating clinical and community social work.* Social workers should consciously try to incorporate into their practice strategies for integrating micro, organizational, and macro modalities.

3. *Sharpen their skills pertaining to such social work roles as advocate, mediator, negotiator, planner, and facilitator.* We discussed strategies and techniques appropriate for these roles in earlier chapters. It is important to have the appropriate skills because most models of community work involve these roles.

4. *Use several methods of needs assessment.* We discussed various approaches to community

needs assessments in an earlier chapter. These are as diverse as analyzing the existing secondary data and contacting people—both key informants and lay. To the extent possible, several methods of needs assessment should be used. If several methods yield the same results, the reliability of those findings is much higher. The process of a community needs assessment itself, when several methods are used, creates the involvement of many community people. This is essential for going beyond the assessment.

5. *Remember that there is a political aspect of needs assessment.* Involvement of those affected by the need should be treated as important principle of needs assessment. "Any needs assessment involves making some judgments about the adequacy (or inadequacy) of existing institutional or organizational arrangements. Such judgments can be threatening to the guardians of those institutions and may lead to inappropriate criticism of the assessor" (Tropman, 1995, p. 568). Therefore, social workers should strive for a balance between the technical and the political aspects of community needs assessment.

6. *Develop a community profile that highlights the various dimensions of the community's life.* For effective work at the community level, a community analysis is essential. The important dimensions include (a) its identification—how the community identifies itself; (b) its location in terms of major geographic characteristics, and accessibility to the different forms of transportation; (c) its history, major events, traditions, and values; (d) its population and the population's characteristics; (e) its economic base and employment and income characteristics of its people; (f) its housing characteristics in terms of the type, ownership, and conditions; (g) its educational facilities, their level, and characteristics; (h) its health and human service resources; (i) its major problems; and (j) an assessment of the community's strengths and liabilities (Devore & Schlesinger, 1981; Siporin, 1975).

7. *Offer their community-related expertise and help their agencies either start new community-level programs or undertake joint projects with other agencies.* The importance of interagency collaboration in different ways will increase in the future. Coordination of interagency activities is an absolute necessity in joint ventures. Social workers should remember that interagency coordination can be of different types and can take different forms. The possibilities include the following:

- *Administrative fiscal integration* encompassing (a) purchase of service, (b) joint budgeting, and (c) joint funding.
- *Administrative support services* such as (a) conducting studies; (b) information processing, dissemination, and exchange;(c) record keeping; (d) grants management and technical assistance; (e) publicity and public relations; (f) procedural integration; (g) joint program or project evaluation; and (h) standards and guidelines.
- *Administrative and programmatic linkages involving agency personnel* through (a) loaner staff; (b) out-stationing; (c) liaison teams and joint use of staff; (d) staff training and development; (e) screening, employment counseling, and placement; (f) volunteer bureaus; and (g) ombudsmen.
- *Programmatic linkages* through development of centralized services such as (a) information and outreach, (b) intake, (c) diagnosis, (d) referral, (e) transportation, (f) follow-up, and (g) grievance machinery.
- *Programmatic coordination* through service integration taking the form of (a) case management, (b) ad hoc case coordination, (c) case conferences, (d) joint program development, and (e) joint projects (Lauffer, 1978).

8. *Ensure that a common mission and a shared view of the problem and its solution are reflected in formal contracts and protocols spelling out the responsibilities of the collaborating parties and the operationalization of those responsibilities.* The essential requisites of interagency coordination are mutual benefits, similarity or complementarity of goals, and mutual respect and communication. "All [collaborations] require certain conditions, commitment, contributions, and competence, and all inherently experience dynamic tensions, which must be expected and managed" (Abramson & Rosenthal, 1995, p. 1481). Social workers' group work knowledge and skills would

enable them to make significant contributions to the building and maintaining of interagency collaboration. We discussed other relevant skills earlier under coalition building.

Culturally Sensitive Practice

The current minorities will constitute a majority of the U.S. population in the future, and public policy will support cultural diversity. The need of health care organizations to deliver their services in culturally sensitive and appropriate ways will be ever present. Social work has a history of concern for such issues as prejudice and discrimination, intergroup relations, and social justice.

> Since the 1960s, social work has strongly supported cultural pluralism and diversity. Social work was one of the first and most consistent supporters of civil rights activity and built the commitment to oppose prejudice and discrimination into its organizational structure and code of ethics. (Guzzetta, 1995, p. 2515)

In 2001, the NASW established Standards for Cultural Competence in Social Work Practice. The Council on Social Work Education (CSWE) standards for accreditation of social work programs also mandate that every program enrich students' educational experience with content on human diversity. The Nondiscrimination and Human Diversity Accreditation Standard of the CSWE Educational Policy and Accreditation Standards states that programs

> make specific and continuous efforts to provide a learning context in which respect for all persons and understanding of diversity (including age, class, color, disability, ethnicity, family structure, gender, marital status, national origin, race, religion, sex, and sexual orientation) are practiced. (CSWE, 2001, Section 6.0)

The aim is to prepare culturally competent social work practitioners. An impressive body of social work literature on understanding and working with ethnic and cultural minorities has grown over the past three decades.

Social workers' professional commitment and training for culturally competent practice should give them an edge over many other health care providers. This is another area with opportunities for their assuming leadership positions. Those positions may involve teaching others through example and orientation, as well as becoming the link between patients and communities on the one hand and other health care providers and organizations on the other. The following suggestions for social workers are likely to enhance culturally sensitive and effective practice.

1. *Keep abreast of the emerging literature on culturally sensitive and multicultural practice and stay aware of the barriers to multicultural practice.* Fong (2008) discussed the evolution of culturally competent practice in social work and described concepts such as ethnic reality, cultural values as strengths, biculturalization of interventions, and multidimensional contextual practice. Ethnic reality highlights the intersection of minority clients' race or ethnicity and their social class. Recognizing minority clients' cultural values as strengths in both assessment and intervention can play an important role in helping those clients effectively. The biculturalization of interventions is a systematic way of assessing the compatibility of Western interventions with the cultural values and indigenous interventions of the client's ethnic group and appropriately mixing the two for maximum impact. A multidimensional contextual practice assumes that people behave differently depending on their experiences in their social environments. Schlesinger (2004) also discussed ideological and theoretical perspectives and practice approaches in ethnic-sensitive and multicultural practice. For an impressive look at the professional efforts in multicultural social work education, see Gutierrez, Zuniga and Lum (2004).

Kirst-Ashman and Hull (1993) listed the following barriers that are still relevant and strong:

- Continued acceptance of the melting pot theory, which can result in blaming people of color for failing to "melt"
- The assumption that everyone who immigrates to this country is overjoyed to be here, which

can lead to ignoring/minimizing clients' losses, fears, and anxieties

- The tendency to explain a person's behavior by reference to his or her culture, which ignores the diversity within a culture and the person's uniqueness
- An attempt to be color-blind and thereby treat everyone alike, which ignores the importance of the person's culture and experience
- A tendency to assume that words carry the same meaning for everyone
- The assumption that clients think as we do, which ignores the fact that everyone has a different frame of reference for viewing reality
- The expectation that clients understand the social worker's role, when their understanding is likely to be conditioned by their experience
- Insufficient self-awareness, which lets the worker's own values, beliefs, and biases color the reality of the client
- The lack of knowledge of the culture and experiences of particular client groups and an absence of a repertoire of appropriate, effective intervention techniques

2. *Know the various models of culturally sensitive practice.* For example, Schlesinger and Devore (1995) conceptualized ethnic-sensitive practice as made up of three components: a professional perspective based on layers of understanding, a series of assumptions, and some practice principles.

The layers of understanding include (1) social work values, (2) knowledge of human behavior, (3) knowledge of social welfare policies and services, (4) self-awareness, (5) knowledge of the impact of ethnic reality, (6) the route to the social worker, and (7) the adaptation and modification of strategies and skills. The impact of ethnic reality determines not only the need for services but also service-related attitudes and abilities. The route to the social worker can be viewed as the path to health care services. Differential approaches are needed for clients taking different paths—those coming on their own and those who are forced, required, or encouraged to come. Regular practice strategies often require rethinking and adaptation for ethnically and culturally effective intervention.

The assumptions of ethnic-sensitive practice include the following: (1) Individual and collective history have a bearing on the generation and solution of problems; (2) the present is the most important; (3) unconscious phenomena affect individual functioning; and (4) ethnicity is a source of cohesion, identity, and strengths, as well as of strain, discordance, and strife (Schlesinger & Devore, 1995, p. 905).

The practice principles include (1) giving simultaneous attention to individual and systemic concerns and (2) modifying the social work cognitive, affective, and behavioral skills in view of the understanding of the client's ethnic reality. Lum (2000) proposed a model of cultural competence, a process-stage approach to social work with members of minority communities that delineates practice process stages, worker-system practice issues, client-system practice issues, and worker-client tasks. It emphasizes the necessity of cultural awareness, knowledge acquisition, skills development, and inductive learning. This approach is applicable at micro, mezzo, and macro levels of practice.

3. *Give attention to both the etic and emic characteristics of the client. Etic* and *emic* refer to cultural commonality and cultural specificity, respectively.

In a real sense, the worker communicates the message that the client is a human being with basic needs and aspirations (etic perspective) and is also a part of a particular cultural and ethnic group (emic perspective). Moving between these two points of reference is a creative experience for both worker and client. (Lum, 1992, p. 90)

4. *Apply the following strategies, which can be used for assessment across all cultural groups:*

- Consider all clients as individuals first, as members of minority status next, and as members of a specific ethnic group last. This will prevent overgeneralization.
- Never assume that a person's ethnic identity tells you anything about his or her cultural values and patterns of behavior. There can be vast within-culture differences.

- Treat all "facts" about cultural values and traits as hypotheses to be tested anew with each client.
- Remember that all minority groups in this society are at least bicultural, living in two cultures—their own and the majority culture. The difficulty of surviving in a bicultural environment may be more important than their cultural background.
- Remember that not all aspects of a client's cultural history, values, and lifestyle are relevant to social work. Only the client can identify which aspects are important.
- Identify and build on the strengths in the client's cultural orientation.
- Be aware of one's own attitude about cultural pluralism.
- Engage the client in the process of learning what cultural content—beliefs, values, and experiences—is relevant for the work together.
- Keep in mind that there is no substitute for professional skills.

5. *With a focus on multicultural counseling, use Dillard's (1983) recommendations for effective interventions*:

- Being aware that the nonverbal component constitutes more of the communication than its verbal component
- Recognizing that eye contact can be a problem for many ethnic groups
- Using both open-ended and closed-ended questions, as they are almost universally acceptable
- Remembering that reflection of feelings does not work with all cultures
- Recalling that paraphrasing is a generally acceptable technique in most cultures
- Using self-disclosure judiciously
- Giving interpretations and advice in cultures expecting a directive helper
- Summarizing from time to time
- Using confrontation carefully with certain racial groups
- Remembering that openness, authenticity, and genuineness are respected in all cultures

6. *Be aware of the following skills for culturally competent practice, which Rogers (1995) considers essential for case management*:

- *Ability to be self-aware:* This challenges one's self-image as an unbiased person and tunes into one's stereotypical thinking.

- *Ability to identify difference as an issue:* This helps in recognizing that both the worker and the client have cultures that cause differential perceptions and possibility of miscommunication.
- *Ability to accept others:* This makes the worker comfortable with a wide range of people and acknowledges that values and behaviors can be understood in relation to a person's culture.
- *Ability to individualize and generalize:* This helps in the application of a generalizable model to any given situation and then the search for its unique elements.
- *Ability to advocate:* This provides for the extra help needed by disadvantaged and nonmainstream clients.

Dealing With Managed Care

Managed care will continue to be the country's major approach to improving access, controlling cost, and ensuring quality of health care. No health care setting—inpatient or outpatient, short-term or long-term—will stay outside the purview of managed care. Already, about 97% of those insured through their employers are under some form of managed care, and most states have introduced managed care practices into their Medicaid systems. Similarly, the majority of those on Medicare are affected by managed care. In Chapter 1, we mentioned the highlights of the history of managed care and its various forms. Vandiver (2008) listed the various federal laws that have influenced the evolution of managed care. Those laws include (1) *Titles XVIII and XIX of the Social Security Act of 1965,* which created the Medicare and Medicaid programs; (2) the *Health Maintenance Organization Act of 1973,* which required businesses with 25 or more employees to provide those employees the optional HMO coverage; (3) the *Omnibus Budget and Reconciliation Act of 1981,* which permitted state-level experimentation with managed care (allowing states to seek federal waivers); (4) the *Tax Equity and Fiscal Responsibility Act of 1982,* which paved the way for HMOs to enroll Medicare beneficiaries; (5) the *Deficit Reduction Act of 1983,* which ushered in the prospective pricing system known as diagnosis-related groups (DRGs); (6) the *Balanced Budget Act of 1997*, which introduced Medicare Part C (also known as Medicare + Choice), encouraging beneficiaries to enroll in managed care health plans; and (7) the *Medicare Prescription Drug, Improvement, and Modernization Act of 2003*, which changed Medicare + Choice to Medicare Advantage, requiring beneficiaries to join a private health plan in order to receive prescription drug coverage.

Managed care is significantly influencing the financing and delivery of health and mental health services. Social workers are working in managed care environments. On the one hand, they are occupying important positions in managed care companies as owners, administrators, supervisors, clinical directors, and case managers (Edinburg & Cottier, 1995). They perform utilization management, network development and management, and operations management functions in those companies (Lopez et al., 1993). On the other hand, they are providing and will continue to provide social work services both as independent providers and as employees of all types of health and mental health care organizations. In those settings, they must deal with managed care companies' case managers on behalf of individual clients.

As pointed out earlier, *managed care* is a collective term used to describe a variety of strategies used by insurers to control health care costs. Overall, those strategies fall along two dimensions. The first entails establishing policies and procedures that regulate benefits, payments, and providers, and the second involves employing gatekeepers to review and authorize services (Wagner, 2001). The philosophy, structure, and procedures of many managed care organizations challenge the fundamental social work values (Neuman & Ptak, 2003). Therefore, it is vitally important that social workers understand the "what" and "how" of the managed care approach. Only then will they be able to make significant contributions to the health care field, their agencies, and their clients.

Managed care is a term that represents many different ideas about health care delivery and resource management. Those ideas have found expression in many different programs. Entities providing managed care have proliferated over the years. These have grown out of utilization review companies, provider groups, insurance companies, employee assistance programs, and independent ventures. They vary on a number of dimensions.

> The variations include their primary corporate client (for example, HMO, commercial insurance, large corporations), the primary service they provide (for example, utilization review, EAPs, direct service delivery), and their use of providers (for example, group practices and solo practitioners). Most of the major companies are now subsidiaries of insurance companies or other corporate health conglomerates. (NASW, 1994a, p. 3)

There is variance in the degree of regulation of managed care companies. They may be regulated by such agencies as insurance, health, or other departments of the local, state, or federal government, or care may not be regulated at all except as profit-making corporations (NASW, 1994b). Most managed care organizations are accredited by such organizations as the Joint Commission on the Accreditation of Health Care Organizations and the National Committee on Quality Assurance.

Social workers will find the following suggestions helpful. Some of these are generic, others are pertinent for those working for managed care organizations, and still others are for those who are service providers—independently or as employees of health care organizations.

- *Look for changes in the current form of managed care.* "At the policy level, the future of managed care will be influenced by a new generation of employees, insurers, politicians, consumers, and voters who are working to eliminate managed care procedures that promote price discrimination for reasons of health or job status," and at a practice level, "consumer groups are working on federal legislation to balance the decision-making power of managed care organizations in areas of provider choice, treatment options, and ability to sue HMOs for denial of care" (Vandiver, 2008). This looking for changes will enable social workers to take a proactive stance.

• *Use advocacy skills against detrimental policies and practices both at the larger systems and individual case levels.* Most managed care programs operate on a "medical model," with its focus primarily on eliminating symptoms of the problem rather than on a "social health model," which views the patient from a biopsychosocial perspective (NASW, 1994b). Thus, there is wide room for denying patients comprehensive needed services. Similarly, efforts to control health care costs can take the form of limiting access to and quality of services. Social workers should work against such policies and practices.

• *Use appropriate approaches for the larger-level social work advocacy,* lobbying for legislation to regulate managed care, making alliances with other health care providers, and using research and analysis of data generated by their practice. Congress has debated and even passed a few versions of a patient's bill of rights, but it has not become a law. The key disagreement has been around the right to sue managed care organizations for punitive damages (Gorin, 2003). Barusch (2006) identified several macro-level social work roles, including (a) negotiating and monitoring each state's contracts with providers, (b) ensuring that needs of consumers are addressed in those processes, (c) advocating for services to address the needs of Medicaid beneficiaries, and (d) increasing the voice of Medicaid recipients in decisions related to managed care.

• *Help in the development and implementation of innovative service delivery models that improve options and quality of care.* In that work, social workers should be guided by the basic values of the social work profession that emphasize the primacy of the individual and a just and equitable social order, its "person-in-environment" perspective, and such concepts as "continuum of care," "optimal functioning of the patient/client," and "least restrictive environment." Successful programs can include educating clients about utilizing the health care system, linking them to a primary case manager or primary care provider, facilitating transportation, and offering more flexible hours of service (Vandivort, 1994).

• *As a part of managed care organizations, function not only within the framework of professional values and standards but also enrich the perspectives of others in the agency with the essentials of social work values and practice principles.* Social workers should become instrumental in managed care programs, working toward the best interest of the consumer of care and not saving costs at the expense of quality of care.

• *Sensitize the managed care establishment to the needs of Medicaid populations and the necessity for adapting services to those populations.* Those on Medicaid will continue being at the bottom in terms of their attractiveness to providers of care, both organizations and individuals, because of the complexity of problems they present and the inadequacy of remuneration to providers for attending to those problems.

• *Be proactive when interfacing with managed care organizations or working in a managed care environment.* Social workers should anticipate and be prepared to deal with conflict. Acker (2010) explored the relationship between the levels of conflict experienced in interfacing with managed care organizations and such outcome variables as job satisfaction, organizational commitment, emotional exhaustion, and turnover intensions for almost 600 social workers in mental health agencies. She found that conflict had statistically significant correlations with emotional exhaustion and organizational commitment. For surviving in managed care environments, they should "develop the business acumen to demonstrate social work's effectiveness in a service industry where demonstrated outcomes predominate" (Schneider, Hyer, & Luptak, 2001, p. 276). This involves translating social work interventions into health care dollars saved and presenting those interventions in corporate language (Dinerman, 1997).

• *Be creative in their case-level advocacy.* Social workers should become familiar with the accreditation standards for managed care organizations.

> To represent patients effectively, social workers need to know the MCO's [managed care organization's] turn-around time for decisions, the credentials of the decision makers, the clinical protocol applied, the rationale for the denial, and the steps of the appeal process. (Neuman & Ptak, 2003)

These authors have provided a wealth of information on how to manage managed care through accreditation standards. "Use every contact with case managers [of managed care companies] to express their priority, that is, meeting the needs of the client" (Cornelius, 1994, p. 59). Similarly, in her book, *Managing Managed Care: Secrets from a Former Case Manager,* Frager (2000) dealt with all dimensions of the working of managed care organizations and provided valuable advice on how to deal with them. For example, when requesting an exception to administrative policies, she suggests that social workers "focus on the clinical reasons why the managed care company should grant the request. If it is not a clinical issue, point out the member satisfaction, financial savings, and/or public relations aspects" (p. 3).

• *Strive to ensure that the following standards are observed.* The standards for managed care plans formulated by the NASW, which will continue to have validity in the future, include (a) a full range of readily available services from emergency to primary care to subspecialty services, including mental health services and hospitalization; (b) clearly maintained safeguards for confidentiality; (c) access to services that meet the needs of families, working people, older people, and people with disabilities; (d) clear agreements with specialty care providers, hospital pharmacies, home care, and other services agencies; (e) appropriate transitions for clients who have to change their health care plans or who have exhausted their benefits to facilitate continuity of treatment; (f) emergency and urgent care procedures available on a 24-hour basis; (g) access to social work services such as crisis intervention, assessment, prevention, health education, rehabilitation, and continuity of care; (h) specialized mental health services provided by social workers, such as psychotherapy and counseling for individuals, families, and groups, and substance abuse prevention and treatment; (i) easy-to-use and readily available complaint and appeal mechanisms; and (j) advisory boards that include consumers and that participate in policy and program development decisions (NASW, 2006).

• *Use their professional knowledge, skills, and value commitments to ensure that managed care serves appropriate ends.* Managed care has the potential to become the strategy for a more equitable distribution of health care resources. There is much about the stated intent of managed care that social workers may wish to support: (a) the control of the use of health care resources for treatments that are efficacious and necessary, (b) the need to control the proportion of private and public resources spent on health care at the expense of other social needs and problems, (c) the use of public monies to improve and maintain the health of the poor and the disabled, rather than an emphasis on treatment of illness alone, and (d) the opportunity to educate the public about the proportionate use of health care services and the distinction between medical need and personal want (Cornelius, 1994, p. 60).

This chapter concludes our discussion of the anticipated changes in the health care system and how social work can continue making significant contributions to the health and progress of that system. The generic strategies suggested in this chapter are not difficult to master and are likely to be helpful to future social work professionals in any work setting. It is hoped that these strategies, combined with basic social work skills and the use of the material presented in preceding chapters, will enable social workers to navigate the waters of the health care system with competence and confidence.

Critical Thinking Questions

1. Grade the approaches suggested in this chapter for thriving in health care according to their importance for you. Critically look at the top three. Can you justify the "why" of their relative positions?

2. Think of the situation/s where merely adding an apostrophe turned *Impossible* into *I'mpossible.* Analyze the process of change, both in terms of the mental and attitudinal shift and the action strategies employed. How can you incorporate the learning from that experience into your professional repertoire?

Note

1. In the community intervention model, steps included in clinical intervention are (a) assessment, (b) diagnosis—problem specification, (c) current status of the problem—baseline, (d) goal setting, (e) controlling conditions—problem causation/the working hypothesis, (f) developing intervention strategies/plans, (g) intervention, (h) evaluation, and (i) maintenance.

Corresponding to these, the steps in the community-level intervention are (a) community needs assessment, (b) identification of community resources, (c) identification of target populations, (d) goal setting, (e) controlling conditions, (f) program planning, (g) program implementation, (h) evaluation of the program impact, and (i) maintenance of the program in the community.

The necessary within-the-agency work involves a process with similar steps, which include (a) needs assessment, including the identification of power bases in the agency; (b) identification of formal and informal rules and norms; (c) building an informal coalition; (d) development of the agency's goals for the community program; (e) modification of the intervention plan in view of the agency goals; (f) development of the final community program plan and its presentation to the agency administration; (g) formalization of agency support; (h) implementation of the community program; (i) evaluation of the program impact on the agency; and (j) maintenance of the program in the agency.

REFERENCES

AAMC policy on the generalist physician. (1993). *Academic Medicine, 68,* 1–5.

Aaronson, W. E., Zinn, J. S., & Rosko, M. D. (1994). Do for-profit and not-for-profit nursing homes behave differently? *The Gerontologist, 34,* 775–786.

Abdul Hamid, W., Wykes, T., & Stansfeld, S. (1993). Homeless mentally ill: Myths and realities. *International Journal of Social Psychiatry, 39*(4), 237–254.

Abrams, M. K., Davis, K., & Haran, C. (2009). *Can patient-centered medical homes transform health care delivery?* Retrieved from http://www.com monwealthfund.org/Content/Form-the-President/ 2009/Can-Patient-Centered

Abramson, J. S., & Rosenthal, B. B. (1995). Interdisciplinary and interorganizational collaboration. In R. L. Edwards (Ed.), *Encyclopedia of social work* (19th ed.). Washington, DC: National Association of Social Workers.

Abramson, M. (1983). A model for organizing an ethical analysis of the discharge planning process. *Social Work in Health Care, 9*(1), 45–51.

Abramson, M. (1984). Collective responsibility in interdisciplinary collaboration: An ethical perspective for social workers. *Social Work in Health Care, 10*(1), 35–43.

Abramson, M. (1990). Ethics and technological advances: Contributions of social work practice. *Social Work in Health Care, 15*(2), 5–17.

Abramson, T. A., & Mendis, K. P. (1990). The organizational logistics of running a dementia group in a skilled nursing facility. *Clinical Gerontologist, 9*(3/4), 111–122.

Acker, G. M. (2010). Influence of managed care on job-related attitudes of social workers. *Social Work in Mental Health, 8*(2), 174–189.

Adelman, M. B., Frey, L. R., & Budz, T. J. (1994). Keeping the community spirit alive. *Journal of Long-Term Care Administration, 22*(2), 4–7.

Adler, G., Alfs, D., Greeman, M., Manske, J., McClellan, T., O'Brien, N., et al. (1993). Social work practitioners as researchers: Is it possible? *Social Work in Health Care, 19*(2), 115–127.

Alper, P. R. (1984). The new language of hospital management. *New England Journal of Medicine, 311,* 1249–1251.

Altepeter, T. S., & Walker, C. E. (1992). Prevention of physical abuse of children through parent training. In D. J. Willis, E. W. Holden, & M. Rosenberg (Eds.), *Prevention of child maltreatment: Developmental and ecological perspectives* (pp. 226–248). New York: John Wiley.

Altman, D. (1987). *AIDS in the mind of America.* New York: Anchor.

Altman, S. H., & Henderson, M. G. (1989). Introduction. In S. H. Altman, C. Brecher, M. G. Henderson, & K. E. Thorpe (Eds.), *Competition and compassion.* Ann Arbor, MI: Health Administration Press.

Amato, P. (2004). Divorce in social and historical context: Changing scientific perspectives on children and marital dissolution. In M. Coleman & L. H. Ganong (Eds.), *Handbook of contemporary families* (pp. 265–280). Thousand Oaks, CA: Sage.

American Medical Association. (1999). *Education for physicians in the end-of-life care.* Chicago: Author.

American Hospital Association. (1989). *Hospitals and older adults: Meeting the challenge.* Chicago: Author.

American Hospital Association. (2009a). *Beyond health care.* Retrieved from http://www.aha.org/ aha/resource-center/index.html

American Hospital Association. (2009b). *Fast facts on U.S. hospitals*. Retrieved from http://www.aha.org/aha/resource-center/Statistics-and-Studies/fast-facts.html

American Society for Microbiology. (1995). Report of the ASM Task Force on antibiotic resistance: Antimicrobial agents and chemotherapy (Suppl., pp. 1–23).

Amputees get back on their feet. (1990, September–October). *The Futurist, 24,* 5.

An ER just for older patients. (2011). *AARP Bulletin, 52*(1), 6.

Anderson, E. A. (1988). AIDS public policy: Implications for families. *New England Journal of Public Policy, 4,* 411–427.

Andrews, F. M., & Withey, S. B. (1976). *Social indicators of well-being: America's perception of life quality*. New York: Plenum.

Andrews, K. (1986). Relevance of readmission of elderly patients discharged from a geriatric unit. *Journal of the American Geriatric Society, 33,* 422–428.

Antonucci, T. C., & Israel, B. A. (1986). Veridicality of social support: A comparison of principal and network members' responses. *Journal of Consulting Clinical Psychology, 54,* 432–437.

Applebaum, R., & Austin, C. (1990). *Long-term care case management: Design and evaluation*. New York: Springer.

Arangua, L., & Gelberg, L. (2007). Homeless persons. In R. M. Andersen, T. H. Rice, & G. F. Kominski (Eds.), *Changing the U.S. health care system: Key issues in health services policy and management* (pp. 491–547). San Francisco: John Wiley.

Archer, J., Probert, B. S., & Gage, L. (1987). College students' attitudes toward wellness. *Journal of College Student Personnel, 28,* 311–317.

Ardell, D. B. (1988). The history and future of the wellness movement. In J. P. Opatz (Ed.), *Wellness promotion strategies: Selected proceedings of the Eighth Annual National Wellness Conference.* Dubuque, IA: Kendall/Hunt.

Arnold, S., Kane, R. L., & Kane, R. A. (1986). Health promotion and the elderly: Evaluating the research. In K. Dychtwald & J. MacLean (Eds.), *Wellness and health promotion for the elderly* (pp. 327–344). Gaithersburg, MD: Aspen.

Aromacology: The psychic effects of fragrances. (1990, September–October). *The Futurist, 24,* 49–50.

A spoonful of hydrogel? (1991, January–February). *The Futurist, 25,* 6.

Astley, W. G., & Sachdeva, P. S. (1984). Structural sources of intraorganizational power: A theoretical synthesis. *Academy of Management Review, 91,* 104–113.

Attkisson, C. C., & Broskowski, A. (1978). Evaluation and the emerging human service concept. In C. C. Attkisson, W. A. Hargreaves, M. J. Horowitz, & J. E. Sorensen (Eds.), *Evaluation of human service programs* (pp. 3–26). San Diego: Academic Press.

Auerbach, C., Mason, S. E., & Laporte, H. H. (2007). Evidence that supports the value of social work in hospitals. *Social Work in Health Care, 44*(4), 17–32.

Auslander, W., & Freedenthal, S. (2006). Social work and chronic disease: Diabetes, heart disease, and HIV/AIDS. In S. Gehlert & T. A. Browne (Eds.), *Handbook of health social work* (pp. 532–567). Hoboken, NJ: John Wiley.

Austin, D. (2003). History of research in social work. In R. English (Ed.), Encyclopedia of social work (19th ed., Suppl.). Washington, DC: National Association of Social Workers.

Bakal, C. (1979). *Charity U.S.A.* New York: Times Books.

Balinsky, W. (1994). *Home care: Current problems and future solutions*. San Francisco: Jossey-Bass.

Bandura, A. (1986). *Social foundations of thought and action*. Upper Saddle River, NJ: Prentice Hall.

Barker, R. L. (1991). *Social work dictionary* (2nd ed.). Silver Spring, MD: National Association of Social Workers.

Barker, R. L. (2003). *Social work dictionary* (5th ed.). Washington, DC: National Association of Social Workers.

Barnes, A. S., Rogers, M., & Tran, C. (2007). Obesity as a clinical and social problem. In T. E. King, Jr., & M. B. Wheeler (Eds.), *Medical management of vulnerable and underserved patients: Principles, practice, and populations* (pp. 319–330). New York: McGraw-Hill.

Barnes, P. M., Adams, P. F., & Powell-Griner, E. (2010, March 9). *Health characteristics of the American Indian or Alaska Native adult population: United States, 2004–2008* (National Health Statistics Report No. 20). Hyattsville, MD: U.S. Department of Health and Human Services, National Center for Health Statistics.

Bartle, E. E., Couchonnal, G., Canda, E. R., & Staker, M. D. (2002). Empowerment as a dynamically developing concept for practice: Lessons learned from organizational ethnography. *Social Work, 47*(1), 32–43.

Barusch, A. (2006). *Foundations of social work* (2nd ed.). Belmont, CA: Thompson Brooks/Cole.

Barzansky, B., Friedman, C. P., Arnold, L., Davis, W. K., Jonas, H. S., Littlefield, J. H., et al. (1993). A view of medical practice in 2020 and its implications for medical school admission. *Academic Medicine, 68,* 31–34.

Baumann, L. J., Young. C. J., & Egan, J. J. (1992). Living with a heart transplant: Long-term adjustment. *Transplant International, 5*(1), 1–8.

Bayer, A.-H., & Harper, L. (2000, May). *Fixing to stay: A national survey on housing and home modification issues.* Washington, DC: AARP. Retrieved from http://assets.aarp.org/rgcenter/il/home_mod.pdf

Bayles, J. (1979). Ambulatory care options: Home care programs. In M. M. Melum (Ed.), *The changing role of the hospital: Options for the future.* Chicago: American Hospital Association.

Be your own big brother. (2009). *The Futurist, 43*(1), 2.

Beauchamp, D. (1976). Public health as social justice. *Inquiry, 13,* 3–14.

Behrens, R. A., & Longe, M. K. (1987). *Hospital-based health promotion programs for children and youth.* Chicago: American Hospital Association.

Beder, J. (2006). *Hospital social work: The interface of medicine and caring.* New York: Routledge.

Beitsch, L. M., Brooks, R. G., Menachemi, N., & Libbey, P. M. (2006). Public health at center stage: New roles, old props. *Health Affairs, 25*(4), 911–922.

Bellin, L. E. (1982). The politics of ambulatory care. In E. F. Pascarelli (Ed.), *Hospital-based ambulatory care* (pp. 95–109). Norwalk, CT: Appleton-Century-Crofts.

Belsky, J. (1980). Child maltreatment: An ecological integration. *American Psychologist, 35,* 320–335.

Bennett, C. (1988). A social worker comments: Some implications for social work practice in health care settings. *Social Work in Health Care, 13*(4), 15–18.

Benton, D., & Marshall, C. (1991). Elder abuse. *Clinical Geriatric Medicine, 7*(4), 831–845.

Berg-Weger, M., Rubio, D. M., & Tebb, S. S. (2000). The Caregiver Well-Being Scale revisited. *Health & Social Work, 25*(4), 255–263.

Berger, C. S. (1990). Enhancing social work influence in the hospital: Identifying sources of power. *Social Work in Health Care, 15*(2), 77–93.

Bergman, A., Wells, L., Bogo, M., Abbey, S., Chandler, V., Embleton, L., et al. (1993). High-risk indicators for family involvement in social work in health care: A review of the literature. *Social Work, 38,* 281–288.

Berkman, B., Bedell, D., Parker, E., McCarthy, L., & Rosenbaum, C. (1988). Pre-admission screening: An efficacy study. *Social Work in Health Care, 13*(3), 35–50.

Berkman, B. J., & Sampson, S. E. (1993). Psychological effects of cancer economics on patients and their families. *Cancer, 72*(Suppl. 9), 2846–2849.

Berkowitz, G., Halfon, N., & Klee, L. (1992). Improving access to health care: Case management for vulnerable children. *Social Work in Health Care, 77*(1), 101–123.

Bern-Klug, M. (2008). State variations in nursing home social worker qualifications. *Journal of Gerontological Social Work, 51*(3–4), 379–409.

Bernard, L. D. (1977). Education for social work. In J. B. Turner (Ed.), *Encyclopedia of social work* (17th ed., pp. 290–300). Washington, DC: National Association of Social Workers.

Bernstein, E., Wallerstein, N., Braithwaite, R., Gutierrez, L., Labonte, R., & Zimmerman, M. (1994). Empowerment forum: A dialogue between guest editorial board members. *Health Education Quarterly, 21,* 281–294.

Berzoff, J., & Silverman, P. R. (Eds.). (2004). *Living with dying: A handbook for end-of-life health care practitioners.* New York: Columbia University Press.

Best-Sigford, B., Bruininks, R. H., Lakin, K. C., Hill, B. K., & Heal, L. W. (1982). Resident release patterns in a national sample of public residential facilities. *American Journal of Mental Deficiency, 87,* 130–140.

Bettman, J. R. (1979). *An information processing theory of consumer choice.* Reading, MA: Addison-Wesley.

Biegel, D. E., Tracy, E. M., & Corvo, K. N. (1994). Strengthening social networks: Intervention strategies for mental health case managers. *Health & Social Work, 19,* 206–216.

Bishop, C. E., Squillace, M. R., Meagher, J., Anderson, W. L., & Weiner, J. M. (2009). Nursing home work practices and nursing assistants' job satisfaction. *The Gerontologist, 49*(5), 611–622.

Bisno, H. (1988). *Managing conflict.* Newbury Park, CA: Sage.

Blacker, S. (2004). Palliative care and social work. In J. Berzoff & R. P. Silverman (Eds.), *Living with dying* (pp. 409–423). New York: Columbia University Press.

Blair, C. E. (1994–1995). Residents who make decisions reveal healthier, happier attitudes. *Journal of Long-Term Care Administration, 22,* 37–39.

Blaisdell, F. W. (1994). Development of the city-county (public) hospital. *Archives of Surgery, 129,* 760–764.

Blanton, T., & Balch, D. C. (1995, September–October). Telemedicine: The health system of tomorrow. *The Futurist, 29,* 14–17.

Blasi, G. (1994). And we are not seen: Ideological and political barriers to understanding homelessness. *American Behavioral Scientist, 37,* 563–586.

Blaustein, M., & Veik, C. (1987). Problems and needs of operators of board and care homes: A survey. *Hospital and Community Psychiatry, 38,* 750–754.

Blazyk, S., & Canavan, M. M. (1985). Therapeutic aspects of discharge planning. *Social Work, 30,* 489–496.

Blazyk, S., & Canavan, M. M. (1986). Managing the discharge crisis following catastrophic illness or injury. *Social Work in Health Care, 11*(4), 19–32.

Bloom, M. (1981). *Primary prevention: The possible science.* Upper Saddle River, NJ: Prentice Hall.

Bloom, M. (1987). Prevention. In A. Minahan (Ed.), *Encyclopedia of social work* (18th ed.). Silver Spring, MD: National Association of Social Workers.

Blumenfield, S. (1986). Discharge planning: Changes for hospital social work in a new health care climate. *Quality Review Bulletin, 12*(2), 51–54.

Blumenfield, S., & Lowe, J. I. (1987). A template for analyzing ethical dilemmas in discharge planning. *Health and Social Work, 12,* 41–56.

Blumenfield, S., & Rosenberg, G. (1988). Toward a network of social health services: Redefining discharge planning and expanding the social work domain. *Social Work in Health Care, 13,* 31–48.

Bodenheimer, T. (2006). Primary care: Will it survive? *New England Journal of Medicine, 355,* 861–864.

Bodenheimer, T. S., & Grumbach, K. (2002). *Understanding health policy: A clinical approach.* New York: McGraw-Hill.

Boes, M., & McDermott, M. (2000). Crisis intervention in the hospital emergency room. In A. R. Roberts (Ed.), *Crisis intervention handbook: Assessment, treatment, and research* (pp. 389–411). New York: Oxford University Press.

Bond, A. F., & Duffle, D. (1995). Forming productive mutually challenging interagency relationships. In J. B. Rauch (Ed.), *Community-based, family-centered services in a changing health care environment.* Arlington, VA: National Maternal and Child Health Clearinghouse.

Bond, G., Miller, L., Krumwied, R., & Ward, R. (1988). Assertive case management in three CMHCs: A controlled study. *Hospital and Community Psychiatry, 39,* 411–417.

Bone substitute. (1994, January–February). *The Futurist, 28,* 6.

Bonuck, K. A. (1993). AIDS and families: Cultural, psychological, and functional impacts. *Social Work in Health Care, 18*(2), 75–89.

Borden, W. (1989). Life review as a therapeutic frame in the treatment of young adults with AIDS. *Health and Social Work, 14,* 253–259.

Bosworth, T. W. (1999). *Community health needs assessment: The health care professional's guide to evaluating the needs in your defined market.* New York: McGraw-Hill.

Bowen, D. E. (1985, November). Taking care of human relations equals taking care of the business. *Human Resources Reporter.*

Bower, B. (1994, January 22). Mental disorders strike about half of U.S. *Science News, 145,* 55.

Boyd, D. R. (1982). Emergency medical services systems. In E. F. Pascarelli (Ed.), *Hospital-based ambulatory care* (pp. 113–140). Norwalk, CT: Appleton-Century-Crofts.

Bracht, N. (1987). Preventive health care and wellness. In A. Minahan (Ed.), *Encyclopedia of social work* (18th ed., pp. 315–321). Silver Spring, MD: National Association of Social Workers.

Bracht, N. (Ed.). (1990). *Health promotion at the community level.* Newbury Park, CA: Sage.

Bracht, N., & Kingsbury, L. (1990). Community organization principles in health promotion. In N. Bracht (Ed.), *Health promotion at the community level* (pp. 66–88). Newbury Park, CA: Sage.

Bracht, N. F. (1978). *Social work in health care: A guide to professional practice.* New York: Haworth.

Brack, G., Jones, E. S., Smith, R. M., White, J., & Brack, C. J. (1993). A primer on consultation theory: Building a flexible worldview. *Journal of Counseling & Development, 71,* 619–628.

Bradshaw, B. R., Vonderharr, W. P., Keeney, V. T., Tyler, L. S., & Harris, S. (1976). Community-based residential care for the minimally impaired elderly: A survey analysis. *Journal of the American Geriatric Society, 24,* 423–428.

Braithwaite, R. L., Taylor, S. E., & Austin, J. N. (2000). *Building health coalitions in the black community.* Thousand Oaks, CA: Sage.

Brandle, B., Dryer, C. B., Heisler, C. J., Otto, J. M., Stiegel, L. A., & Thomas, R. W. (2007). *Elder abuse detection and intervention: A collaborative approach*. New York: Springer.

Brault, M. (2008). Americans with disabilities: 2005. In *Current population reports* (pp. 70–117). Washington, DC: U.S. Census Bureau.

Brawley, E. A. (1983). *Mass media and human services: Getting the message across*. Beverly Hills. CA: Sage.

Brecken, D. J., Harvey, J. R., & Lancaster, R. B. (1985). *Community health education: Settings, roles, and skills*. Gaithersburg, MD: Aspen.

Breslow, L., & Fielding, J. E. (2007). Public health and personal health services. In R. M. Andersen, T. H. Rice, & G. F. Kominski (Eds.), *Changing the U.S. health care system: Key issues in health services policy and management* (pp. 591–608). San Francisco: John Wiley.

Brickner, P. W. (1978). *Home health care for the aged*. Norwalk, CT: Appleton-Century-Crofts.

Brill, N. I. (1976). *Teamwork: Working together in the human services*. Philadelphia: J. B. Lippincott.

Brockett, R. G. (1981). The use of reality orientation in adult foster care homes: A rationale. *Journal of Gerontological Social Work, 3,* 3–13.

Brockington, C. F. (1975). The history of public health. In W. Hobson (Ed.), *The theory and practice of public health*. London: Oxford University Press.

Brody, E. M. (1977). *Long-term care of older people: A practical guide*. New York: Human Science Press.

Brooks, M. K. (2010). Hospice services: The technology at the end of life. In T. S. Kerson, J. L. M. McCoyd, & Associates (Eds.), *Social work in health care settings: Practice in context* (3rd ed., pp. 235–245). New York: Routledge.

Brown, B. B. (1978). Social and psychological correlates of help-seeking behavior among urban adults. *American Journal of Community Psychology, 6,* 425–439.

Brown, D., Pryzwansky, W. B., & Schultz, A. C. (1987). *Psychological consultation: Introduction to theory and practice*. Needham Heights, MA: Allyn & Bacon.

Brown, E. R., & Lavarreda, S. A. (2007). Public policies to extend health care coverage. In R. M. Anderson, T. H. Rice, & G. F. Kominski (Eds.), *Changing the U.S. health care system: Key issues in health services policy and management* (pp. 81–114). San Francisco: John Wiley.

Brown, J. S. T., & Furstenberg, A. (1992). Restoring control: Empowering older patients and their families during health crisis. *Social Work in Health Care, 17*(4), 81–101.

Brown, T. M. (1982). A historical view of health care teams. In G. J. Agich (Ed.), *Responsibility in health care*. Boston: D. Reidel.

Buada, L., Pomeranz, W., & Rosenberg, S. (1986). *Developing long-term care services: Product lines for the rural elderly* (Rural hospitals: Strategies for survival monograph series). Kansas City, MO: National Rural Health Care Association.

Buchanan, A., Brock, D. W., Daniels, N., & Wikler, D. (2000). *From chance to choice: Genetics and justice*. New York: Cambridge University Press.

Buck, S. (2006, July–August). Who pays for Hospice? *Medicare Patient Management,* 31–33.

Buie, V. C., Owings, M. F., DeFrances, C. J., & Golosinksiy, A. (2010, December). National hospital discharge survey: 2006 annual summary. *Vital Health Statistics, 13*(168). Hyattsville, MD: National Center of Health Statistics. Retrieved from http://www.cdc.gov/nchs/data/series/sr_13/sr13_168.pdf

Burg, M. A., Zebrack, B., Walsh, K., Maramaldi, P., Lim, J., Smolinski, K. M., et al. (2010). Barriers to accessing quality health care for cancer patients: A survey of members of the Association of Oncology Social Work. *Social Work in Health Care, 49,* 38–52.

Burling, T., Lentz, E. M., & Wilson, R. N. (1956). *The give and take in hospitals: A study of human organization in hospitals*. New York: Putnam.

Burman, L. E., & Johnson, R. W. (2007). *A proposal to finance long-term care services through Medicare with an income tax surcharge*. Washington, DC: Urban Institute.

Burr, J. A., Mutchler, J. E., & Warren, J. P. (2005). State commitment to home- and community-based services effects on independent living for older unmarried women. *Journal of Aging and Social Policy, 17*(1), 1–18.

Burr, J. T. (1990, November). The tools of quality: Part VI; Pareto charts. *Quality Progress,* 59–61.

Burt, M. R., Aron, L. Y., Douglas, T., Valente, J., Lee, E., & Iwen, B. (1999, December). *Homelessness: Programs and people they serve; Summary report*. Washington, DC: Interagency Council on Homelessness.

Bussolari, C. J., & Goodell, J. A. (2009). Chaos theory as a model for life transitions counseling: Nonlinear dynamics and life's changes. *Journal of Counseling & Development, 87*(1), 98–107.

Butcher, S. (1995). Promoting maternal and child health social work in a changing health care environment. In J. B. Rauch (Ed.), *Community-based, family-centered services in a changing health care environment.* Arlington, VA: National Maternal and Child Health Clearinghouse.

Butler, R. N. (1963). The life review: An interpretation of reminiscence in the aged. *Psychiatry, 26*(3), 65–76.

Byrd, W. M., & Clayton, L. A. (1993). The African-American cancer crisis: Part II; A prescription. *Journal of Health Care for the Poor and Underserved, 4*(2), 102–116.

Cable, E. P., & Mayers, S. P. (1983). Discharge planning effect on length of hospital stay. *Archives of Physical Medicine and Rehabilitation, 64*(2), 57–60.

Cabot, R. C. (1915). *Social service and the art of healing.* New York: Moffat, Yard.

Cagle, J. G., & Kovacs, P. J. (2009). Education: A complex and empowering social work intervention at the end of life. *Health & Social Work, 34,* 17–27.

Calista, M. R. (1989). *Implications of empowerment concept and strategies for social work education and practice.* Paper presented at the Annual Program Meeting of the Council on Social Work Education, Chicago.

Callahan, D. (2000). *The troubled dream of life: In search of a peaceful death.* Washington, DC: Georgetown University Press.

Campbell, D. T., & Stanley, J. C. (1966). *Experimental and quasi-experimental designs for research.* Chicago: Rand McNally.

Cannon, I. M. (1913). *Social work in hospitals.* New York: Russell Sage.

Cannon, I. M. (1952). *On the social frontier of medicine: Pioneering in medical social service.* Cambridge, MA: Harvard University Press.

Cantor, M., & Chichin, E. (1990). *Stress and strain among home care workers of the frail elderly.* New York: Fordham University, Third Age Center, Brookdale Research Institute on Aging.

Caplan, G., & Caplan, R. (1993). *Mental health consultation and collaboration.* San Francisco: Jossey-Bass.

Capuzzi, D., Gross, D., & Friel, S. E. (1990, Winter). Recent trends in group work with elders. *Generations,* 43–48.

Carlett, C. (1993). Teams and teamwork. *American Speech-Language-Hearing Association, 35,* 30–31.

Carling, P. J. (1984). *Developing family foster care programs in mental health: A resource guide.* Boston: Boston University Center for Rehabilitation Research & Training in Mental Health.

Carlton, T. O. (1984). *Clinical social work in health settings: A guide to professional practice with exemplars.* New York: Springer.

Carlton, T. O. (1989). Stand up and cheer. *Health and Social Work, 14,* 227–230.

Caro, F. G. (1990). The world of home care: What does it look like? In C. Zuckerman, N. N. Dubler, & B. Collopy (Eds.), *Home health care options: A guide for older persons and concerned families.* New York: Plenum.

Caroff, P. (1988). Clinical social work: Present role and future challenge. *Social Work in Health Care, 13*(3), 21–33.

Caroff, P., & Mailick, M. D. (1985). The patient has a family: Reaffirming social work's domain. *Social Work in Health Care, 10*(4), 17–34.

Casey, M., Moscovice, I., Virnig, B. A., & Durham, S. (2005). Providing hospice care in rural areas: Challenges and strategies to address them. *American Journal of Hospice & Palliative Care, 22,* 363–368.

Cassel, J. (1976). The contribution of social environment to host resistance. *American Journal of Epidemiology, 104,* 107–123.

Centers for Disease Control and Prevention. (2001). Compendium of HIV prevention intervention with evidence of effectiveness. Atlanta, GA: Author. Retrieved from http://www.cdc.gov/hiv/resources/reports/hiv_compendium/pdf/HIVcompendium.pdf

Centers for Disease Control and Prevention. (2007). A glance at the HIV/AIDS epidemic: *CDC HIV/AIDS fact sheet, revised.* Retrieved from http://www.cdc.gov/hiv/resources/factsheets/PDF/At-A-Glance.pdf

Centers for Disease Control and Prevention. (2010a). *Heart disease and stroke prevention: Time for action.* Retrieved from http://www.cdc.gov/dhdsp/action_plan/pdfs/action_plan_3of7.pdf

Centers for Disease Control and Prevention. (2010b). *NHIS arthritis surveillance.* Retrieved from www.cdc.gov/arthritis/data_statistics/national_nhis.htm

Chapman, M. (1989, Spring). Making peace with the media. *Public Welfare,* 35–36.

Checkoway, B. (1995). Six strategies of community change. *Community Development Journal, 30,* 220.

Cheek, L. B. (1987). Alzheimer's families. *Aging, 335,* 17–19.

Chell, B. (1988). But murderers can have all the children they want: Surrogacy and public policy. *Theoretical Medicine, 9,* 3–21.

Chen, H., & Landefeld, C. S. (2007). The hidden poor: Care of the elderly. In T. E. Kin & M. B. Wheeler (Eds.), *Medical management of vulnerable and underserved patients: Principles, practice, and populations* (pp. 119–209). New York: McGraw-Hill.

Chen, M. S., Kuun, P., Guthrie, R., Wen, L., & Zaharlick, A. (1991). Promoting heart health for Southeast Asians: A database for planning interventions. *Public Health Reports, 106,* 304–309.

Cheng, M. (2010, January 14). Doctors give injured woman a new windpipe. *Lexington Herald-Leader.*

Cherlin, E., Fried, T., Prigerson, H. S., Schulman-Green, D., Hohnson-Hurzeler, R., & Bradley, E. H. (2006). Communication between physicians and family caregivers about care at the end of life: When do discussions occur and what is said? *Journal of Palliative Medicine, 8,* 1176–1185.

Children's Defense Fund. (2010). *The state of America's children.* Washington, DC: Author. Retrieved from http://www.childrensdefense.org/

Christen, A. G., & Christen, J. A. (1994). Why is cigarette smoking so addicting? An overview of smoking as a chemical and process addiction. *Health Values: The Journal of Health Behavior, Education, & Promotion, 18,* 17–24.

Chung, I. (2005). The sociocultural reality of the Asian immigrant elderly: Implications for group work practice. *Journal of Gerontological Social Work, 44*(1–2), 81–93.

Ciotti, M., & Watt, S. (1992). Discharge planning and the role of the social worker. In M. J. Holosko & P. A. Taylor (Eds.), *Social work practice in health care settings.* Toronto: Canadian Scholars' Press.

Claiborne, N. (2006). Effectiveness of a care coordination model for stroke survivors: A randomized study. *Health & Social Work, 31*(2), 87–96.

Clapp, R. L. (1993, November/December). Health care continuum. *Nursing Homes,* 7–9.

Clark, D., & Connelly, T. (1979). *Developing interdisciplinary education in allied health programs: Issues and decisions.* Atlanta, GA: Southern Regional Education Board.

Clark, E. (1971). Nursing homes. In R. Morris (Ed.), *Encyclopedia of social work* (16th ed., pp. 886–890). New York: National Association of Social Workers.

Clark, R. E., & LaBeff, E. E. (1982). Death telling: Managing the delivery of bad news. *Journal of Health and Social Behavior, 23,* 366–380.

Clement, J. L., & Durgin, J. S. (1987). Emergency health services. In A. Minahan (Ed.), *Encyclopedia of social work* (18th ed.). Silver Spring, MD: National Association of Social Workers.

Coates, J. (1994, July–August). The highly probable future: 83 assumptions about the year 2025. *The Futurist, 28,* 1–7.

COBRA: The Emergency Medical Treatment and Active Labor Act. 42 USC 1395 (1986). (Pub. No. 99-272.9121, 1986). Washington, DC: Government Printing Office.

Cohen, A. M. (2009). Child homelessness on the rise. *The Futurist, 43*(4), 7.

Cohen, A. M. (2010). Digital bandage monitors vital signs: Wireless technology for early detection. *The Futurist, 44*(2), 9.

Cohen, J. (1980). Nature of clinical social work. In P. L. Ewalt (Ed.), *Toward a definition of clinical social work.* Washington, DC: National Association of Social Workers.

Cohen, L. L. (2008). Racial/ethnic disparities in hospice care: A systematic review. *Journal of Palliative Medicine, 11,* 763–768.

Coile. R. C., Jr. (1990). *The new medicine: Reshaping medical practice and health care management.* Gaithersburg, MD: Aspen.

Coleman, T. M., Looney, S., O'Brien, J., Ziegler, C., Pastorino, C. A., & Turner, C. (2002). The Eden alternative: Findings after 1 year of implementation. *Journal of Gerontology: Medical Sciences, 57A,* M422–M427.

Colerick, E. J., & George, L. K. (1986). Predictors of institutionalization among caregivers of patients with Alzheimer's disease. *Journal of the American Geriatrics Society, 34,* 493–498.

Collins, A., Pancoast, D., & Dunn, J. (1977). *Consultation workbook.* Portland, OR: Portland State University.

Collins, F. S. (2010, June 20). The cancer you can beat. *Parade,* p. 8.

Collins, S. R., Davis, K., Nicholson, J. L., & Stremikis, K. (2010, September 1). Realizing health reform's potential: Small businesses and the Affordable Care Act of 2010. *Issue Brief (Commonwealth Fund), 97,* 1–18.

Collins, S. R., & Nicholson, J. L. (2010, May 1). Rite of passage: Young adults and the Affordable Care Act of 2010. *Issue Brief (Commonwealth Fund), 97,* 1–24.

Collins, S. R., Rustgi, S., & Doty, M. M. (2010, July 1). Realizing health reform's potential: Women and the Affordable Care Act of 2010. *Issue Brief (Commonwealth Fund), 97*, 1–18.

Colon, M. (2005). Hospice and Latinos: A review of the literature. *Journal of Social Work in End-of-Life & Palliative Care, 1*, 27–43.

Committee on Aging of the Group for the Advancement of Psychiatry. (1971). *The aged and community mental health: A guide to program development* (Report No. 80). New York: Group for the Advancement of Psychiatry.

Committee on Cost of Medical Care. (1932). *Medical care for the American people: The final report of the committee.* Chicago: University of Chicago Press.

Committee on Violence. (2004). *Partner violence: How to recognize and treat victims of abuse; A guide for physicians and other health care professionals.* Waltham: Massachusetts Medical Society. Retrieved from www.massmed.org

Community-State Partnerships to Improve End-of-Life Care. (2001, January). How end-of-life care can be a positive issue for policy leaders. *State Initiatives in End-of-Life Care* (Issue 9). Kansas City, MO: Author. Retrieved from http://www.rwjf.org/files/publications/other/State_Initiatives_EOL9.pdf

Community-State Partnerships to Improve End-of-Life Care. (2002, November). Barriers to hospice care and some proposed policy solutions. *State Initiatives in End-of-Life Care* (Issue 17). Kansas City, MO: Author. Retrieved from http://www.rwjf.org/files/publications/other/State_Initiatives_EOL17.pdf

Community-State Partnerships to Improve End-of-Life Care. (2003, June). Championing end-of-life care policy change. *State Initiatives in End-of-Life Care* (Issue 19). Kansas City, MO: Author. Retrieved from http://www.rwjf.org/files/publications/other/State_Initiatives_EOL19.pdf

Conference. (1994, November–December). *Nursing Homes,* 10–15.

Conger, S. A., & Moore, K. D. (1988). Chronic illness and the quality of life: The social worker's role. In J. S. McNeil & S. E. Weinstein (Eds.), *Innovations in health care practice* (pp. 102–115). Washington, DC: National Association of Social Workers.

Connaway, R. S., & Gentry, M. E. (1988). *Social work practice.* Upper Saddle River, NJ: Prentice Hall.

Conroy, A. M. (1994). Bringing family members into the community. *Journal of Long-Term Care Administration, 22*(2), 8.

Cooper, C. L., & Dewe, P. (2004). *Stress: A brief history.* Malden, MA: Blackwell.

Cornelius, D. S. (1994). Managed care and social work: Constructing a context and a response. *Social Work in Health Care, 20*(1), 47–63.

Cornish, E. (1994, May–June). Responsibility for the future. *The Futurist, 28,* 60.

Coulton, C. J. (1985). Research and practice: An ongoing relationship. *Health & Social Work, 10,* 282–291.

Council on Social Work Education. (2001). *Educational policy and accreditation standards.* Alexandria, VA: Author.

Cowles, L. A. F. (2003). *Social work in the health field: A care perspective* (2nd ed.). Binghamton, NY: Haworth.

Cox, C. (1992). Expanding social work's role in home care: An ecological perspective. *Social Work, 37,* 97–192.

Crawford, J. M. (1999, May–June). Co-parent adoptions by same-sex couples: From loophole to law. *Families in Society, 80,* 271–278.

Crawley, L. M. (2007). Care of the dying patient. In T. E. King & M. B. Wheeler (Eds.), *Medical management of vulnerable and underserved patients: Principles, practice, and populations* (pp. 223–233). New York: McGraw-Hill.

Crossman, L. (1992, August). *A history of rape in American society prior to 1990.* Paper presented at the Annual Meeting of the American Psychological Association, Washington, DC.

Crouch, D. J., Birky, M. M., Gust, S. W., Rollins, D. E., Walsh, J. M., Moulden, J. V., et al. (1993). The prevalence of drugs and alcohol in fatally injured truck drivers. *Journal of Forensic Science, 38*(6), 1342–1353.

Csikai, E. L. (2004). Social workers' participation in the resolution of ethical dilemmas in hospice care. *Health & Social Work, 29,* 67–76.

Currie, B. F., & Beasley, J. W. (1982). Health promotion in the medical encounter. In R. B. Taylor, J. R. Ureda, & J. W. Denham (Eds.), *Health promotion: Principles and clinical applications* (pp. 143–160). Norwalk, CT: Appleton-Century-Crofts.

Czeizel, A. E., Kodaj, I., & Lenz, W. (1994). Smoking during pregnancy and congenital limb deficiency. *British Medical Journal, 308*(6942), 1473–1476.

Dalton. H. L. (1989). AIDS in black face. *Daedalus, 118,* 205–227.

Daro, D., & Donnelly, A. C. (2002). Charting the waves of prevention: Two steps forward, one step back. *Child Abuse & Neglect, 26,* 731–742.

Davey, T. L., & Ivery, J. M. (2009). Using organizational collaboration and community partnerships to transition families from homelessness to home ownership: The HomeBuy5 Program. *Journal of Prevention & Intervention in the Community, 37*(2), 155–156.

Davidson, K. W. (1978). Evolving social work roles in health care: The case of discharge planning. *Social Work in Health Care, 4*(1), 43–54.

Davis, A. J. (2000). Bioethically constructed ideal dying patient in USA. *Medical Law, 19,* 161–164.

Davis, E. M., & Millman, M. L. (1983). *Health care for the urban poor: Directions for policy.* Totowa, NJ: Rowman & Allanheld.

Davis, M. A. (1991). On nursing home quality: A review and analysis. *Medical Care Review, 48,* 129–166.

Davis, N. J. (1988). Shelters for battered women: Social policy response to interpersonal violence. *Social Science Journal, 25,* 401–419.

Davis, N. M. (1988, November). Fundraising success: Knowing why people give. *Association Management,* 120–127.

Deming, E. W. (1986). *Out of the crisis.* Cambridge: MIT, Center for Advanced Engineering Study.

Demographics of the United States. (2010). Retrieved October 20, 2010, from http://en.wikipedia.org/wiki/Demographics_of_the_United_States

DeSpiegler, G. (1979). The South Dakota experimental swing-bed program. In M. M. Melum (Ed.), *The changing role of the hospital: Options for the future.* Chicago: American Hospital Association.

Deutsch, M. (1973). *The resolution of conflict: Constructive and destructive processes.* New Haven, CT: Yale University Press.

Deutsch, M. (2006). Cooperation and competition. In M. Deutsch, P. T. Coleman, & E. C. Marcus (Eds.), *The handbook of conflict resolution* (pp. 23–42). San Francisco: Jossey-Bass.

Devore, W., & Schlesinger, E. G. (1981). *Ethnic-sensitive social work practice.* St. Louis, MO: C. V. Mosby.

DeWald, S. L., & Moe, A. M. (2010). Like a prison: Homeless women's narratives of surviving shelter. *Journal of Sociology and Social Welfare, 37*(1), 115–135.

Dhooper, S. S. (1983). Coping with the crisis of heart attack. *Social Work in Health Care, 9*(1), 1531.

Dhooper, S. S. (1984). Social networks and support during the crisis of heart attack. *Health and Social Work, 9,* 294–303.

Dhooper, S. S. (1990). Identifying and mobilizing social supports for the cardiac patient's family. *Journal of Cardiovascular Nursing, 5*(1), 65–73.

Dhooper, S. S. (1991). Caregivers of Alzheimer's disease patients: A review of the literature. *Journal of Gerontological Social Work, 18,* 19–37.

Dhooper, S. S. (1994a). *Social work and transplantation of human organs.* New York: Praeger.

Dhooper, S. S. (1994b, May). *Social work contributions to interdisciplinary teamwork in the field of disabilities.* Paper presented at the Conference on Social Work and Disabilities, Young Adult Institute, New York.

Dhooper, S. S. (2003). Health care needs of foreign-born Asian Americans. *Health & Social Work, 28*(1), 63–73.

Dhooper, S. S., Green, S. M., Huff, M. B., & Austin-Murphy, J. (1993). Efficacy of a group approach to reducing depression in nursing home elderly residents. *Journal of Gerontological Social Work, 20,* 87–100.

Dhooper, S. S., & Moore, S. E. (2001). *Social work practice with culturally diverse people.* Thousand Oaks, CA: Sage.

Dhooper, S. S., Royse, D. D., & Rihm, S. J. (1989). Adults with mental retardation in community residential settings: An exploratory study. *Adult Residential Care Journal, 3,* 33–51.

Dillard, J. M. (1983). *Multicultural counseling.* Chicago: Nelson-Hall.

Dillon, C. (1985). Families, transitions, and health: Another look. *Social Work in Health Care, 10*(4), 35–44.

Dillon, C. (1990). Managing stress in health social work roles today. *Social Work in Health Care, 14*(4), 91–108.

Dimant, J. (1991). From quality assurance to quality management in long-term care. *Quality Review Bulletin, 17,* 207–215.

DiMatteo, M., Giordani, P., Lepper, H., & Croghan, T. (2002). Patient adherence and medical treatment outcomes: A meta-analysis. *Medical Care, 40*(9), 794–811.

Dinerman, M. (1997). Social work roles in America's changing health care. *Social Work in Health Care, 25*(1/2), 23–33.

DiNitto, D. M., & McNeece, C. A. (1990). *Social work: Issues and opportunities in a changing profession.* Upper Saddle River, NJ: Prentice Hall.

Dluhy, M. J. (1990). *Building coalitions in the human services.* Newbury Park, CA: Sage.

Dobrof, R., & Litwak, E. (1977). *Maintenance of family ties of long-term care patients: Theory and guide to practice.* Rockville, MD: National Institute of Mental Health.

Doss-Martin, L., & Stokes, D. J. (1989). Historical development of social work in primary care. In M. L. Henk (Ed.), *Social work in primary care* (pp. 17–30). Newbury Park, CA: Sage.

Douglass, A., & Winterfeld, A. (1995). *Helping children and families through legislative activism: A guide to the legislative process.* Englewood, CO: American Humane Association.

Drew, J. A. (1979). A Connecticut hospital's experience with satellite clinics. In M. M. Melum (Ed.), *The changing role of the hospital: Options for the future* (pp. 107–114).Chicago: American Hospital Association.

Drinka, T. J., & Clark, P. G. (2000). *Health care teamwork: Interdisciplinary practice teaching.* Westport, CT: Auburn House.

Drubach, D. A., Kelly, M. P., Winslow, M. M., & Flynn, J. P. (1993). Substance abuse as a factor in the causality, severity, and recurrence rate of traumatic brain injury. *Maryland Medical Journal, 42,* 989–993.

Dunham, W., Bolden, J., & Kvale, E. (2003). Obstacles to the delivery of acceptable standards of care in rural home hospices. *American Journal of Hospice and Palliative Care, 20,* 259–261.

Dunkel, J., & Hatfield, S. (1986). Countertransference issues in working with persons with AIDS. *Social Work, 31,* 114–117.

Durkin, M. S., Davidson, L. L., Kuhn, L., O'Connor, P., & Barlow, B. (1994). Low-income neighborhoods and the risk of severe pediatric injury: A small-area analysis in northern Manhattan. *American Journal of Public Health, 84,* 587–592.

Dworkin, S. H., & Pincu, L. (1993). Counseling in the era of AIDS. *Journal of Counseling & Development, 71,* 275–281.

Edelman, M., & Mihaly, L. (1989). Homeless families and the housing crisis in the United States. *Children and Youth Services Review, 11,* 91–108.

Edinburg, G. M., & Cottier, J. M. (1995). Managed care. In R. L. Edwards (Ed.), *Encyclopedia of social work* (19th ed.). Washington, DC: National Association of Social Workers.

Edlis, N. (1993). Rape crisis: Development of a center in an Israeli hospital. *Social Work in Health Care, 18*(3/4), 169–178.

Egan, G. (1990). *The skilled helper: A systematic approach to effective helping.* Pacific Grove, CA: Brooks/Cole.

Ehrlich, P., & Anetzberger, G. (1991). Survey of state public health departments on procedures for reporting elder abuse. *Public Health Reports, 106*(2), 151–154.

Eisdorfer, C., & Maddox, G. L. (1988). A distinctive role for hospitals in caring for older adults: Issues and opinions. In C. Eisdorfer & G. L. Maddox (Eds.), *The role of hospitals in geriatric care* (pp. 1–18). New York: Springer.

Elder, J. P., Schmid, T. L., Dower, P., & Hedlund, S. (1993, Winter). Community heart health programs: Components, rationale, and strategies for effective interventions. *Journal of Public Health Policy, 14,* 463–479.

Ellis, L. (1991). A synthesized (biosocial) theory of rape. *Journal of Consulting and Clinical Psychology, 59,* 631–642.

Emerson, H. (1945). *Local health units for the nation.* New York: Commonwealth Fund.

Epstein, I. (2001). Using available clinical information in practice-based research: Mining for silver while dreaming of gold. Social Work in Health Care, *33*(3/4), 15–32.

Epstein, I., & Blumenfield, S. (Eds.). (2001). Clinical data mining in practice-based research: Social work in hospital settings. Binghamton, NY: Haworth.

Epstein, I., & Kapp, S. A. (2008). Agency-based research. In T. Mizrahi & L. E. Davis (Eds.), Encyclopedia of social work (20th ed.). Washington, DC: National Association of Social Workers and Oxford University Press. Retrieved from http://www.oxford-naswsocialwork.com

Epstein, J., Turgeman, A., Rotstein, Z., Horoszowski, H., Honig, P., Baruch, L., et al. (1998). Preadmission psychosocial screening of older orthopedic surgery patients. *Social Work in Health Care, 27*(2), 1–25.

Erdmann, E., & Stover, D. (1993, September–October). Drowning in preconceptions. *The Futurist, 27,* 60.

Erickson, R., & Erickson, G. (1992). An overview of social work practice in health settings. In M. J. Holosko & P. A. Taylor (Eds.), *Social work in health care settings* (pp. 5–19). Toronto: Canadian Scholars' Press.

Ervin, S. L. (2000). Fourteen forecasts for an aging society. *The Futurist, 34*(6), 24–28.

Eskildson, L., & Yates, G. R. (1991). Lessons from industry: Revising organizational structure to improve health care quality assurance. *Quality Review Bulletin, 17,* 38–41.

Estes, C. L. (1999). Critical gerontology and the new political economy of aging. In M. Minkler &

C. L. Estes (Eds.), *Critical gerontology: Perspectives from political and moral economy* (pp. 17–35). New York: Baywood.

Evans, R., Stone, D., & Elwyn, G. (2004). Organizing palliative care for rural populations: A systematic review of the evidence. *Family Practice, 21,* 114–115.

Evans, R. W. (1991). Quality of life assessment and the treatment of end-stage renal disease. In R. W. Evans, D. L. Manninen, & F. B. Dong (Eds.), *The National Cooperative Transplantation Study: Final report* (BHARC-100-91-020). Seattle, WA: Battelle-Seattle Research Center.

Evashwick, C. J., & Branch, L. G. (1987). Clients of the continuum of care. In C. J. Evashwick & L. J. Weiss (Eds.), *Managing the continuum of care* (pp. 45–56). Gaithersburg, MD: Aspen.

Ewing, R. S. (1979). Future of the trustee. In M. M. Melum (Ed.), *The changing role of the hospital: Options for the future* (pp. 11–14). Chicago: American Hospital Association.

Ezell, M. (1994). Advocacy practice of social workers. *Families in Society: The Journal of Contemporary Social Services, 75*(1), 36–46.

Fagan, R. M., Williams, C. C., & Burger, S. G. (1997). *Meeting of pioneers in nursing home culture change.* Rochester, NY: Lifespan of Greater Rochester.

Fallcreek, S., Warner-Reitz, A., & Mettler, M. H. (1986). Designing health promotion programs for elders. In K. Dychtwald (Ed.), *Wellness and health promotion for the elderly* (pp. 219–233). Gaithersburg, MD: Aspen.

Family Violence Prevention Fund. (2002, September). *National consensus guidelines: On identifying and responding to domestic violence victimization in health care settings.* San Francisco: Author. Retrieved from http://www.futureswithoutviolence.org/userfiles/file/Consensus.pdf

Feather, J. (1993). Factors in perceived hospital discharge planning effectiveness. *Social Work in Health Care, 19*(1), 1–14.

Feigenbaum, A. V. (1983). *Total quality control.* New York: McGraw-Hill.

Fenske, V., & Roecker, M. (1971). Finding foster homes for adults. *Public Welfare, 29,* 404–410.

Ferguson, T. (1992, January–February). Patient, heal thyself: Health in the information age. *The Futurist, 26,* 9–13.

Fergusson, D. M., Horwood, J., & Lynskey, M. T. (1993). Maternal smoking before and after

pregnancy: Effects on behavioral outcomes in middle childhood. *Pediatrics, 92,* 815–822.

Fernie, B., & Fernie, G. (1990). Organizing group programs for cognitively impaired elderly residents of nursing homes. *Clinical Gerontologist, 9,* 123–134.

Field, D. M. (1993, January–February). Highlights from "Creating the 21st Century." *The Futurist, 27,* 35.

Fields, G. (1978). Editorial. *Social Work in Health Care, 4*(1), 5–6.

Fine, M., & Asch, A. (1988). Disability beyond stigma: Social interaction, discrimination, and activism. *Journal of Social Issues, 44,* 3–21.

Finkelhor, D. (1979). *Sexually victimized children.* New York: Free Press.

Finkelhor, D., & Baron, L. (1986). High-risk children. In D. Finkelhor (Ed.), *A sourcebook on child sexual abuse* (pp. 60–88). Beverly Hills, CA: Sage.

Finkelhor, D., & Strapko, N. (1992). Sexual abuse prevention education: A review of evaluation studies. In D. J. Willis, E. W. Holden, & M. Rosenberg (Eds.), *Prevention of child maltreatment: Developmental and ecological perspectives* (pp. 150–167). New York: John Wiley.

Finley, W., Mutran, E., Zeitler, R., & Randall, C. (1990). Queues and care: How medical residents organize their work in a busy clinic. *Journal of Health and Social Behavior, 31,* 292–305.

Fisher, H. (2010). The new monogamy: Forward to the past. *The Futurist, 44*(6), 26–28.

Fisher, J. A. (1992). *Rx 2000: Breakthroughs in health, medicine, and longevity in the next five to forty years.* New York: Simon & Schuster.

Fisher, R., & Ury, W. (1981). *Getting to yes: Negotiating agreement without giving in.* Boston: Houghton Mifflin.

Fiske, A., O'Riley, A. A., & Widoe, R. K. (2008). Physical health and suicide in late life: An evaluative review. *Clinical Gerontologist, 31*(4), 31–50.

Flora, J. A., & Cassady, D. (1990). Role of media in community-based health promotion. In N. Bracht (Ed.), *Health promotion at the community level* (pp. 143–157). Newbury Park, CA: Sage.

Flynn, B. C., Ray, D. W., & Rider, M. S. (1994). Empowering communities: Action research through health cities. *Health Education Quarterly, 21,* 395–405.

Flynn, J. P. (1995). Social justice in social agencies. In R. L. Edwards (Ed.), *Encyclopedia of social work* (19th ed., pp. 2173–2179). Washington, DC: National Association of Social Workers.

Fong, R. (2008). Culturally competent social work practice. In D. M. DiNitto & C. A. McNeece (Eds.), *Social work issues and opportunities in a challenging profession* (pp. 79–98). Chicago: Lyceum.

Foods that bring better health. (1991, September–October). *The Futurist, 25,* 52–53.

Foreman, M. D., Theis, S. L., & Anderson, M. A. (1993). Adverse events in the hospitalized elderly. *Clinical Nursing Research, 2*(3), 360–370.

Forste, R., & Heaton, T. B. (2004). The divorce generation: Well-being, family attitudes, and socioeconomic consequences of marital disruption. *Journal of Divorce and Remarriage, 41*(1/2), 95–114.

Frager, S. (2000). *Managing managed care: Secrets from a former case manager.* New York: John Wiley.

Frankel, A. J. (1989, March). *Clinical social work and community organization: A re-marriage made in heaven.* Paper presented at the 35th Annual Program Meeting, Council on Social Work Education, Chicago.

Frankenberg, R. (Ed.). (1992). *Time, health, and medicine.* Newbury Park, CA: Sage.

Frankish, C. J., Lovato, C. Y., & Poureslami, I. (2007). Models, theories, and principles of health promotion: Revisiting their use with multicultural populations. In M. V. Kline & R. M. Huff (Eds.), *Health promotion in multicultural populations: A handbook for practitioners and students* (pp. 57–101). Thousand Oaks, CA: Sage.

Frazier, P. A., & Cohen, B. B. (1992). Research on the sexual victimization of women: Implications for counselor training. *Counseling Psychologist, 20,* 141–158.

Freddolino, P. P., Moxley, D. P., & Hyduk, C. A. (2004). A differential model of advocacy in social work practice. *Families in society: The journal of contemporary social services, 85*(1), 119–128.

Freedman, S. A. (2009). Psychological effects of terror attacks. In S. C. Shapira, J. S. Hammond, & L. A. Cole (Eds.), *Essentials of terror medicine* (pp. 405–424). New York: Springer.

French, J. R. P., & Raven, B. (1959). The bases of social power. In D. Cartwright (Ed.), *Studies in social power* (pp. 150–167). Ann Arbor: University of Michigan, Institute for Social Research.

Freudenberg, N., Eng, E., Flay, B., Parcel, G., Rogers, T., & Wallerstein, N. (1995). Strengthening individual and community capacity to prevent disease and promote health: In search of relevant theories and principles. *Health Education Quarterly, 22,* 290–306.

Friedman, E. (1991). Patients as partners: The changing health care environment. *Social Work in Health Care, 17,* 31–46.

Friesen, B. (1987). Administration: Interpersonal aspects. In A. Minahan (Ed.), *Encyclopedia of social work* (18th ed.). Silver Spring, MD: National Association of Social Workers.

Friesen, B. J. (1993). Overview: Advances in child mental health. In H. C. Johnson (Ed.), *Child mental health in the 1990s: Curricula for graduate and undergraduate professional education* (pp. 12–19). Washington, DC: Government Printing Office.

Fulmer, T. T. (1984). Elder abuse assessment tool. *Dimensions of Critical Care Nursing, 10*(12), 16–20.

Fuqua, D. R., & Kurpius, D. J. (1993). Conceptual models in organizational consultation. *Journal of Counseling & Development, 71,* 607–618.

Furlong, R. M. (1986). The social worker's role on the institutional ethics committee. *Social Work in Health Care, 11*(4), 93–100.

Furstenberg, A. (1984). Social work in medical care settings. In R. J. Estes (Ed.), *Health care and the social services: Social work practice in health care* (pp. 23–77). St. Louis, MO: Warren H. Green.

Furstenberg, A., & Mezey, M. D. (1987). Mental impairment of elderly hospitalized hip fracture patients. *Comprehensive Gerontology, 1,* 80–85.

Furstenberg, A., & Olson, M. M. (1984). Social work and AIDS. *Social work in health care, 9*(4), 45–62.

Futurist update: Laptop "doctors" will monitor our vital signs on the go. (2005). *The Futurist, 39*(6), 8.

Gabard, D. L., & Martin, M. W. (2003). *Physical therapy ethics.* Philadelphia: F. A. Davis.

Gage, B., Miller, S. C., Coppola, K., Harvell, J., Laliberte, L., Mor, V., et al. (2000, March). *Important questions for hospice in the next century: Executive Summary.* Retrieved from http://aspe.hhs.gov/daltcp/reports/impquees.htm

Galanter, M., Egelko, S., & Edwards, H. (1993). Rational recovery: Alternative to AA for addiction? *American Journal of Alcohol Abuse, 19,* 499–510.

Galewitz, P. (2011, May 5). Health care law draws many older dependents: Outpacing predictions, young adults flock to parents' plans. *Lexington Herald-Leader,* p. C-12.

Gallessich, J. (1982). *The profession and practice of consultation.* San Francisco: Jossey-Bass.

Gallo-Silver, L., Raveis, V. H., & Moynihan, R. (1993). Psychosocial issues in adults with transfusion-related HIV infection and their families. *Social Work in Health Care, 18*(2), 63–74.

Gambrill, E. (2006). Evidence-based practice and policy: Choices ahead. *Research* in Social Work Practice, *16*(3), 338–357.

Gance-Cleveland, B. (2005). Family-centered care: Motivational interviewing as a strategy to increase families' adherence to treatment regimes. *Journal for Specialists in Pediatric Nursing, 10*(3), 151–155.

Ganikos, M. L., McNeil, C., Braslow, J. B., Arkin, E. B., Klaus, D., Oberley, E. E., et al. (1994). A case study in planning for public health education: The organ and tissue donation experience. *Public Health Reports, 109,* 626–631.

Ganz, P. A., Litwin, M. S., Hays, R. D., & Kaplan, R. M. (2007). Measuring outcomes and health-related quality of life. In R. M. Anderson, T. H. Rice, & G. F. Kominski (Eds.), *Changing the U.S. health care system: Key issues in health services policy and management* (pp. 185–211). San Francisco: John Wiley.

Garbarino, J. (1992). Preventing adolescent maltreatment. In D. J. Willis, E. W. Holden, & M. Rosenberg (Eds.), *Prevention of child maltreatment: Developmental and ecological perspectives* (pp. 94–114). New York: John Wiley.

Garibaldi, R. A., Popkave, C., & Bylsma, W. (2005). Career plans for trainees in internal medicine residency programs. *Academic Medicine, 80,* 507–512.

Garrett, K. J. (1994). Caught in a bind: Ethical decision making in schools. *Social Work in Education, 16*(2), 97–105.

Gaugler, J. E. (2005). *Promoting family involvement in long-term care settings: A guide to programs that work.* Baltimore, MD: Health Professions Press.

Gaugler, J. E., Kane, R. L., Kane, R. A., & Newcomer, R. (2005). Early community-based service utilization and its effects on institutionalization in dementia caregiving. *The Gerontologist, 45*(2), 177–185.

Gelberg, L., & Leake, B. D. (1993). Substance use among impoverished medical patients: The effect of housing status and other factors. *Medical Care, 31,* 757–766.

Gelberg, L., Leake, B. D., Lu, M. C., Andersen, R. M., Wenzel, S. L., Morgenstern, H., et al. (2001). Use of contraceptive methods among homeless women for protection against unwanted pregnancies and STDs: Prior use and willingness to use in the future. *Contraception, 63,* 277–281.

Gellert, G. A. (1993). U.S. health care reform and the economy of prevention. *Archives of Family Medicine, 2,* 563–567.

Gelman, S. R. (1986). Life vs. death: The value of ethical uncertainty. *Health & Social Work, 12,* 118–125.

Gerbino, S., & Henderson, S. (2004). End-of-life bioethics in clinical social work practice. In J. Berzoff & P. R. Silverman (Eds.), *Living with dying* (pp. 593–608). New York: Columbia University Press.

Gerhart, U. C. (1990). *Caring for the chronically mentally ill.* Itasca, IL: F. E. Peacock.

Germain, C. B. (1984). *Social work practice in health care: An ecological perspective.* New York: Free Press.

Germain, C. B., & Gitterman, A. (1980). *The life model of social work practice.* New York: Columbia University Press.

Gerson, S. M., & Chassler, D. (1995). Advancing the state of the art: Establishing guidelines for long-term care case management. *Journal of Case Management, 4*(1), 9–13.

Getzel, G. S. (1992). AIDS and social work: A decade later. *Social Work in Health Care, 17*(2), 1–9.

Gillies, D. A. (1989). *Nursing management: A systems approach.* Philadelphia: W. B. Saunders.

Gitterman, A. (1988). The social worker as educator: An educator's view. In *Health care practice today: The social worker as educator* (Conference proceedings). New York: Columbia University School of Social Work.

Glanz, K., & Rimer, B. K. (1995). *Theory at a glance: A guide for health promotion practice.* Washington, DC: U.S. Public Health Service, National Institute of Health.

Gleick, J. (1987). *Chaos: Making a new science.* New York: Viking.

Gock, T. S. (1994). Acquired immunodeficiency syndrome. In N. W. S Zane, D. T. Takeuchi, & K. N. J. Young (Eds.), *Confronting critical health issues of Asian and Pacific Islander Americans* (pp. 247–265). Thousand Oaks, CA: Sage.

Goering, P., Wasylenki, D., Farkas, M., & Ballantyne, R. (1988). What difference does case management make? *Hospital and Community Psychiatry, 39,* 272–276.

Golan, N. (1969). When is a client in crisis? *Social Casework, 50,* 389–394.

Goldberger, A. L., Rigney, R. D., & West, B. J. (1990). Chaos and fractals in human physiology. *Scientific American,* 43–49.

Goldstein, H. (1987). The neglected moral link in social work practice. *Social Work, 32,* 181–186.

Goldwater, S. S. (1943). Concerning hospital origins. In A. C. Bachmeyer & G. Hartman (Eds.), *The hospital in modern society.* New York: Commonwealth Fund.

Gordon, L. (1993). Public health is more important than health care [Guest editorial]. *Journal of Public Policy, 14,* 261–264.

Gorin, S. H. (2003). Unraveling of managed care: Recent trends and implications. *Health & Social Work, 28*(3), 241–246.

Gotou, J., et al. (1994). Evaluation of the effective use of the "health notebook." *Nippon Koshu Eisei Zasshi, 41,* 1090–1098.

Gottlieb, B. (1995). *New choices in natural healing: Over 1,800 of the best self-help remedies from the world of alternative medicine.* Emmaus, PA: Rodale.

Gottlieb, B. H. (1985). Assessing and strengthening the impact of social support on mental health. *Social Work, 30,* 293–300.

Goudsblom, J. (1986). Public health and the civilizing process. *Milbank Quarterly, 64,* 161–188.

Grant, L. A., & Harrington, C. (1989). Quality of care in licensed and unlicensed home care agencies: A California case study. *Home Health Care Services Quarterly, 10,* 115–138.

Grant, M. (1987). *Handbook of community health.* Philadelphia: Lea & Febiger.

Graves, J. R., & MacDowell, N. M. (1994–1995, Winter). Mapping out the road to quality. *Journal of Long-Term Care Administration,* 12–17.

Gray, B. H. (1991). *The profit motive and patient care.* Cambridge, MA: Harvard University Press.

Gray, L. A., & House, R. M. (1989). AIDS and adolescents. In D. Capuzzi & D. Gross (Eds.), *Working with at-risk youth: Issues and interventions* (pp. 231–270). Alexandria, VA: American Association for Counseling and Development.

Gray, N. L. (1993). The relationship of cigarette smoking and other substance use among college students. *Journal of Drug Education, 23,* 117–124.

Green, A. (1993, March–April). The fragrance revolution: The nose goes to new lengths. *The Futurist, 27,* 13–17.

Green, D. L., & Roberts, A. R. (2008). *Helping victims of violent crime: Assessment, treatment, and evidence-based practice.* New York: Springer.

Green, L. W., & Kreuter, M. W. (1991). *Health promotion planning: An educational and environmental approach.* Mountain View, CA: Mayfield.

Green, L. W., & Raeburn, J. (1990). Contemporary developments in health promotion: Definitions and challenges. In N. Bracht (Ed.), *Health promotion at the community level* (pp. 29–44). Newbury Park, CA: Sage.

Greenberg, M., Schneider, D., & Martell, J. (1995). Health promotion priorities of economically stressed cities. *Journal of Health Care for the Poor and Underserved, 6*(1), 10–22.

Greenberg, S., Motenko, A. K., Roesch, C., & Embleton, N. (2000). Friendship across the life cycle: A support group for older women. *Journal of Gerontological Social Work, 32*(4), 7–23.

Greene, G., Kruse, K. A., & Arthurs, R. J. (1985). Family practice social work: A new area of specialization. *Social Work in Health Care, 10*(3), 53–73.

Greene, R. R. (1982). Families and the nursing home social worker. *Social Work in Health Care, 7*(3), 57–67.

Greer, D. S., Bhak, K. N., & Zenker, B. M. (1994). Comments on the AAMC policy statement recommending strategies for increasing the production of generalist physicians. *Academic Medicine, 69,* 245–260.

Grinnell, R. M., Jr. (1985). *Social work research and evaluation.* Itasca, IL: F. E. Peacock.

Grossman, L. (2010, December 15). Person of the year 2010: Mark Zuckerberg. *Time, 176*(26), 59.

Grover, R. M. (1982). The impact of resident councils. *Journal of Long-Term Care Administration, 10,* 2–6.

Grumbach, K., Braveman, P., Adler, N., & Bindman, A. B. (2007). Vulnerable populations and health disparities: An overview. In T. E. King, Jr., & M. B. Wheeler (Eds.), *Medical management of vulnerable and underserved patients: Principles, practice, and populations* (pp. 3–11). New York: McGraw-Hill.

Gummer, B. (1985). Power, power—who's got the power. *Administration in Social Work, 9*(2), 99–111.

Guterman, N. B., & Taylor, C. A. (2005). Prevention of physical child abuse and neglect. In G. P. Mallon & P. M. Hess (Eds.), *Child welfare* for the 21st century: A handbook of practice, policies, and programs* (pp. 270–289). New York: Columbia University Press.

Gutierrez, L. (1992, October). *Macro practice for the 21st century: An empowerment perspective.* Paper presented at the First Annual Conference on the Integration of Social Work and Social Science, School of Social Work, University of Michigan, Ann Arbor.

Gutierrez, L., Zuniga, M. E., & Lum, D. (2004). *Education for multicultural social work practice: Critical viewpoints and future directions.* Alexandria, VA: Council on Social Work Education.

Guzzetta, C. (1995). White ethnic groups. In R. L. Edwards (Ed.), *Encyclopedia of social work* (19th ed.). Washington, DC: National Association of Social Workers.

Gwyther, L. P. (1995). When "the family" is not one voice: Conflict in caregiving families. *Journal of Case Management, 4*(4), 150–155.

Haber, P. A. (1983). The Veterans Administration community care setting. *Psychiatry Quarterly, 55,* 187–191.

Haggard, W. K. (1991). The feminist theory of rape: Implications for prevention programming targeted at male college students. *College Student Affairs Journal, 11,* 13–20.

Hall, H. D. (1985). Historical perspective: Legislative and regulatory aspects of discharge planning. In E. McClellan, K. Kelly, & K. C. Buckwalter (Eds.), *Continuity of care: Advancing the concept of discharge planning* (pp. 11–20). New York: Grune & Stratton.

Hall, M. J., DeFrances, C. J., Williams, S. N., Golosinskiy, A., & Schwartzman, A. (2010). Patient and hospital characteristics. *National hospital discharge survey: 2007 summary* (National Hospital Statistics Report No. 29). Hyattsville, MD: National Center for Health Statistics. Retrieved from http://www.cdc.gov/nchs/data/nhsr/nhsr029.pdf

Halper, A. S. (1993). Teams and teamwork: Health care settings. *American Speech-Language-Hearing Association, 35,* 34–35, 48.

Handy, J. (1995). Alternative organizational models in home care. *Journal of Gerontological Social Work, 24*(3/4), 49–65.

Haney, P. (1988). Providing empowerment to the person with AIDS. *Social Work, 33,* 251–253.

Hanlon, J., & Pickett, G. (1984). *Public health administration and practice.* St. Louis, MO: Times Mirror/Mosby.

Harbert, A. S., & Ginsberg, L. H. (1990). *Human services for older adults: Concepts and skills.* Columbia: University of South Carolina Press.

Harrington, M. (1987). *Who are the poor?* Washington, DC: Justice for All National Office.

Harris, L. I. (1919). The epidemic of influenza. *Hospital Social Service Quarterly, 1,* 1–14.

Harris, S. N., Mowbray, C. T., & Solarz, A. (1994). Physical health, mental health, and substance abuse problems of shelter users. *Social Work, 19,* 37–45.

Hasenfeld, Y. (1983). *Human service organizations.* Upper Saddle River, NJ: Prentice Hall.

Hasenfeld, Y. (1987). Power in social work. *Social Service Review, 61,* 469–483.

Hastings, G., Devlin, E., & MacFadyen, L. (2005). Social marketing. In J. Kerr, R. Weitkunat, & M. Moretti (Eds.), *ABC of behavior change: A guide to successful disease prevention and health promotion* (pp. 315–334). Philadelphia: Elsevier.

Haub, C. (2008). *U.S. population could reach 438 million by 2050, and immigration is key.* Retrieved from www.prb.org/Articles/2008/pewprojections.aspx

Haughton, J. G. (1972). Federal government and the poor; why has it failed? In L. C. Corey, S. E. Saltman, & M. F. Epstein (Eds.), *Medicine in a changing society.* St. Louis, MO: C. V. Mosby.

Haxton, J. E., & Boelk, A. Z. (2010). Serving families on the frontline: Challenging and creative solutions in rural hospice social work. *Social Work in Health Care, 49*(6), 526–550.

Hay, D., & Oken, D. (1972). The psychological stresses of intensive care unit nursing. *Psychosomatic Medicine, 34*(2), 109–118.

Hayden, J. (2009). *Introduction to health behavior theory.* Sudbury, MA: Jones & Bartlett.

Hayes, J. A. (1991). Psychosocial barriers to behavior change in preventing human immunodeficiency virus (HIV) infection. *Counseling Psychologist, 19,* 585–602.

Health & medicine: Doctors use sonar to detect bone fractures. (2007). *The Futurist, 41*(6), 6.

Health & medicine: Repairing injuries to nervous system. (2007). *The Futurist, 41*(6), 6.

Heartbeat monitor by phone. (2010). *The Futurist, 44*(1), 10.

Heckler, M. M. (1984). Preface. In P. J. Carling, *Developing family foster care programs in mental health: A resource guide.* Boston: Boston University Center for Rehabilitation Research and Training in Mental Health.

Heger, R. L., & Hunzeker, J. M. (1988). Moving toward empowerment-based practice in public child welfare. *Social Work, 33,* 499–502.

Henry, R. S. (1993, November–December). Considerations in opening an adult day center. *Nursing Homes,* 16–17.

Hepworth, D. H., & Larsen, J. A. (1986). *Direct social work practice: Theory and practice.* Belmont. CA: Dorsey.

Herman, S. P. (1990, November). Special issues in child custody evaluations. *Journal of the American Academy of Child and Adolescent Psychiatry, 29,* 969–974.

Herson, J. (2007). The coming osteoporosis epidemic. *The Futurist, 41*(2), 32.

Hess, P. M. (1994). Supporting roster famines in their support of families. *Journal of Emotional and Behavioral Problems, 2*(4), 24–27.

Hessing, M. (1994). More than clockwork: Women's time management in their combined workloads. *Sociological Perspective, 37,* 611–633.

Hettler, B. (1984). Wellness: Encouraging a lifetime pursuit of excellence. *Health Values, 8*(4), 13–17.

Hiatt, K., Stelle, C., Mulsow, M., & Scott, J. P. (2007). The importance of perspective: Evaluation of hospice care from multiple stakeholders. *American Journal of Hospice and Palliative Care, 24,* 376–382.

Hick, S., & McNutt, J. G. (2002). *Advocacy, activism, and the Internet: Community organization and social policy.* Chicago: Lyceum.

Hill, P. (1973). *A theory of political coalitions in simple and policymaking situations.* Beverly Hills, CA: Sage.

Hirschwald, J. F. (1984). Social work in physical rehabilitation. In R. J. Estes (Ed.), *Health care and the social services: Social work practice in health care* (pp. 165–205). St. Louis, MO: Warren H. Green.

History of reform. (2010, Spring/Summer). *Think: The Magazine of Case Western Reserve University,* 33.

Hoffman, L. (1988). The family life cycle and discontinuous change. In B. Carter & M. McGoldrick (Eds.), *The changing family life cycle: A framework for family therapy* (pp. 91–106). New York: Gardner.

Holosko, M. J. (1992). Social work practice roles in health care: Daring to be different. In M. J. Holosko & P. A. Taylor (Eds.), *Social work practice in health care settings* (pp. 21–31). Toronto: Canadian Scholars' Press.

Hospital of the future. (1990, November–December). *The Futurist, 24,* 46–47.

Hospitals and patients seek alternatives. (2009). *The Futurist, 43*(2), 2.

House, R. M., & Walker, C. M. (1993). Preventing AIDS via education. *Journal of Counseling & Development, 71,* 282–289.

Houser, A. N., Fox-Grage, W., & Gibson, M. J. (2006). Across the states: Profiles of long-term care and independent living. Washington, DC: AARP Public Policy Institute. Retrieved from http://www.aarp.org/acrossthestates

Howard, G., Burke, G. L., Szklo, M., Tell, G. S., Eckfeldt, J., Evans. G., et al. (1994). Active and passive smoking are associated with increased carotid wall thickness: The Atherosclerosis Risk in Communities Study. *Archives of Internal Medicine, 154,* 1277–1282.

Howell, M. (1987). Clients who are mentally retarded and also old: Developmental, emotional, and medical needs. In S. F. Gilson, T. L. Goldsbury, & E. H. Faulkner (Eds.), *Three populations of primary focus: Persons with mental retardation and mental illness, persons with mental retardation who are elderly, persons with mental retardation and complex medical needs* (pp. 95–102). Omaha: University of Nebraska Medical Center.

Howell, S., Silberberg, M., Quinn, W. V., & Lucas, J. A. (2007). Determinants of remaining in the community after discharge: Results from New Jersey's nursing home transition program. *The Gerontologist, 47*(4), 535–547.

Hubbard, P., Werner, P., Cohen-Mansfield, A., & Shusterman, R. (1992). Seniors for justice: A political and social action group for nursing home residents. *The Gerontologist, 32,* 856–858.

Hudson, A. L., Wright, K., Bhattacharya, D., Sinha, K., Nyamathi, A., & Marfisee, M. (2010). Correlates of adult assault among homeless women. *Journal of Health Care for the Poor and Underserved, 21,* 1250–1262.

Hudson, C. G. (2000). At the edge of chaos: A new paradigm for social work? *Journal of Social Work Education, 36*(2), 215–230.

Hudson, R. B. (1990). Home care policy: Loved by all, feared by many. In C. Zuckerman, N. N. Dubler, & B. Collopy (Eds.), *Home health care options: A guide for older persons and concerned families* (pp. 271–301). New York: Plenum.

Huff, M. (2010). What do I need to know to work with people with disabilities? In D. Royse, S. S. Dhooper,

& E. L. Rompf (Eds.), *Field instruction: A guide for social work students* (6th ed., pp. 130–132). Boston: Allyn & Bacon.

Huff, R. M., & Yasharpour, S. (2007). Cross-cultural concepts in health and disease. In M. V. Kline & R. M. Huff (Eds.), *Health promotion in multicultural populations: A handbook for practitioners and students* (pp. 23–39). Thousand Oaks, CA: Sage.

Hughes, S. L., Ulasevich, A., Weaver, F. M., Henderson, W., Manheim, L., Kubal, J. D., et al. (1997). Impact of home care on hospital days: A meta-analysis. *Health Services Research, 32*(4), 415–532.

Humar, A., Matas, A. J., & Payne, W. D. (2006). *Atlas of organ transplantation.* London: Springer.

Huntington, J. (1986). The proper contributions of social workers in health practice. *Social Science and Medicine, 22,* 1151–1160.

Hutchins, V. L. (1985). Celebrating a partnership: Social work and maternal and child health. In A. Gitterman, R. B. Black, & F. Stein (Eds.), *Public health social work in maternal and child health: A forward plan* (Report of the Working Conference of the Public Health Social Work Advisory Committee for the Bureau of Health Care Delivery and Assistance). New York: Columbia University School of Social Work.

Hyduk, C. A. (2002). Community-based long-term care case management models for older adults. *Journal of Gerontological Social Work, 37*(1), 19–47.

Hyer, L., Swanson, G., Lefkowitz, R., Hillesland, D., Davis, H., & Woods. M. G. (1990). The application of the cognitive behavioral model to two older stressor groups. *Clinical Gerontologist, 9*(3/4), 145–189.

Ignani, K. (1995, Spring). Navigating the health care marketplace. *Health Affairs, 14,* 221–225.

Iles, P., & Auluck, R. (1990). Team building, interagency team development, and social work practice. *British Journal of Social Work, 20,* 151–164.

Institute for the Advancement of Social Work Research. (2003). *1993–2003: A decade of linking policy, practice, and education through advancement of research.* Washington, DC: Author.

Institute of Family-Centered Care. (2004, September 26–28). *Hospitals moving forward with patient and family-centered care.* Annual national seminar of the Institute of Family-Centered Care.

Institute of Medicine. (1978). *Report of a study: A manpower policy for primary health care.* Washington, DC: National Academy of Sciences.

Institute of Medicine. (1986). *Improving the quality of care in nursing homes.* Washington, DC: National Academy Press.

Institute of Medicine. (1988a). *The future of public health.* Washington, DC: National Academy Press.

Institute of Medicine. (1988b). *Homelessness, health, and human needs.* Washington, DC: National Academy Press.

Institute of Medicine. (2001). *Improving the quality of long-term care.* Washington, DC: National Academy Press.

Invisible scalpel. (1989, September–October). *The Futurist, 23,* 5.

Irvin, N., II. (2007). The U.S. is headed for a "demographic singularity." *The Futurist, 41*(6), 57.

Israel, B. A., Checkoway, B., Schulz, A., & Zimmerman, M. (1994). Health education and community empowerment: Conceptualizing and measuring perceptions of individual, organizational, and community control. *Health Education Quarterly, 21,* 149–170.

Jacobsen, P. (2005). The Cleo Eulau Center Resiliency Consultation Program: Development, practice, challenges, and efficacy of a relationship-based consultation for challenged schools. *Smith College Studies in Social Work, 75*(4), 7–23.

James, B. C. (1989). *Quality management for health care delivery.* Chicago: American Hospital Association.

Jansson, B. S., & Simmons, J. (1984). Building departmental or unit power within human service organizations: Empirical findings and theory building. *Administration in Social Work, 8*(3), 41–56.

Jenkins, R., Carder, P. C., & Maher, L. (2004). The Coming Home Program: Creating a state road map for affordable assisted living policy, programs, and demonstrations. *Journal of Housing for the Elderly, 18*(3/4), 165–178.

Johns Hopkins University. (2004). *Partnership for solutions: Better lives for people with chronic conditions.* Retrieved from http://www.partnershipforsolutions.org/

Johnson, A. K. (1998). The revitalization of community practice: Characteristics, competencies, and curricula for community-based services. *Journal of Community Practice, 5*(3), 37–62.

Johnson, D. L., et al. (1993, March). *Tobacco smoke in the home and child intelligence.* Paper presented at the 60th Biennial Meeting of the Society for Research in Child Development, New Orleans.

Johnson, D. R., Agresti, A., Jacob, M. C., & Nies, K. (1990). Building a therapeutic community through specialized groups in a nursing home. *Clinical Gerontologist, 9*(3/4), 203–217.

Johnson, K., Kuchibhatla, M., & Tulsky, J. A. (2009). Racial differences in self-reported exposure to information about hospice care. *Journal of Palliative Medicine, 12,* 921–927.

Johnson, K. A. (1990). Medical technology and public meaning: The case of viable organ transplantation. In J. Shanteau & R. J. Harris (Eds.), *Organ donation and transplantation: Psychological and behavioral factors* (pp. 161–178). Washington, DC: American Psychological Association.

Johnson, L. C. (1989). *Social work practice: A generalist approach.* Needham Heights, MA: Allyn & Bacon.

Jones, A. L., Dwyer, L. L., Bercovitz, A. R., & Strahan, G. W. (2009, June). The national nursing home survey: 2004 overview. *Vital Health Statistics, 13*(167). Hyattsville, MD: National Center for Health Statistics. Retrieved from http://www.cdc.gov/nchs/data/series/sr_13/sr13_167.pdf

Jones, M. (1953). *The therapeutic community.* New York: Basic Books.

Jones, W. J. (1979). Selecting and implementing specific role options. In M. M. Melum (Ed.), *The changing role of the hospital: Options for the future* (pp. 31–42). Chicago: American Hospital Association.

Joslyn-Scherer, M. S. (1980). *Communication in the human services: A guide to therapeutic journalism.* Beverly Hill, CA: Sage.

Jost, T. S. (2010). Pro & con: State lawsuits won't succeed in overturning the individual mandate. *Health Affairs, 29*(6), 1225–1228.

Joubert, L. (2006). Academic-practice partnerships in practice research: A cultural shift for health social workers. *Social Work in Health Care, 43*(2–3), 151–161.

Justins, D. (1994). Hospital pain clinics: An invaluable resource. *Practitioner, 238,* 278, 281–282.

Kachingwe, A. F. (2000). *Interculturalization and the education of professionals: A grounded theory investigation of diversity, multiculturalism, and conviction in the physical therapy profession.* Unpublished dissertation, Northern Illinois University, DeKalb.

Kachingwe, A. F., & Huff, R. M. (2007). The ethics of health promotion intervention in culturally diverse populations. In M. V. Kline & R. M. Huff (Eds.), *Health promotion in multicultural populations: A handbook for practitioners and students* (pp. 40–56). Thousand Oaks, CA: Sage.

Kagan, R., & Schlossberg, S. (1989). *Families in perpetual crisis.* New York: Norton.

Kahn, S. (1995). Community organization. In R. L. Edwards (Ed.), *Encyclopedia of social work* (19th ed.). Washington DC: National Association of Social Workers.

Kaiser Family Foundation. (2007). HIV/AIDS policy fact sheet. Retrieved from http://www.kff.org/hivaids/upload/3029-071.pdf

Kalichman, S. C., Rompa, D., Cage, M., DiFonzo, K., Simpson, D., Austin, J., et al. (2001). Effectiveness of an intervention to reduce HIV transmission risks in HIV-positive people. American Journal of Preventive Medicine, *21*(2), 84–92.

Kaluzny, A. D., & McLaughlin, C. P. (1992). Managing transitions: Assuring the adoption and impact of TQM. *Quality Review Bulletin, 18,* 380–384.

Kane, R. A. (1984). Toward a science of hospital social work. In T. O. Carlton (Ed.), *Clinical social work in health settings: A guide to professional practice with exemplars.* New York: Springer.

Kane, R. A. (1987). Long-term care. In A. Minahan (Ed.), *Encyclopedia of social work* (18th ed.). Silver Spring, MD: National Association of Social Workers.

Kane, R. A. (2001). Long-term care and a good quality of life: Bringing them closer together. Gerontologist, 41(3), 293–304.

Kane, R. A., & Kane, R. L. (1981). *Assessing the elderly: A practical guide to measurement.* Lexington, MA: D. C. Heath.

Kane, R. A., & Kane, R. L. (1987). *Long-term care: Principles, programs, and policies.* New York: Springer.

Kane, R. L. (1988). The hospital and geriatrics: Can a medical center be happy at the periphery? In C. Eisdorfer & G. L. Maddox (Eds.), *The role of hospitals in geriatric care* (pp. 19–34). New York: Springer.

Kane, R. L. (1994). Making aging a public health priority. *American Journal of Public Health, 84,* 1213-1214.

Kane, R. L. (2011). Finding the right level of posthospital care: "We didn't realize there was any other option for him." *Journal of the American Medical Association, 305*(3), 284–293.

Kaplan, K. O. (1995). End of life decisions. In R. L. Edwards (Ed.), *Encyclopedia of social work* (19th ed., Vol. 1, pp. 856–868). Washington, DC: National Association of Social Workers Press.

Kapp, M. B. (1990). Home care service deliverers: Options for consumers. In C. Zukerman, N. N. Dubler,

& B. Collopy (Eds.), *Home health care options: A guide for older persons and concerned families.* New York: Plenum.

Kapust, L. R. (1982). Living with dementia: The ongoing funeral. *Social Work in Health Care, 7*(4), 82.

Kaufman, J., & Forman, W. B. (2005). Hospice and palliative care: An educational intervention for health care professionals in a rural community. *American Journal of Hospice and Palliative Medicine, 22,* 415–418.

Kaufman, K. L., Johnson, C. F., Cohn, D., & McCleery, J. (1992). Child maltreatment prevention in the health care and social service system. In D. J. Willis, E. W. Holden, & M. Rosenberg (Eds.), *Prevention of child maltreatment: Developmental and ecological perspectives* (pp. 193–225). New York: John Wiley.

Kaufman, K. L., & Zigler, E. (1992). The prevention of child maltreatment: Programming, research, and policy. In D. J. Willis, E. W. Holden, & M. Rosenberg (Eds.), *Prevention of child maltreatment: Developmental and ecological perspectives* (pp. 269–296). New York: John Wiley.

Kaye, H. S., Harrington, C., & LaPlante, M. P. (2010). Long-term care: Who gets it, who provides it, who pays, and how much? *Health Affairs, 29*(1), 11–21.

Kelly, J. A., & Kalichman, S. C. (2002). Behavioral research in HIV/AIDS primary and secondary prevention: Recent advances and future directions. Journal of Consulting and Clinical Psychology, *70*(3), 626–639.

Kelly, M. P., Charlton, B. G., & Hanlon, P. (1993). The four levels of health promotion: An integrated approach. *Public Health, 107,* 319–326.

Kelly, R. J. (2001). Status report on the homeless. *Journal of Social Distress and the Homeless, 10*(3), 229–233.

Kemler, B. (1985). Family treatment in the health setting: The need for innovation. *Social Work in Health Care, 10*(4), 45–53.

Kenny, J. J. (1990). Social work management in emerging health care system. *Health and Social Work, 15,* 22–31.

Kermis, M. D. (1986). *Mental health in late life: The adaptive process.* Boston: Jones & Bartlett.

Kerson, T. S. (1979). Sixty years ago: Hospital social work in 1918. *Social Work in Health Care, 4*(3), 331–343.

Kerson, T. S. (1985). Responsiveness to need: Social work's impact on health care. *Health and Social Work, 10,* 300–307.

Kerson, T. S., DuChainey, D., & Schmid, W. W. (1989). Maternal and child health: Teen mother-well baby clinic. In T. S. Kerson & Associates (Eds.), *Social work in health settings: Practice in context* (pp. 215–230). New York: Haworth.

Kessler, R. C., Mickelson, K. D., & Zhao, S. (1997). Patterns and correlates of self-help group membership in the United States. *Social Policy, 27,* 27–46.

Keys, P. R. (1995). Quality management. In R. L. Edwards (Ed.), *Encyclopedia of social work* (19th ed.). Washington, DC: National Association of Social Work.

Kieffer, C. (1984). Citizen empowerment: A developmental perspective. In J. Rappaport, C. Swift, & R. Hess (Eds.), *Studies in empowerment: Steps toward understanding and action.* New York: Haworth.

Kimberg, L. (2007). Intimate partner violence. In T. E. King, Jr., & M. B. Wheeler (Eds.), *Medical management of vulnerable and underserved patients: Principles, practice, and populations* (pp. 307–317). New York: McGraw-Hill.

Kindig, D. A., Asada, Y., & Booske, B. A. (2008). A population health framework for setting national and state goals. *Journal of the American Medical Association, 299*(17), 2081–2083.

King, T. E., Jr., Wheeler, M. B., Bindman, A. B., Fernandez, A., Grumbach, K., Shillinger, D., et al. (2007). Preface. In T. E. King, Jr., & M. B. Wheeler (Eds.), *Medical management of vulnerable and underserved patients: Principles, practice, and populations* (pp. xvii–xviii). New York: McGraw-Hill.

Kirk, A. (2002). The effects of divorce on young adults' relationship competence: The influence of intimate friendships. *Journal of Divorce and Remarriage, 38*(1/2), 61–90.

Kirsch, A., & Donovan, S. (1992, August). Quality issues: The journey to quality improvement in health care. *Caring, 46*–51.

Kirst-Ashman, K. K. (1994, March). *A generalist approach to macro practice: Integrating micro, mezzo, and macro perspectives.* Paper presented at the 40th Annual Program Meeting of the Council on Social Work Education, Atlanta, GA.

Kirst-Ashman, K. K., & Hull, G. H., Jr. (1993). *Understanding generalist practice.* Chicago: Nelson-Hall.

Kitchen, A., & Brook, J. (2005). Social work at the heart of the medical team. Social Work in Health Care, 40(4), 1–18.

Kitchen, B. E. (2005). Family-centered care: A case study. *Journal for Specialists in Pediatric Nursing, 10*(2), 93–97.

Kitchner, M., Ng, T., & Harrington, C. (2005). *Medicaid home- and community-based program data, 1992–2002.* San Francisco: University of California.

Klein, T., & Danzig, F. (1985). *Publicity: How to make the media work for you.* New York: Scribner.

Klima, D. E. (1992). Incremental change: Community hospital reaction. In B. J. Jaeger (Ed.), *Hospitals in the year 2000: Three scenarios* (Report of the 1991 National Forum on Hospital and Health Affairs held in Durham, NC, May 15–17; pp. 49–56). Durham. NC: Duke University.

Kline, M. V., & Huff, R. M. (2007). Tips for students and practitioners: Foundations of multicultural health promotion. In M. V. Kline & R. M. Huff (Eds.), *Health promotion in multicultural populations: A handbook for practitioners and students* (pp. 175–184). Thousand Oaks, CA: Sage.

Koenig, B. A. (1997). Cultural diversity in decision making about care at the end of life. In M. J. Field & C. K. Cassel (Eds.), *Approaching death: Improving care at the end of life* (pp. 363–382). Washington, DC: National Institute of Medicine.

Kogak, L. (1999). *Smart guide to managing your time.* New York: John Wiley.

Kokkinos, J., & Levine, S. R. (1993). Stroke. *Neurology Clinician, 11*(3), 577–590.

Kolata, G. (2010, February 14). Doctors feel push for robot-assisted surgery. *Lexington Herald-Leader,* p. A14.

Kominski, G. F., & Melnick, G. A. (2007). Managed care and the growth of competition. In R. M. Anderson, T. H. Rice, & G. F. Kominski (Eds.), *Changing the U.S. health care system: Key issues in health services policy and management* (pp. 551–568). San Francisco: John Wiley.

Komisar, H. L., & Thompson, L. S. (2007). National spending for long-term care. Washington, DC: Georgetown University.

Koplin, A. N. (1993). A national program to restructure local public health agencies in the United States. *Journal of Public Health Policy, 14,* 393–402.

Kossman, H. D., Lamb, J. M., O'Brien, M. W., Predmore, S. M., & Prescher, M. J. (2008). Measuring productivity in medical social work. *Social Work in Health Care, 42*(1), 1–16.

Kotler, P. (1982). *Marketing for nonprofit organizations.* Upper Saddle River, NJ: Prentice Hall.

Kramer, A. M., Fox, P. D., & Morgenstern, N. (1992). Geriatric care approaches in health maintenance organizations. *Journal of the American Geriatrics Society, 40,* 1055–1067.

Kraus, W. A. (1980). *Collaboration in organizations: Alternatives to hierarchy.* New York: Human Sciences Press.

Ku, L. (2010). Ready, set, plan, implement: Executing the expansion of Medicaid. *Health Affairs, 29*(6), 1173–1177.

Kurlowicz, L. H. (1994). Depression in hospitalized medically ill elders: Evolution of the concept. *Archives of Psychiatric Nursing, 3*(2), 124–136.

Kurpius, D. J. (1978). Consultation theory and process: An integrated model. *Personnel and Guidance Psychologist, 13,* 368–389.

Kurpius, D. J., & Fuqua, D. R. (1993). Fundamental issues in defining consultation. *Journal of Counseling & Development, 71,* 598–600.

Kurpius, D. J., Fuqua, D. R., & Rozecki, T. (1993). The consulting process: A multidimensional approach. *Journal of Counseling & Development, 71,* 601–606.

Kushel, M., & Iezzoni, L. I. (2007). Disability and patients with disability. In T. E. King, Jr., & M. B. Wheeler (Eds.), *Medical management of vulnerable and underserved patients: Principles, practice, and populations* (pp. 383–395). New York: McGraw-Hill.

Lakein, A. (1973). *How to get control of your time and your life.* New York: New American Library.

Lakey, J. F. (1992). Myth information and bizarre beliefs of male juvenile sex offenders. *Journal of Addictions and Offender Counseling, 13*(1), 2–10.

Landers, S. H. (2010). Why health care is going home. *New England Journal of Medicine, 363,* 1690–1691.

Lane, W. G., & Dubowitz, H. (2009). Primary care pediatricians' experience, comfort, and competence in the evaluation and management of child maltreatment: Do we need child abuse experts? *Child Abuse & Neglect, 33*(2), 76–83.

Larkin, G. L., & Woody, J. (2005). Psychological impact of terrorism. In D. C. Keyes, J. L. Burstein, R. B. Schwartz, & R. E. Swienton (Eds.), *Medical response to terrorism* (pp. 389–400). Philadelphia: Lippincott Williams & Wilkins.

Latinos on the rise. (1993, January–February). *The Futurist, 27,* 48–49.

Latkin, C., Mandell, W., Vlahov, D., Oziemkowska, M., Knowlton, A., & Celentano, D. (1994). My place, your place, and no place: Behavior settings as a risk factor for HIV-related injection practices of drug users in Baltimore, Maryland. *American Journal of Community Psychology, 22,* 415–430.

Lattanzi, J. B., & Purnell, L. D. (2006). Exploring cultural health care practices and roles of health care practitioners. In J. B. Lattanzi & L. D. Purnell (Eds.), *Developing cultural competence in physical therapy practice* (pp. 136–160). Philadelphia: F. A. Davis.

Lauffer, A. (1978). *Social planning at the community level.* Upper Saddle River, NJ: Prentice Hall.

Law, S. (1976). *Blue Cross: What went wrong?* New Haven, CT: Yale University Press.

Lawrence, F., & Volland, P. J. (1988). The community care program: Description and administration. *Adult Foster Care Journal, 2,* 26–37.

Lawrence, T. (1980, September). Your self-image determines your success as a leader *Leadership,* 17–19.

Lawton, M. P. (1986). Functional assessment. In L. Teri & P. M. Lewinson (Eds.), *Geropsychological assessment and treatment.* New York: Springer.

Lazarus, R. S., & Folkman, S. (1984). *Stress, appraisal, and coping.* New York: Springer.

Leavell, H. R., & Clark, E. G. (1965). *Preventive medicine for the doctor in his community.* New York: McGraw-Hill.

Lechman, C., & Duder, S. (2009). Hospital length of stay: Social work services as an important factor. *Social Work in Health Care, 48*(5), 495–504.

Lee, P. R. (1994). Reinventing the Public Health Service: A look in a 50-year-old mirror [Editorial]. *Public Health Reports, 109,* 466–467.

Lee, P. R., & Toomey, K. E. (1994). Epidemiology in public health in the era of health care reform. *Public Health Reports, 109,* 1–3.

Lee, T. H., & Mongan, J. J. (2009). *Chaos and organization in health care.* Cambridge: MIT Press.

Lehman, D. R., Ellard, J. H., & Wortman, C. B. (1986). Social support for the bereaved: Recipients' and providers' perspectives on what is helpful. *Journal of Consulting and Clinical Psychology, 54,* 438–446.

Lehning, A. J., & Austin, M. J. (2010). Long-term care in the United States: Policy themes and promising practices. *Journal of Gerontological Social Work, 53,* 43–63.

Lehr, H., & Strosberg, M. (1991). Quality improvement in health care: Is the patient still left out? *Quality Review Bulletin, 17,* 326–329.

Lessler, D. S., & Dunn, C. (2007). Promoting behavior change. In T. E. King, Jr., & M. B. Wheeler (Eds.), *Medical management of vulnerable and underserved patients: Principles, practice, and populations* (pp. 69–79). New York: McGraw-Hill.

Leukefeld, C., Godlaski, T., Clark, J., Brown, C., & Hays, L. (2000). *Behavioral therapy for rural substance abusers.* Lexington: University of Kentucky Press.

Leukefeld, C. G., & Welsh, R. (1995). Health care systems policy. In R. L. Edwards (Ed.), *Encyclopedia of social work* (19th ed.). Washington, DC: National Association of Social Workers.

Levine, C. (1984). Questions and (some very tentative) answers about hospital ethics committees. *Hastings Center Report, 14*(3), 9–12.

Levine, C. (1991). Commentary: AIDS prevention and education; Reframing the message. *AIDS Education and Prevention, 3,* 147–163.

Levine, S. (1987). The changing terrains of medical sociology: Emergent concern with quality of life. *Journal of Health and Social Behavior, 28,* 1–6.

Levitas, A. S., & Gilson, S. F. (1987). Emotional and developmental needs of mentally retarded people. In S. F. Gilson, T. L. Goldsbury, & E. H. Faulkner (Eds.), *Three populations of primary focus* (pp. 139–140). Omaha: University of Nebraska & Creighton University.

Lewis, D., Das, N. K., Hopper, C. L., & Jencks, M. (1991). A program of support for AIDS research in the social/behavioral sciences. *Quarterly Journal of Minority Community AIDS Research, 5*(3), 2–5.

Lewis, V. S. (1971). Charity organization society. In R. Morris (Ed.), *Encyclopedia of social work* (16th ed., pp. 94–98). New York: National Association of Social Workers.

Lichter, D. T., Graefe, D. R., & Brown, J. B. (2003). Is marriage a panacea? Union formation among economically disadvantaged unwed mothers. *Social Problems, 50*(1), 60–86.

Lightfoot, M., Rotheram-Borus, M. J., & Tevendale, H. (2007). An HIV-preventive intervention for youth living with HIV. Behavior Modification, 31(3), 345–363.

Lindgren, C. L., & Linton, A. D. (1991). Problems of nursing home residents: Nurse and resident perceptions. *Applied Nursing Research, 4,* 113–121.

Linhorst, D. M., & Eckert, A. (2002). Involving people with severe mental illness in evaluation and performance improvement. Evaluation and the Health Professions, 25, 285–301.

Linn, M. W., Caffey, E. M., Klett, J., & Hogarty, G. (1977). Hospital vs. community (foster) care for psychiatric patients. *Archives of General Psychiatry, 34*, 78–83.

Lippitt, R., & Lippitt, G. (1978). *The consulting process in action*. La Jolla, CA: University Associates.

Litwak, E., & Meyer, H. F. (1966). A balanced theory of coordination between bureaucratic organizations and community primary groups. *Administrative Science Quarterly, II*, 31–58.

Litwak, E., & Meyer, H. J. (1974). *School, family, and neighborhood: The theory and practice of school-community relations*. New York: Columbia University Press.

Lo, B. (2007). Principles of ethical care of underserved patients. In T. E. King, Jr., & M. B. Wheeler (Eds.), *Medical management of vulnerable and underserved patients: Principles, practice, and populations* (pp. 47–55). New York: McGraw-Hill.

Locke, N. H. (1993). Hospitals and raising funds. *Canadian Medical Association Journal, 149*(3), 260.

Lockhart, L. L., & Wodarski, J. S. (1989). Facing the unknown: Children and adolescents with AIDS. *Social Work, 34*, 215–222.

London. H. I. (1988, July–August). The phenomenon of change. *The Futurist, 22,* 64.

Long, C. E., Artis, N. E., & Dobbins, N. J. (1993). The hospital: An important site for family-centered early intervention. *Topics in Early Childhood Special Education, 13*(1), 106–119.

Longe, M. E., & Wolf, A. (1983). *Promoting community health through innovative hospital-based programs*. Chicago: American Hospital Association.

Longer-lived artificial hips. (1994, July–August). *The Futurist, 28,* 5.

Loomis, J. (1988). Case management in health care. *Health and Social Work, 13*, 219–225.

Lopez, S. A., et al. (1993). *The social work perspective on managed care for mental health and substance abuse treatment*. Washington, DC: National Association of Social Workers.

Lorber, J. (1975). Good patients and problem patients: Conformity and deviance in a general hospital. *Journal of Health and Social Behavior, 16*, 213–225.

Louria, D. B. (1989). *Your body, your healthy life: How to take control of your medical destiny*. New York: Master Media Limited.

Lowe, J. I., & Herranen, M. (1981). Understanding teamwork: Another look at the concepts. *Social Work in Health Care, 7*(2), 1–11.

Lum, D. (1992). *Social work practice and people of color: A process-stage approach* (2nd ed.). Pacific Grove, CA: Brooks/Cole.

Lum, D. (2000). *Social work practice and people of color: A process-stage approach* (4th ed.). Belmont, CA: Brooks/Cole.

Lundberg, G. D. (1994). United States health care system reform: An era for shared sacrifice and responsibility begins. *Journal of the American Medical Association, 271*, 1530–1533.

Luptak, M. (2004). Social work and end-of-life care for older people: A historical perspective. *Health & Social Work, 29*(1), 7–15.

Lurie, N., Wasserman, J., & Nelson, C. D. (2006). Public health preparedness: Evolution or revolution? *Health Affairs, 25*(4), 935–945.

Luscombe, B. (2010). Marriage: What is it good for? *Time, 176*(22), 48–56.

Lynn, J., Arkes, H., Stevens, M., Cohn, F., Koenig, B., Fox, E., et al. (2000). Rethinking fundamental assumptions: SUPPORT's implications for future reform. *Journal of the American Gerontological Society, 48*, S214–S221.

MacAdam, M., & Yee, D. (1990). *Providing high-quality services to the frail elderly: A study of homemaker services in greater Boston*. Boston: Brandeis University, Bigel Institute for Health Policy.

MacGillis, A. (2010, February 15). Federal vs. state: Who should fix health care? *Lexington Herald-Leader*, p. A11.

Macias, C., Kinney, R., Farley, O. W., Jackson, R., & Vos, B. (1994). The role of case management with a community support system: Partnership with psychosocial rehabilitation. *Community Mental Health Journal, 30*, 323–339.

Mackelprang, R. W., & Mackelprang, R. D. (2005). Historical and contemporary issues in end-of-life decisions: Implications for social work. *Social Work, 50*, 315–324.

Madara, E. J. (1997). The mutual-aid self-help online revolution. *Social Policy, 27*, 20–27.

Maguire, L. (1983). *Understanding social networks*. Beverly Hills, CA: Sage.

Mainstream takes new look at alternative medicine. (1994, September 22). *Lexington Herald-Leader*, pp. A3, A8.

Malamuth, N. M. (1991). Characteristics of aggressors against women: Testing a model using a national sample of college students. *Journal of Consulting and Clinical Psychology, 59*, 670–681.

Malench, S. S. (2004). Family and social work roles in the long-term care facility. *Journal of Gerontological Social Work, 43*(1), 49–60.

Malone-Rising, D. (1994). The changing face of long-term care. *Nursing Clinics of North America, 29*, 417–429.

Mandel, I. (1994). Smoke signals: An alert for oral disease. *Journal of American Dental Association, 125,* 872–878.

Mantell, J. E. (1984). Social work in public health. In R. J. Estes (Ed.), *Health care and the social services: Social work practice in health care* (pp. 207–259). St. Louis, MO: Warren H. Green.

Maple, M. F. (1992). STEAMWORK: An effective approach to team building. *Journal of Specialists in Group Work, 17,* 144–150.

Marcenko, M. O., & Smith, L. K. (1992). The impact of a family-centered case management approach. *Social Work in Health Care, 17*(1), 87–99.

Martin, P. A. (1995). Finding time for research. *Applied Nursing Research, 8*(3), 151–153.

Martin, P. Y., & O'Connor, G. (1988). *The social environment: Open systems applications.* New York: Longman.

Martinez-Brawley, E. E. (1995). Community. In R. L. Edwards (Ed.), *Encyclopedia of social work* (19th ed.). Washington, DC: National Association of Social Workers.

Marx, J. (1993). Up in smoke: The effects of second-hand smoke on children's health. *PTA Today, 19*(2), 10–11.

Mathews, T. J., & MacDorman, M. F. (2010). Infant mortality statistics from the 2006 period: Linked birth/infant death data set. National Vital Statistics Reports, 58(17). Retrieved from http://www.cdc.gov/nchs/data/nvsr/nvsr58/nvsr58_17.pdf

Matthews, D. (2003). *AIDS sourcebook* (3rd ed.). Detroit, MI: Omnigraphics.

Maus, S. L. (2010). Geriatric social work in a community hospital: High-touch, low tech working a high-tech, low-touch environment. In T. S. Kerson, J. L. M. McCoyd, & Associates (Eds.), *Social work in health care settings: Practice in context* (3rd ed., pp. 225–234). New York: Routledge.

Mayer, B. (2008). Conflict resolution. In T. Mizrahi & L. E. Davis (Eds.), *Encyclopedia of social work* (20th ed.). Washington, DC: National Association of Social Workers and Oxford University Press. Retrieved from http://www.oxford-naswsocialwork.com

Mayer, B. S. (1995). Conflict resolution. In R. L. Edwards (Ed.), *Encyclopedia of social work* (19th ed.). Washington, DC: National Association of Social Workers.

McCabe, W. J. (1992). Total quality management in a hospital. *Quality Review Bulletin, 18,* 134–140.

McCarty, M. (2010, October 29). Face transplant recipient urges Ohioans to donate organs. *Dayton Daily News.*

McCoin, J. M. (1983). *Adult foster homes.* New York: Human Sciences Press.

McCoin, J. M. (1995). Editorial observations: What is adult residential care? *Adult Residential Care Journal, 9,* 1–11.

McDonnell, J. R., Abell, N., & Miller, J. (1991). Family members' willingness to care for people with AIDS: A psychosocial assessment model. *Social Work, 35,* 43–53.

McFarland, S. (1995, April). *Government by special interest: The Children's Defense Fund lobby.* Paper presented at the Annual Meeting of the Central States Communication Association, Indianapolis, IN.

McGinnis, J. M. (1982). Future directions of health promotion. In R. B. Taylor, J. R. Ureda, & J. W. Denham (Eds.), *Health promotion: Principles and clinical applications.* Norwalk, CT: Appleton-Century-Crofts.

McGowan, B. G. (1987). Advocacy. In A. Minahan (Ed.), *Encyclopedia of social work* (18th ed.). Silver Spring, MD: National Association of Social Workers.

McInerney, S. L. (1979). Inpatient options: Summary of hospice. In M. M. Melum (Ed.), *The changing role of the hospital: Options for the future* (pp. 43–60). Chicago: American Hospital Association.

McKay, M., Block, M., Mellins, C., & Traube, D. E. (2005). Adapting a family-based HIV prevention program for HIV infected preadolescents and their families: Youth, families, and health care providers coming together to address complex needs. *Social Work in Mental Health, 5*(3/4), 349–372.

McLean, D. (2004). Asthma among homeless children: Undercounting and undertreating the underserved. *Archives of Pediatric and Adolescent Medicine, 158,* 244–249.

McMahon, B. (1993). Time for a change in direction: Effects of poverty on ill health and service provision. *Professional Nurse, 8,* 610–613.

McNally, P. C. (1990). Expanding the public mind. *Justice Horizons, 11*(2).

McNeece, C. A., & Thyer, B. A. (2004). Evidence-based practice and social work. *Journal of Evidence-Based Social Work, 1,* 7–25.

McNutt, J. (2000). Organizing by cyberspace: Strategies for teaching about community practice and technology. *Journal of Community Practice, 7,* 96–109.

Mechanic, D. (1980). The management of psychosocial problems in primary care: A potential role for social work. *Journal of Human Stress, 6,* 16–21.

Medicaid Access Study Group. (1994). Access of Medicaid recipients to outpatient care. *New England Journal of Medicine, 330,* 1426–1430.

Meichenbaum, D., & Jaremko M. E. (1983). *Stress reduction and prevention.* New York: Plenum.

Melamed, S., Shalit-Kenig, D., Gelkopf, M., Lerner, A., & Kodesh, A. (2004). Mental homelessness: Locked within, locked without. *Social Work in Health Care, 39*(1/2), 209–223.

Melton, G. B. (1992). The improbability of prevention of sexual abuse. In D. J. Willis, E. W. Holden, & M. Rosenberg (Eds.), *Prevention of child maltreatment: Developmental and ecological perspectives* (pp. 168–192). New York: John Wiley.

Merrill, J. (1992). A test of our society: How and for whom we finance long-term care. *Inquiry, 29,* 176–187.

Merrill, J. C. (1994). *The road to health care reform: Designing a system that works.* New York: Plenum.

Meyer, C. H. (1984). The perils and promises of the health practice domain. *Social Work in Health Care, 10*(2), 1–11.

Miller, C. A., Brooks, E. F., DeFriese, G. H., Gilbert, B., Jain, S. C., & Kavaler, F. (1977). A survey of local public health departments and their directors. *American Journal of Public Health, 67,* 931–939.

Miller, L. (1986). The making of a home. *Nursing Times, 82,* 40–41.

Miller, L. (2004). Psychotherapeutic interventions for survivors of terrorism. *American Journal of Psychotherapy, 58,* 1–16.

Miller, R. H., & Luft, H. S. (1994). Managed care plan performance since 1980: A literature analysis. *Journal of the American Medical Association, 271,* 1512–1519.

Miller, R. H., & Luft, H. S. (2002). HMO plan performance update: An analysis of the literature, 1997–2001. *Health Affairs, 21*(4), 63–86.

Milton, T. (1983). What is primary care? *Journal of Public Health Policy, 4,* 129–130.

Minkler, M., & Pasick, R. J. (1986). Health promotion and the elderly: A critical perspective on the past and future. In K. Dychtwald (Ed.), *Wellness and health promotion for the elderly* (pp. 39–54). Gaithersburg, MD: Aspen.

Mintz, S. G. (1994, November–December). Family outreach: Image upgrade. *Nursing Homes,* 22–24.

Mironov, V. (2011, January–February). The future of medicine: Are custom-printed organs on the horizon? *The Futurist, 45,* 21–24.

Mishel, M. M., & Murdaugh, C. L. (1987). Family adjustment to heart transplantation: Redesigning the dream. *Nursing Research, 36*(6), 332–338.

Misiorski, S. (2003). Pioneering culture change. *Nursing Homes: Long-Term Care Management, 52*(10), 24–31.

Mizrahi, T. (1993). Managed care and managed competition: A primer for social work. *Health & Social Work, 18,* 86–91.

Mizrahi, T., & Rosenthal, B. B. (2001). Complexities of coalition building: Leaders' successes, strategies, struggles, and solutions. *Social Work, 46*(1), 63–78.

Mondros, J., & Staples, L. (2008). Community organization. In T. Mizrahi & L. E. Davis (Eds.), Encyclopedia of social work (20th ed.). Washington, DC: National Association of Social Workers and Oxford University Press. Retrieved from http://www.oxford-naswsocialwork.com

Monk, A. (1981, January). Social work with the aged: Principles of practice. *Social Work, 26,* 61–68.

Moon, S. S., & DeWeaver, K. L. (2005). Electronic advocacy and social welfare policy education. *Journal of Teaching in Social Work, 25*(1/2), 57–68.

Moonilal, J. M. (1982). Trauma centers: A new dimension for hospital social work. *Social Work in Health Care, 7*(4), 15–25.

Moore, C. W. (1986). *The mediation process: Practical strategies for resolving conflict.* San Francisco: Jossey-Bass.

Morey, M. A., & Friedman, L. S. (1993). Health care needs of homeless adolescents. *Current Opinion in Pediatrics, 5*(4), 395–399.

Morgado, P. B., Chen, H. C., Patel, V., Herbert, L., & Kohner, E. M. (1994). The acute effect of smoking on retinal blood flow in subjects with and without diabetes. *Ophthalmology, 101,* 1220–1226.

Morgan, A., & Zimmerman, M. (1990). Easing transition to nursing homes: Identifying the needs of spousal caregivers at the time of institutionalization. *Clinical Gerontologist, 9*(3/4), 1–17.

Morrice, J. K. W. (1976). *Crisis intervention: Studies in community care.* Elmsford, NY: Pergamon.

Morris, R. (Ed.). (1971). *Encyclopedia of social work* (16th ed.). New York: National Association of Social Workers.

Morrow-Howell, N., Proctor, E., & Mui, A. (1991). Adequacy of discharge plans for elderly patients. *Social Work Research and Abstracts, 27,* 6–13.

Morton, C. J. (1985). Public health social work priorities in maternal and child health. In A. Gitterman,

R. B. Black, & F. Stein (Eds.), *Public health social work in maternal and child health: A forward plan* (Report of the Working conference of the Public Health Social Work Advisory Committee for the Bureau of Health Care Delivery and Assistance). New York: Columbia University School of Social Work.

Moynihan, R., Christ, G., & Gallo-Silver, L. (1988). AIDS and terminal illness. *Social Casework, 6,* 380–387.

Mukamel, D. B., Spector, W. D., Zinn, J. S., Huang, L., Weimer, D. L., & Dozier, A. (2007). Nursing homes' response to the nursing home compare report card. *Journal of Gerontology (Series B: Psychological Sciences & Social Sciences), 62*(4), S218–S225.

Mukamel, D. B., Weimer, D. L., Spector, W. D., & Zinn, J. S. (2008). Publication of quality report cards and trends in reported quality measures in nursing homes. *Health Services Research, 43*(4), 1244–1262.

Mullaney, J. W., & Andrews, B. J. (1983). Legal problems and principles in discharge planning: Implications for social work. *Social Work in Health Care, 9*(1), 53–62.

Munley, A., Powers, C., & Williamson, J. B. (1982). Humanizing nursing home environments: The relevance of hospice principles. *International Journal of Aging and Human Development, 15,* 263–284.

Myers, A. M., Pfeiffle, P., & Hinsdale, K. (1994). Building a community-based consortium for AIDS patient services. *Public Health Reports, 109,* 555–562.

Myers, V. (1995, April). *Offering a pragmatic approach to State Speech Association involvement in advocacy efforts—Or lessons learned, unlearned, and relearned the hard way in seeking to influence education policy in Texas.* Paper presented at the Annual Meeting of the Central State Speech Communication Association, Oklahoma City.

Nacman, M. (1977). Social work in health settings: A historical review. *Social Work in Health Care, 2*(4), 407–418.

Nason, F. (1983). Diagnosing the hospital team. *Social Work in Health Care, 9*(2), 25–45.

National Academy of Sciences. (1966). *Accidental death and disability: The neglected disease of modern society.* Washington, DC: U.S. Department of Health, Education, & Welfare.

National Advisory Committee on Rural Health and Human Services. (2008). *The 2008 report to the secretary: Rural health and human services issues.* Washington, DC: Author.

National Association for Home Care & Hospice. (2010). *Basic statistics about home care.* Retrieved from http://www.nahc.org

National Association of Social Workers. (1981). *Guidelines for the selection and use of social workers.* Silver Spring, MD: Author.

National Association of Social Workers. (1991). *Standards of practice for social work mediators.* Silver Spring, MD: Author.

National Association of Social Workers. (1992). *Standards for social work case management.* Washington, DC: Author.

National Association of Social Workers. (1994a). *A brief look at managed mental health care.* Washington, DC: Author.

National Association of Social Workers. (1994b). Managed care. In *Social work speaks* (pp. 169–174). Washington, DC: Author.

National Association of Social Workers. (2000). *Code of ethics.* Washington, DC: Author.

National Association of Social Workers. (2004). *NASW standards for social work practice in palliative and end-of-life care.* Washington, DC: Author.

National Association of Social Workers. (2006). *Social work speaks: National Association of Social Workers policy statements 2006–2009* (7th ed.). Washington, DC: Author.

National Center on Elder Abuse. (1998, September). *The national elder abuse incidence study.* Retrieved from http://aoa.gov/AoA_Programs/Elder_Rights/Elder_Abuse/docs/ABuseReport_Full.pdf

National Center for Health Statistics. (2010a). *Health, United States, 2009.* Hyattsville, MD: U.S. Department of Health and Human Services, Centers for Disease Control and Prevention, National Center for Health Statistics. (DHHS Publication No. 2010-1232)

National Center for Health Statistics. (2010b). Table 126 (Personal health care expenditures by source of funds and type of expenditure). *Health, United States, 2009.* Hyattsville, MD: U.S. Department of Health and Human Services, Centers for Disease Control and Prevention, National Center for Health Statistics.

National Center for Injury Prevention and Control. (2003). *Costs of intimate partner violence against women.* Atlanta, GA: Centers for Disease Control and Prevention. Retrieved from http://www.cdc.gov/violenceprevention/pdf/IPVBook-a.pdf

National Hospice and Palliative Care Organization. (2005). *Hospice standards of practice.* Alexandria, VA: Author.

National Hospice and Palliative Care Organization. (2010). *NHPCO facts and figures: Hospice care in America.* Retrieved from www.nhpco.org/files/public/Statistics_Research/Hospice_Facts_Figures_Oct-2010.pdf

Neigh, G. N., Gillespie, C. F., & Nemeroff, C. B. (2009). The neurobiological toll of child abuse and neglect. *Trauma, Violence, & Abuse, 10*(4), 389–410.

Neighbors, H. W., Braithwaite, R. L., & Thompson, E. (1995). Health promotion and African Americans: From personal empowerment to community action. *American Journal of Health Promotion, 9,* 281–286.

Netting, F. E. (2008). Macro social work practice. In T. Mizrahi & L. E. Davis (Eds.), Encyclopedia of social work (20th ed.). Washington, DC: National Association of Social Workers and Oxford University Press. Retrieved from http://www.oxford-naswsocialwork.com

Netting, F. E., & Williams, F. G. (2000). Expanding the boundaries of primary care for elderly people. *Health & Social Work, 25*(4), 233–242.

Neuman, K. M., & Ptak, M. (2003). Managing managed care through accreditation standards. *Social Work, 48*(30), 384–391.

Neville, K., Bromberg, A., Ronk, S., Hanna, B. A., & Rom, W. N. (1994). The third epidemic: Multidrug-resistant tuberculosis. *Chest, 105*(1), 45–48.

Newcomer, R., Kang, T., & Graham, C. (2006). Outcomes in a nursing home transition case-management program targeting new admissions. *The Gerontologist, 46*(3), 385–390.

Ng, P., & Chan, K. (2008). Integrated group program for improving sleep quality of elderly people. *Journal of Gerontological Social Work, 51*(3–4), 366–378.

Nickelsberg, B. (1988, November). Getting a grant. *Association Management,* 126–129.

Nolte, W. W., & Wilcox, D. L. (1984). *Effective publicity: How to reach people.* New York: John Wiley.

Norris, F. H. (1992). Epidemiology of trauma: Frequency and impact of different potentially traumatic events on different demographic groups. *Journal of Consulting and Clinical Psychology, 60,* 409–418.

Norris, V. (2010). Group intervention for adults with HIV/AIDS: Meeting the needs of Latino patients living with HIV/AIDS at a comprehensive care center in New York City. In T. S. Kerson, J. L. M. McCoyd, & Associates (Eds.), *Social work in health care settings: Practice in context* (3rd ed., pp. 269–279). New York: Routledge.

Nunez, R. D. (1998). Homeless families today: Our challenge tomorrow; A regional perspective. *Journal of Children & Poverty, 4*(2), 71–83.

O'Brien, J., Saxberg, B., & Smith, H. (1983). For-profit or not-for-profit: Does it matter? *The Gerontologist, 23,* 229–248.

O'Donnell, P. (2004). Ethical issues in end-of-life care: Social work facilitation and proactive intervention. In J. Berzoff & P. R. Silverman (Eds.), *Living with dying* (pp. 171–187). New York: Columbia University Press.

O'Donovan, T. R. (1976). *Ambulatory surgical centers: Development and management.* Gaithersburg, MD: Aspen.

O'Hare, P. A., Malone, D., Lusk, E., & McCorkle, R. (1993). Unmet needs of black patients with cancer posthospitalization: A descriptive study. *Oncology Nurses Forum, 20*(4), 659–664.

Oktay, J. S. (1987). Foster care for adults. In A. Minahan (Ed.), *Encyclopedia of social work* (18th ed., pp. 634–638). Silver Spring, MD: National Association of Social Workers.

Oktay, J. S., & Palley, H. A. (1988). The frail elderly and the promise of foster care. *Adult Foster Care Journal, 2,* 8–25.

Oktay, J. S., & Volland, P. J. (1981). Community care programs for the elderly. *Health & Social Work, 6,* 41–47.

Oktay, J. S., & Volland, P. J. (1987). Foster home care for the frail elderly as an alternative to nursing home care: An experimental evaluation. *American Journal of Public Health, 77,* 1505–1510.

Olds, D. L., Henderson, C., & Tatelbaum, R. (1994). Intellectual impairment in children of women who smoke cigarettes during pregnancy. *Pediatrics, 93,* 221–227.

O'Leary, D. S. (1991a). Accreditation in the quality improvement mold: A vision for tomorrow. *Quality Review Bulletin, 17,* 72–77.

O'Leary, D. S. (1991b). CQI: A step beyond QA. *Quality Review Bulletin, 17,* 4–5.

Olesen, D. E. (1995, September–October). The top 10 technologies for the next 10 years. *The Futurist, 29,* 9–13.

Olinde, J. F., & McCard, H. (2005). Understanding the boundaries of the HIPPA preemption analysis. *Defense Counsel Journal, 72,* 158–169.

Olson, D. H. (1989). Circumplex model of family systems: Part VIII; Family assessment and intervention. In D. H. Olson, C. S. Russell, & D. H. Sprenkle (Eds.), *Circumplex model: Systemic assessment and treatment of families* (pp. 7–50). New York: Haworth.

Olson, D. H., & Hanson. M. K. (1990). *2001: Preparing families for the future.* Minneapolis, MN: National Council on Family Relations.

Organ Procurement and Transplantation Network. (2010). *Data.* Retrieved from http://optn.transplant.hrsa.gov/data/

Osman, H., & Becker, M. A. (2003). Complexity of decision making in a nursing home: The impact of advance directives on end-of-life care. *Journal of Gerontological Social Work, 42*(1), 27–40.

Ostrow, D. G. (1989). AIDS prevention through effective education. *Daedalus, 118,* 229–253.

O'Toole, T. P. (2007). Advocacy. In T. E. King, Jr., & M. B. Wheeler (Eds.), *Medical management of vulnerable and underserved patients: Principles, practice, and populations* (pp. 429–436). New York: McGraw-Hill.

Owens, A. (1988, September). How much did your earnings grow last year? *Medical Economics, 65,* 159–180.

Pagana, K. D. (1995). Teaching students time management strategies. *Journal of Nursing Education, 35*(8), 381–383.

Pagelow, M. D. (1981). *Woman-battering: Victims and their experiences.* Beverly Hills, CA: Sage.

Pagelow, M. D. (1992). Adult victims of domestic violence: Battered women. *Journal of Interpersonal Violence, 7,* 87–120.

Pande, A., Laditka, S. B., Laditka, J. N., & Davis, D. R. (2007). Aging in place? Evidence that a state Medicaid waiver program helps frail older persons avoid institutionalization. *Home Health Care Services Quarterly, 26*(3), 39–60.

Park, A. (2010a). A blood test to predict heart attack. *Time, 176*(16), 26.

Park, A. (2010b). Predicting IVF success on film. *Time, 176*(16), 26.

Parsons, R. J. (1988). Empowerment for role alternatives for low-income minority girls: A group work approach. *Social Work with Groups, 11*(4), 27–45.

Parsons, R. J. (2008). Empowerment practice. In T. Mizrahi & L. E. Davis (Eds.), Encyclopedia of social work (20th ed.). Washington, DC: National Association of Social Workers and Oxford University Press. Retrieved from http://www.oxford-naswsocialwork.com

Pascarelli, E. F. (Ed.). (1982). *Hospital-based ambulatory care.* Norwalk, CT: Appleton-Century-Crofts.

Passel, J. S., & Cohn, D. (2008). *U.S. population projections: 2005–2050.* Washington, DC: Pew Research Center.

Patrick, D. L., & Erickson, P. (1993). *Assessing health-related quality of life for clinical decision in the 1990s.* Dordrecht, Netherlands: Kluwer Academic.

Patterson, J. (1995). Pediatric and maternal HIV/AIDS: Social work intervention. In J. B. Rauch (Ed.), *Community-based, family-centered services in a changing health care environment.* Arlington, VA: National Maternal and Child Health Clearinghouse.

Paul, A. M. (2010). Cancer. Heart disease. Obesity. Depression. Scientists can now trace adult health to the 9 months before birth. *Time, 174*(14), 51–55.

Pear, R. (2010, September). GOP determined to unravel health care law. *Lexington Herald-Leader,* p. A-8.

Pearman, L. U., & Searles, J. (1978). Unmet social service needs in skilled nursing facilities. In N. F. Bracht (Ed.), *Social work in health care: A guide to professional practice* (pp. 184–197). New York: Haworth.

Pepper, C. (1986). *Statement at the hearings before the Subcommittee on Health and Long-Term Care of the Select Committee on Aging, House of Representatives, 99th Congress on September 18, 1985* (Comm. Pub. No. 99-543). Washington, DC: Government Printing Office.

Petersdorf, R. G. (1993). The doctor is in. *Academic Medicine, 68,* 113–117.

Peterson, M. (2010, November 10). Smoking's harm to lungs, DNA called immediate. *Lexington Herald-Leader,* p. B12.

Pickering, P. (2000). *How to manage conflict: Turn conflicts into win-win outcomes.* Franklin Lakes, NJ: Career Press.

Pietgen, H. O., & Richter, P. H. (1986). *The beauty of fractals: Images of complex dynamical systems.* New York: Springer.

Piliavin, I., Westerfelt, A., Yin-Ling, I., & Afflerbach, A. (1994). Health status and health-care utilization among the homeless. *Social Service Review, 68*(2), 236–253.

Pinderhughes, E. B. (1983). Empowerment for our clients and for ourselves. *Social Casework, 64,* 331–338.

Pleis, J. R., Ward, B. W., & Lucas, J. W. (2010). Summary health statistics for U.S. adults: National health interview survey, 2009. *Vital*

Health Statistics, 10(249). Hyattsville, MD: National Center for Health Statistics. Retrieved from http://www.cdc.gov/nchs/data/series/sr_10/sr10_249.pdf

Plichta, S. (1992). The effects of woman abuse on health care utilization and health status: A literature review. *Women's Health Issues, 2*(3), 154–163.

Ponte, P. R., Connor, M., DeMarco, R., & Price, J. (2004). Patient safety: Linking patient- and family-centered care and patient safety: The next leap. *Nursing Economics, 22*(4), 211–213.

Pratt, C., Schmall, V., Wright, S., & Hare, J. (1987). The forgotten client: Family caregivers to institutionalized dementia patients. In T. Brubaker (Ed.), *Aging, health, and family: Long-term care* (pp. 197–285). Newbury Park, CA: Sage.

Prentky, R. A., & Knight, R. A. (1991). Identifying critical dimensions for discriminating among rapists. *Journal of Consulting and Clinical Psychology, 59,* 643–661.

President's Commission for the Study of Ethical Problems in Medicine and Biomedical and Behavioral Research. (1983). *Deciding to forgo life-sustaining treatment: A report of the ethical, medical, and moral issues in treatment decisions.* Washington, DC: Government Printing Office.

Preventing sudden cardiac death. (1990, July–August). *The Futurist, 24,* 6.

Prochaska, J. O., DiClemente, B., & Norcross, J. C. (1992). In search of how people change: Applications to addictive behaviors. *American Psychologist, 47,* 1102–1114.

Prochaska, J. O., & DiClemente, C. C. (1983). Stages and processes of self-change of smoking: Towards an integrated model of change. *Journal of Consulting and Clinical Psychology, 51,* 350.

Proctor, E. K. (2003). Research to inform the development of social work interventions. Social Work *Research, 27*(1), 3–6.

Proctor, E., & Morrow-Howell, N. (1990). Complications in discharge planning with Medicare patients. *Health and Social Work, 8,* 45–54.

Proton therapy. (1989, November–December). *The Futurist, 23,* 5.

Public Health Service. (1979). *Healthy people: The Surgeon General's report on health promotion and disease prevention.* Washington, DC: Government Printing Office.

Public Health Service. (1980). *Promoting health/preventing disease: Objectives for the nation.* Washington, DC: Government Printing Office.

Pugh, G. L. (2009). Exploring HIV/AIDS case management and client quality of life. *Journal of HIV/AIDS & Social Services, 8*(2), 202–218.

Quam, J. K. (2008). Devine, Edward Thomas. In T. Mizrahi & L. E. Davis (Eds.), *Encyclopedia of social work* (20th ed.). Washington, DC: National Association of Social Work and Oxford University Press. Retrieved July 3, 2011, from http://www.oxford-naswsocialwork.com

Quinn, J., Segal, J., Raisz, H., & Johnson, C. (Eds.). (1982). *Coordinating community services for the elderly: The triage experience.* New York: Springer.

Raffel, M. W., & Raffel, N. K. (1989). *The U.S. health system: Origin and functions.* New York: John Wiley.

Rainey, J., & Lindsay, G. (1994). 101 questions for community health promotion program planning. *Journal of Health Education, 25,* 309–312.

Randall, H., & Csikai, E. (2004). Issues affecting utilization of hospice services by rural Hispanics. *Journal of Ethnic and Cultural Diversity in Social Work, 12,* 79–94.

Randall, T. (1990). Domestic violence intervention calls for more than treating injuries. *Journal of the American Medical Association, 264,* 939–940.

Randall, V. R. (1994). Impact of managed care organizations on ethnic Americans and underserved populations. *Journal of Health Care for the Poor and the Underserved, 5*(3), 224–236.

Rapaport, L. (1967). Crisis-oriented short-term casework. *Social Service Review, 41,* 31–43.

Rathbone-McCuan, E. (1995). Agency-based research. In R. L. Edwards (Ed.), *Encyclopedia of social work* (19th ed., pp. 136–142). Washington, DC: National Association of Social Workers.

Rauch, J. B. (1988). Social work and the genetics revolution: Genetic services. *Social Work, 33,* 389–394.

Raymer, M., & Reese, D. J. (2008). Hospice. In T. Mizrahi & L. E. Davis (Eds.), *Encyclopedia of social work* (20th ed.). Washington, DC: National Association of Social Workers and Oxford University Press. Retrieved from http://www.oxford-naswsocialwork.com

Re, R. N., & Krousel-Wood, M. A. (1990). How to use continuous quality improvement theory and statistical quality control tools in a multispecialty clinic. *Quality Review Bulletin, 16,* 391–397.

Reamer, F. G. (1986). The emergence of bioethics in social work. *Health & Social Work, 10*(4), 271–281.

Reamer, F. G. (1998). The evolution of social work ethics. *Social Work, 43*(6), 488–500.

Reardon, G. T., Blumenfield, S., Weissman, A. L., & Rosenberg, G. (1988). Findings and implications from preadmission screening of elderly patients waiting for elective surgery. *Social Work in Health Care, 13*(3), 51–63.

Reece, R. L. (2007). Innovation-driven health care: 34 key concepts for transformation. Sudbury, MA: Jones & Bartlett.

Reese, D. (2000). The role of primary caregiver denial in inpatient placement during home hospice care. Hospice Journal, 15(1), 15–33.

Reese, D., & Raymer, M. (2004). Relationship between social work services and hospice outcomes: Results of the National Hospice Social Work Survey. *Social Work*, 49(3), 415–422.

Reese, D. J., Ahern, R. E., Nair, S., O'Faire, J. D., & Warren, C. (1999). Hospice access and the use by African Americans: Addressing cultural and institutional barriers through participatory research. *Social Work*, 44(6), 549–559.

Rehr, H. (1986). Discharge planning: An ongoing function of quality care. *Quality Review Bulletin, 72*(2), 47–50.

Rehr, H. (1991). Introduction: The changing context of social-health care. *Social Work in Health Care, 17*, 3–16.

Rehr, H., & Rosenberg, G. (1991). Social health care: Problems and predictions. *Social Work in Health Care, 15*(4), 97–120.

Reid, W. J. (1995). Research overview. In R. L. Edwards (Ed.), *Encyclopedia of social work* (19th ed.). Washington, DC: National Association of Social Workers.

Reinhard, S. C. (2010). Diversion, transition programs target nursing homes' status quo. *Health Affairs, 29*(1), 44–48.

Resnick, C., & Dziegielewski, S. F. (1996). The relationship between therapeutic termination and job satisfaction among medical social workers. *Social Work in Health Care, 23*, 17–35.

Reynolds, R. E. (1975). Primary care, ambulatory care, and family medicine: Overlapping but not synonymous. *Journal of Medical Education, 50*(9), 893–895.

Rice, E. P. (1957, November). *Social work in public health.* Paper presented at a meeting of the National Association of Social Workers, Cleveland Chapter, Cleveland, OH.

Richards, T. N., Garland, T. S., Bumphus, V. W., & Thompson, R. (2010). Personal or political? Exploring the feminization of the American homeless population. *Journal of Poverty*, *14*(1), 97–115.

Richardson, J. L., Milam, J., McCutchan, A., Stoyanoff, S., Bolan, R., Weiss, J., et al. (2004). Effect of brief provider safer-sex counseling of HIV-1 seropositive patients: A multi-clinic assessment. AIDS, *18*, 1179–1186.

Richman, D. (1987, June 5). PPOs outstripped HMOs last year in number of locations and enrollment. *Modern Health Care,* 130–136.

Riessman, F. (1994). Alternative health movements. *Social Policy, 24*(3), 53–57.

Roberts, A. R. (2000). An overview of crisis theory and crisis intervention. In A. R. Roberts (Ed.), *Crisis intervention handbook: Assessment, treatment, and research* (pp. 3–30). New York: Oxford University Press.

Roberts, A. R., & Roberts, B. S. (2000). A comprehensive model for crisis intervention with battered women and their children. In A. R. Roberts (Ed.), *Crisis intervention handbook: Assessment, treatment, and research* (pp. 177–208). New York: Oxford University Press.

Roberts, C. S., Severinsen, C., Kuehn, C., Straker, D., & Fritz, C. J. (1992). Obstacles to effective case management with AIDS patients: The clinician's perspective. *Social Work in Health Care, 17*(2), 27–40.

Roberts, M. C. (1994). Prevention/promotion in America: Still spitting on the sidewalk. *Journal of Pediatric Psychology, 19*, 267–281.

Roberts-DeGennaro, M. (2004). Using technology for grassroots organizing. In L. Staples (Ed.), Roots to power: A manual for grassroots organizing (2nd ed., pp. 270–281). Westport, CT: Praeger.

Robinson, J. C. (1994). The changing boundaries of the American hospital. *Milbank Quarterly, 72*, 259–275.

Robinson, M. A. (1982). Telephone notification of relatives of emergency and critical care patients. *Annals of Emergency Medicine, 11*, 616–618.

Rochman, B. (2010). Oncofertility: Saving for a family. *Time, 176*(15), Wellness 1–5.

Rock, B. D., Haymes, E., Auerbach, C., & Beckerman, A. (1992). Helping patients in the supportive milieu of a community residence program for the chronically mentally ill: Conceptual model and initial evaluation. *Social Work in Health Care, 16*(3), 97–114.

Rockwood, G. F. (1993). Edgar Schein's process versus content consultation models. *Journal of Counseling & Development, 71,* 636–638.

Rodwell, M. K., & Chambers, D. E. (1992). Primary prevention of child abuse: Is it really possible? *Journal of Sociology and Social Welfare, 19*(3), 159–176.

Roemer, M. I. (1986). *Introduction to the health care system.* New York: Springer.

Roessler, R. T., & Rubin, S. (1982). *Case management and rehabilitation counseling.* Baltimore, MD: University Park Press.

Rogak, L. (1999). *Smart guide to managing your time.* New York: John Wiley.

Rogers, G. (1995). Educating case managers for culturally competent practice. *Journal of Case Management, 4*(2), 60–65.

Role of the social worker in discharge planning: Position statement of the Society for Hospital Social Work Directors of the American Hospital Association. (1986). *Quality Review Bulletin, 12*(2), 76.

Rose, S. M., & Moore, V. L. (1995). Case management. In R. L. Edwards (Ed.), *Encyclopedia of social work* (19th ed.). Washington, DC: National Association of Social Workers.

Rosen, A. (2003). Evidence-based social work practice: Challenges and promises. *Social Work Research, 27,* 197–208.

Rosen, B., Locke, B., Goldberg, I., & Babigian, H. (1972). Identification of emotional disturbance in patients seen in general medical clinics. *Hospital and Community Psychiatry, 23,* 12.

Rosen, G. (1974). *From medical police to social medicine: Essays on the history of health care* (pp. 112–116). New York: Science History Publications.

Rosenberg, C. E. (1989). *Caring for the working man: The rise and fall of the dispensary; An anthology of sources.* New York: Garland.

Rosenberg, G., & Clarke, S. (Eds.). (1987). Social workers in health care management: The move to leadership [Special issue]. *Social Work in Health Care, 12*(3), 1–3.

Rosenberg, M. S., & Sonkin, D. J. (1992). The prevention of child maltreatment in school-aged children. In D. J. Willis, E. W. Holden, & M. Rosenberg (Eds.), *Prevention of child maltreatment: Developmental and ecological perspectives* (pp. 78–93). New York: John Wiley.

Rosenfeld, L. S. (1971). *Ambulatory care: Planning and organization.* Rockville, MD: U.S. Department of Health, Education, and Welfare, Health Services and Mental Health Administration.

Rosenkrantz, B. G. (1972). *Public health and the state.* Cambridge, MA: Harvard University Press.

Rosenstock, I. M., Strecher, V. J., & Becker, M. H. (1988). Social learning theory and health belief model. *Health Education Quarterly, 15,* 175–183.

Rosenthal, B. B., & Mizrahi, T. (2004). Coalitions: Essential tools for organizing. In L. Staples, *Roots to power: A manual for grassroots organizing* (pp. 316–330). Westport, CT: Praeger.

Ross, A., & Williams, S. J. (1991). Epilogue: A new world. In A. Ross, S. J. Williams, & E. L. Schafer (Eds.), *Ambulatory care management* (pp. 398–401). Albany, NY: Delmar.

Ross, J. W. (1993). Taking responsibility. *Health and Social Work, 16,* 3–5.

Rothman, J. (1970). Three models of community organization practice. In F. M. Cox, J. L. Erlich, J. Rothman, & J. E. Tropman (Eds.), *Strategies of community organization* (pp. 20–36). Beverly Hills, CA: Sage.

Rothman, J. (2001). Approaches to community intervention. In J. Rothman, J. L. Erlich, & J. E. Tropman (Eds.), Strategies of *community* intervention (6th ed., pp. 27–64). Itasca, IL: F. E. Peacock.

Royse, D., Dhooper, S. S., & Rompf, E. L. (2010). *Field instruction: A guide for social work students* (6th ed.). Boston: Allyn & Bacon.

Rubin, A., & Babbie, E. (1993). *Research methods for social work.* Pacific Grove, CA: Brooks/Cole.

Rubin, F. H., & Black, J. S. (1992). Health care and consumer control: Pittsburgh's town meeting for seniors. *The Gerontologist, 32,* 853–855.

Rubin, H. J., & Rubin, I. S. (2001). *Community organizing and development* (3rd ed.). Boston: Allyn & Bacon.

Rukmana, D. (2008). Where the homeless children and youth come from: A study of the residential origins of the homeless in Miami-Dade County, Florida. *Children and Youth Services Review, 30*(9), 1009–1021.

Sabatino, C. A. (2009). School social work consultation models and response to intervention: A perfect match. *Children & Schools, 31*(4), 197–206.

Sahney, V. K., & Warden, G. L. (1991). The quest for quality and productivity in health service. *Frontiers of Health Services Management, 7*(4), 2–40.

Salamon, M. J. (1986). *A basic guide to working with elders.* New York: Springer.

Salinsky, E., & Gursky, E. A. (2006). The case for transforming governmental public health. *Health Affairs, 25*(4), 1017–1028.

Sanborn, C. J. (Ed.). (1983). *Case management in mental health services.* New York: Haworth.

Sarazan, S. J. (1990, July). The tools of quality: Part II; Cause-and-effect diagrams. *Quality Progress,* 59–62.

Satcher, D., & Pamies, R. (2006). *Multicultural medicine and health differences.* Columbus, OH: McGraw-Hill.

Scherzer, T., Wong, A., & Newcomer, R. (2007). Financial management services in consumer-directed programs. *Home Health Care Services Quarterly, 26*(1), 29–42.

Schlesinger, E. (2004). Historical perspectives on education for ethnic-sensitive and multicultural practice. In L. Gutierrez, M. E. Zuniga, & D. Lum (Eds.), *Education for multicultural social work practice: Critical viewpoints and future directions* (pp. 31–52). Alexandria, VA: Council on Social Work Education.

Schlesinger, E. G., & Devore, W. (1995). Ethnic-sensitive practice. In R. L. Edwards (Ed.), *Encyclopedia of social work* (19th ed.). Washington, DC: National Association of Social Workers.

Schillinger, D., Villela, T. J., & Saba, J. W. (2007). Creating a context for effective intervention in the clinical care of vulnerable patients. In T. E. King, Jr., & M. B. Wheeler (Eds.), *Medical management of vulnerable and underserved patients: Principles, practice, and populations* (pp. 59–67). New York: McGraw-Hill.

Schmitz, C. L., Wagner, J. D., & Menke, E. M. (2001). The interconnection of childhood poverty and homelessness: Negative impact/points of access. *Families in Society: The Journal of Contemporary Social Services, 82*(1), 69–77.

Schneider, A. W., Hyer, K., & Luptak, M. (2001). Suggestions to social workers for surviving in managed care. *Health & Social Work, 25*(4), 276–279.

Schneiderman, L. J., Jecker, N. S., & Jonsen, A. R. (1990). Medical futility: Its meaning and ethical implications. *Annals of Internal Medicine, 112,* 949–954.

Schroeder, S. A. (1993). Training an appropriate mix of physicians to meet the nation's needs. *Academic Medicine, 68,* 118–122.

Schultz, J. A., Fawcett, S. B., Francisco, V. T., Wolff, T., Berkowitz, B. R., & Nagy, G. (2000). The Community Tool Box: Using the Internet to support the work of community health and development.

Journal of Technology in Human Services, 17(2/3), 193–215.

Searight, H. R., & Gafford, J. (2005). Cultural diversity at the end of life: Issues and guidelines for family practitioners. *American Family Practitioner, 71*(3), 515–522.

Sears, R., Rudisill, J., & Mason-Sears, C. (2006). *Consultation skills for mental health professionals.* Hoboken, NJ: John Wiley.

Sedgeman, J. A. (2005). Health realization/innate health: Can a quiet mind and a positive feeling state be accessible over the life span without stress-relief techniques? *Medical Science Monitor, 22*(12), HY47–HY52.

Seligman, M. E. P. (1975). *Helplessness: On depression, development, and death.* New York: Freeman.

Seward, P. J., & Todd, J. S. (1995). Health system reform: Whither or whether? *Journal of the American Medical Association, 273*(3), 246–247.

Shachter, B., & Seinfeld, J. (1994). Personal violence and the culture of violence. *Social Work, 39,* 347–350.

Shainin, P. D. (1990, August). The tools of quality: Part III; Control charts. *Quality Progress,* 79–82.

Shapira, S. C., Hammond, J. S., & Cole, L. A. (Eds.). (2009). *Essentials of terror medicine.* New York: Springer.

Sharara, F. I., Beatse, S. N., Leonardi, M. R., Navot, D., & Scott, R. T., Jr. (1994). Cigarette smoking accelerates the development of diminished ovarian reserve as evidenced by the clomiphene citrate challenge test. *Fertility and Sterility, 62,* 257–262.

Sheafor, B. W., Horejsi, C. R., & Horejsi, G. A. (1988). *Techniques and guidelines for social work practice.* Needham Heights, MA: Allyn & Bacon.

Sheehan, N. W., & Oakes, C. E. (2004). Public policy initiatives addressing supportive housing: The experience of Connecticut. *Journal of Housing for the Elderly, 18*(3/4), 81–113.

Sheldon, P., & Bender, M. (1994). High-technology in-home care. *Community Health Nursing and Home Health Nursing, 3,* 507–519.

Shelton, T. L., Jeppson, E. S., & Johnson, B. H. (1987). *Family-centered care for children with special health care needs.* Washington, DC: Association for the Care of Children's Health.

Sheridan, J. E., White, J., & Fairchild, T. J. (1992). Ineffective staff, ineffective supervision, or ineffective administration? Why some nursing homes fail to provide adequate care. *The Gerontologist, 32,* 334–341.

Sheridan, M. S. (1988). Time management in health care social work. *Social Work in Health Care, 75*(3), 91–99.

Sherman, S. R., & Newman, E. S. (1988). *Foster families for adults: A community alternative in long-term care.* New York: Columbia University Press.

Shevlin, K. M. (1983). Why a social service department in a hospital? In I. Hubschman (Ed.), *Hospital social work practice* (pp. 1–14). New York: Praeger.

Shippee, T. P. (2009). "But I am not moving": Residents' perspective on transitions within a continuing care retirement community. *The Gerontologist, 49*(3), 418–427.

Shulman, N. M., & Shewbert, A. L. (2000). A model of crisis intervention in critical and intensive care units of general hospitals. In A. R. Roberts (Ed.), *Crisis intervention handbook: Assessment, treatment, and research* (pp. 412–429). New York: Oxford University Press.

Sickman, J. N., & Dhooper, S. S. (1991). Characteristics and competence of care providers in a Veterans Affairs community residential care home program. *Adult Residential Care Journal, 5,* 171–184.

Siefert, K. (1983). An exemplar of primary prevention in social work: The Sheppard-Towner Act of 1921. *Social Work in Health Care, 9*(1), 87–103.

Siegel, K., & Krauss, B. (1991). Living with HIV infection: Adaptive tasks of seropositive gay men. *Journal of Health and Social Behavior, 32,* 17–32.

Siegel, L. M., Attkisson, C. C., & Carlson, L. G. (1995). Need identification and program planning in the community context. In J. E. Tropman, J. Erlich, & J. Rothman (Eds.), *Tactics and techniques of community intervention* (3rd ed.). Itasca, IL: F. E. Peacock.

Sigerist, H. E. (1946). *The university at the crossroads.* New York: Henry Schuman.

Silverman, E. (1986). The social worker's role in shock-trauma units. *Social Work, 31,* 311–313.

Silverman, P. R. (2004). Dying and bereavement in historical perspective. In J. Berzoff & P. R. Silverman (Eds.), *Living with dying* (pp. 128–149). New York: Columbia University Press.

Simmons, J. (2004). Financing end-of-life care. In J. Berzoff & P. R. Silverman (Eds.), *Living with dying* (pp. 815–824). New York: Columbia University Press.

Simmons, L., & Wolff, H. (1954). *Social science and medicine.* New York: Russell Sage.

Simmons, R. J., & Abress, L. (1990). Quality-of-life issues for end-stage renal disease patients. *American Journal of Kidney Diseases, 15,* 311–318.

Simon, B. L. (1994). *The empowerment tradition in American social work: A history.* New York: Columbia University Press.

Simon, R. L., & Aigner, S. M. (1985). *Practice principles: A problem-solving approach to social work.* New York: Macmillan.

Simons, K., Shepherd, N., & Munn, J. (2008). Advancing the evidence base for social work in long-term care: The disconnect between practice and research. *Social Work in Health Care, 47*(4), 392–415.

Siporin, M. (1975). *Introduction to social work practice.* New York: Macmillan.

Smart cane will help visually impaired. (2009). *The Futurist, 43*(6), 2.

Smid, M., Bourgois, P., & Auerswald, C. L. (2010). The challenge of pregnancy among homeless youth: Reclaiming a lost opportunity. *Journal of Health Care for the Poor and Underserved, 21,* 140–156.

Smirnow, V. (1994, June). News and commentary from the nation's capital. *Dialysis & Transplantation.*

Smith, B. S., & Feng, Z. (2010). The accumulated challenges of long-term care. *Health Affairs, 29*(1), 29–34.

Smith, D. R. (1979). Hospice: Lessons of a Wisconsin hospital. In M. M. Melum (Ed.), *The changing role of the hospital: Options for the future* (pp. 61–64). Chicago: American Hospital Association.

Smith, H. Y., Loppnow, D. M., & Davis, L. E. (1995, March). *Community management: A postmodern response to traditional social work education and practice.* Paper presented at the 41st Annual Program Meeting of the Council on Social Work Education, San Diego, CA.

Smith, L. L. (1977). Crisis intervention theory and practice. *Community Mental Health Review, 2,* 4–13.

Snow, D. L., & Gordon, J. B. (1980). Social network analysis and intervention with the elderly. *The Gerontologist, 20,* 463–467.

Soap sniffer monitors hygiene. (2009). *The Futurist, 43*(5), 2.

Soloman, B. (1976). *Black empowerment: Social work in oppressed communities.* New York: Columbia University Press.

Solomon, R. (1983). Serving families of the institutionalized aged: The four crises. In G. S. Getzel & M. J. Mellor (Eds.), *Gerontological social work practice in long-term care* (pp. 83–96). New York: Haworth.

Sondik, E., Huang, D. T., Klein, R. J., & Satcher, D. (2010). Progress toward the *Healthy People 2010* goals and objectives. *Annual Review of Public Health, 31*(1), 271–281.

Sosin, M., & Caulum, S. (1983). Advocacy: A conceptualization for social work practice. *Social Work, 28,* 12–17

Soskis, C. W. (1980). Emergency room on weekends: The only game in town. *Health and Social Work, 5*(3), 37–43.

Soskis, C. W. (1985). *Social work in the emergency room.* New York: Springer.

Spain opens world's first organ-growing laboratory for human transplants. (2010). Retrieved from http://thereader.es/en/spain-news-stories/4907-spain-opens-world

Spitzer, W. J., & Neely, K. (1992). Critical incident stress: The role of hospital-based social work in developing a statewide intervention system for first responders delivering emergency services. *Social Work in Health Care, 18*(1), 39–58.

Staples, L. (1987). Can't ya hear me knocking: An organizing model. In F. M. Cox, J. L. Erlich, J. Rothman, & J. E. Tropman (Eds.), *Strategies of community organization.* Itasca, IL: F. E. Peacock.

Staples, L. (2004). *Roots to power: A manual for grassroots organizing.* Westport, CT: Praeger.

Staples, L. H. (1990). Powerful ideas about empowerment. *Administration in Social Work, 14,* 29–42.

Stark, E., Flitcraft, A., Zuckerman, D., Gray, A., Robinson, J., & Frazier, W. (1981). *Wife abuse in the medical setting: An introduction for health personnel* (Domestic Violence Monograph Series No. 7). Washington, DC: National Clearinghouse on Domestic Violence, Government Printing Office.

Steckler, A., Allegrante, J. P., Altman, D., Brown, R., Burdine, J. N., Goodman, R. M., et al. (1995). Health education intervention strategies: Recommendations for future research. *Health Education Quarterly, 22,* 307–328.

Steckler, A., Dawson, L., Goodman, R. M., & Epstein, N. (1987). Policy advocacy: Three emerging roles for health education. In W. Ward (Ed.), *Advances in health education and promotion* (Vol. 2, pp. 5–27). Greenwich, CT: JAI.

Steinberg, R. M., & Carter, G. W. (1983). *Case management and the elderly.* Lexington, MA: Lexington Books.

Steinberg, T. N. (1991). Rape on college campuses: Reform through Title IX. *Journal of College and University Law, 18,* 39–71.

Stephens, G. (1994, July–August). The global crime wave: And what we can do about it. *The Futurist, 28,* 22–28.

Stevens, R. (1989). *In sickness and in wealth: American hospitals in the twentieth century.* New York: Basic Books.

Stewart, V. (1990). *The David solution.* Brookfield, VT: Gower.

Stobbe, M. (2010, October 23). By 2005, 1 in 3 adults could have diabetes. *Lexington Herald-Leader,* p. A10.

Stoil, M. J. (1994, November–December). Patient self-determination: A good idea that needs work. *Nursing Homes,* 8–9.

Stone, R. I., & Reinhard, S. C. (2007). The place of assisted living in long-term care and related service systems. *The Gerontologist, 47*(Special Issue III), 23–32.

Stones, M. J., Rattenbury, C., Taichman, B., Kozma, A., & Stones, L. (1990). Effective selection of participants for group discussion intervention. *Clinical Gerontologist, 9*(3/4), 135–143.

Street, D., Burge, S., & Quadagno, J. (2009). The effect of licensure type on the policies, practices, and resident composition of Florida assisted living facilities. *The Gerontologist, 49*(2), 211–223.

Stroh, L., & Johnson, H. (2006). *The basic principles of effective consulting.* Mahwah, NJ: Erlbaum.

Suchman, E. (1967). *Evaluative research.* New York: Russell Sage.

Suddenly breathless. (1990, July–August). *The Futurist, 24,* 6.

Suicide in the elderly. (2009). *Depression and anxiety.* Retrieved from http://www.johnshopkinshealthalerts.com/alerts_index/depression_anxiety/16-1.html

Sulman, J., Kanee, M., Stewart, P., & Savage, D. (2007). Does difference matter? Diversity and human rights in a hospital workplace. *Social Work in Health Care, 44*(3), 1–16.

Sultz, H. A., & Young, K. M. (2001). *Health care USA: Understanding its organization and delivery.* Gaithersburg, MD: Aspen.

Sutherland, B. S., & Oktay, J. S. (1987). Adult foster programs: Different strokes for different folks? *Adult Foster Care Journal, 1,* 226–131.

Swartz, W. B. (1999). The conquest of disease: It's almost within sight. *The Futurist, 33*(1), 51.

Sylvester, C., & Sheppard, F. (1988). Health and social services in the community care program. *Adult Foster Care Journal, 2,* 38–51.

Tabone, C., et al. (1992, April). *Why do women accept the rape myth?* Paper presented at the 63rd

Annual Meeting of the Eastern Psychological Association, Boston.

Talmadge, H., & Murphy, D. F. (1983). Innovative home care program offers appropriate alternative for elderly. *Hospital Progress, 64,* 50–51, 72.

Task Force on Social Work Research. (1991). *Building social work knowledge for effective service and policies: A plan for research development.* Austin: School of Social Work, University of Texas.

Taylor, R. B., Denham, J. W., & Ureda, J. R. (1982). Health promotion: A perspective. In R. B. Taylor, J. R. Ureda, & J. W. Denham (Eds.), *Health promotion: Principle and clinical applications* (pp. 1–18). Norwalk, CT: Appleton-Century-Crofts.

Terris, M. (1975). Approaches to an epidemiology of health. *American Journal of Public Health, 65,* 1037–1044.

Terris, M. (1983). The cost-effective national health program. *Journal of Public Health Policy, 5*(3).

Thomas. J. (1992, September 14–15). *Protecting children and animals: Agenda for a non-violent future.* Summary of the American Humane Association Conference, Herndon, VA.

Thompson, D. H., Fawley-Huss, K., Miller, C., Modrzynski, J., Morrison, M., Pieh, M., et al. (1989). *Adult foster care in Michigan: A descriptive study.* Kalamazoo: Western Michigan University, School of Social Work.

Tilson, H., & Berkowitz, B. (2006). The public health enterprise: Examining our twenty-first-century policy challenges. *Health Affairs, 25*(4), 900–910.

Tiny hearing aid developed. (1995, January–February). *The Futurist, 29,* 5.

Tiny needles deliver medicine painlessly. (1998). *The Futurist, 32*(9), 9.

Tiny pumps for drugs. (1988, March–April). *The Futurist, 22,* 4.

Tomorrow in brief: Nanotubes may deliver drugs. (2005). *The Futurist, 39*(6), 2.

Tomorrow in brief: Plastic blood. (2007). *The Futurist, 41*(6), 2.

Tomorrow in brief: Producing artificial skin, factory style. (2009). *The Futurist, 43*(3), 2.

Tompsett, C. J., Toro, P. A., Guzicki, M., Manrique, M., & Zatakia, J. (2006). Homelessness in the United States: Assessing changes in prevalence and public opinion, 1993–2001. *American Journal of Community Psychology, 37*(1/2), 47–61.

Torabi, M. R., Bailey, W. J., & Majd-Jabbari, M. (1993). Cigarette smoking as a predictor of alcohol and other drug use by children and adolescents: Evidence of the "gateway drug effect." *Journal of School Health, 63,* 302–306.

Tow, B. L., & Gilliam, D. A. (2009, May–June). Synthesis: An interdisciplinary discipline. *The Futurist, 43,* 43.

Townsend, A. L. (1990). Nursing home care and family caregiver's stress. In M. A. P. Stephens, J. H. Crowther, S. E. Hobfoll, & D. L. Tennenbaum (Eds.), *Stress and coping in later-life families* (pp. 267–285). New York: Hemisphere.

Trabold, N. (2007). Screening for intimate partner violence within a health care setting: A systematic review of the literature. *Social Work in Health Care, 45*(1), 1–31.

Tracy, E. M., & Biegel, D. E. (1994). Preparing social workers for social network interventions in mental health practice. *Journal of Teaching in Social Work, 70*(1/2), 19–41.

Tripodi, T., Lalayants, M., & Zlotnik, J. L. (2008). Research. In T. Mizrahi & L. E. Davis (Eds.), Encyclopedia of social work (20th ed.). Washington, DC: National Association of Social Workers and Oxford University Press. Retrieved from http://www.oxford-naswsocialwork.com

Trocchio, J. (1993, November–December). Community partnerships for nursing homes. *Nursing Homes,* 18–19, 24.

Trocchio, J. (1994). Oldest and newest promise is responding to community needs. *Journal of Long-Term Care Administration, 22*(3), 22–24.

Tropman, J. E. (1995). Community needs assessment. In R. L. Edwards (Ed.), *Encyclopedia of social work* (19th ed.). Washington, DC: National Association of Social Workers.

Tucker, K., & McNerney, S. L. (1992, January). Building coalitions to initiate change. *Public Relations Journal,* 28–30.

Tucker, P. (2010, November–December). Gene therapy gets a big boost. *The Futurist, 44,* 11.

Tumulty, K., Pickert, K., & Park, A. (2010). America, the doctor will see you now. *Time, 175*(13), 25–32.

Turnock, B. J., Handler, A., Hall, W., Potsic, S., Nalluri, R., & Vaughn, E. H. (1994). Local health department effectiveness in addressing the core functions of public health. *Public Health Reports, 109,* 653–658.

Ullman, D. (1988, July–August). Homeopathy: Medicine for the 21st century. *The Futurist, 22,* 43–47.

Umoren, J. A. (1992). Maslow's hierarchy of needs and OBRA 1987: Toward need satisfaction by nursing home residents *Educational Gerontology, 18,* 657–670.

Underwood, S. M., Hoskins, D., Cummins, T., & Williams, A. (1994). Obstacles to cancer care: Focus on the economically disadvantaged. *Oncology Nurses Forum, 27*(1), 47–52.

U.S. Bureau of Labor Statistics. (2008). *Labor force statistics from the current population survey.* Washington, DC: U.S. Department of Labor, U.S. Bureau of Labor Statistics.

U.S. Census Bureau. (2010). *An older and more diverse nation by mid-century.* Retrieved from http://PIO@census.gov

U.S. Department of Health, Education, and Welfare. (1975). *Emergency medical services systems program guidelines* (DHEW Pub. No. [HSA] 75-2013). Hyattsville, MD: Author.

U.S. Department of Health and Human Services. (1990). *Child abuse and neglect: Critical first steps in response to a national emergency.* Washington, DC: Government Printing Office.

U.S. Department of Health and Human Services. (2003). *Summary of HIPPA privacy rules.* Washington, DC: Office of Civil Rights.

U.S. Department of Health and Human Services. (2010, November). *Health People 2020.* Washington, DC: Author. Retrieved from http://www.healthy people.gov/2020/topicsobjectives2020/pdfs/hp2020_brochure.pdf

U.S. Department of Justice, Federal Bureau of Investigation. (2010, September). *Crime in the United States, 2009.* Retrieved from http://www.fbi.gov/ucr/09cius.htm

U.S. Senate Special Committee on Aging. (1991). *Aging America: Trends and projections.* Washington, DC: Government Printing Office.

Usatine, R. P., Gelberg, L., Smith, M. H., & Lesser, J. (1994). Health care for the homeless: A family medicine perspective. *American Family Physician, 49,* 139–146.

Vandiver, V. L. (2008). Managed care. In T. Mizrahi & L. E. Davis (Eds.), Encyclopedia of social work (20th ed.). Washington, DC: National Association of Social Workers and Oxford University Press. Retrieved from http://www.oxford-naswsocial work.com

Vandivort, R. E. (1994). Advanced social work practice update paper: Report of the 1994 National Managed Care Congress. In *Social work practice update.* Washington, DC: National Association of Social Workers.

Vandivort, R., Kurren, G. M., & Braun, K. (1984). Foster family care for frail elderly: A cost-effective quality care alternative. *Journal of Gerontological Social Work, 7,* 101–114.

Veatch, R. M. (2009). *Patient, heal thyself: How the new medicine puts the patient in charge.* New York: Oxford University Press.

Velecky, M. (1995). An evaluation of preadmission assessment for elective surgery. *Australian Social Work, 48*(4), 33–40.

Velleman, R. A. (1990). *Meeting the needs of people with disabilities: A guide for librarians, educators, and other service professionals.* Phoenix, AZ: Oryx.

Viney, L. L., & Westbrook, M. T. (1981). Psychological reactions to chronic illness-related disability as a function of its severity and type. *Journal of Psychosomatic Research, 25,* 513–523.

Virnig, B. A., Ma, H., Hartman, L. C., Moscovice, I., & Carlin, B. (2006). Access to home-based hospice care for rural populations: Identification of areas lacking service. *Journal of Palliative Medicine, 9,* 1292–1299.

Virnig, B. A., Moscovice, I. S., Durham, S. B., & Casey, M. M. (2004). Do rural elders have limited access to Medicare hospice services? *Journal of the American Geriatrics Society, 52,* 731–735.

Vladeck, B. C. (1980). *Unloving care: The nursing home tragedy.* New York: Basic Books.

Vladeck, B. C. (1988). Hospitals, the elderly, and comprehensive care. In C. Eisdorfer & G. L. Maddox (Eds.), *The role of hospitals in geriatric care* (pp. 35–48). New York: Springer.

Vonk, M. E., Tripodi, T., & Epstein, I. (2006). *Research* techniques for clinical social workers (2nd ed.). New York: Columbia University Press.

Vourlekis, B., & Ell, K. (2007). Best practice case management for improved medical adherence. *Work in Health Care, 44*(3), 166–171.

Vourlekis, B. S., Gelfand, D. E., & Greene, R. R. (1992). Psychosocial needs and care in nursing homes: Comparison of views of social workers and home administrators. *The Gerontologist, 32,* 113–119.

Wade, K., & Neuman, K. (2007). Practice-based research: Changing the professional culture and language of social work. *Social Work in Health Care, 44*(4), 49–64.

Wagner, C. (2010). Homosexuality and family formation. *The Futurist, 44*(3), 6–7.

Wagner, E. R. (2001). Types of managed care organizations. In P. R. Kongstvedt (Ed.), *The managed care handbook* (pp. 33–45). Gaithersburg, MD: Aspen.

Wall, S. (1998). Transformation in public health systems. *Health Affairs, 17*(3), 65.

Wallace, S. R., Goldberg, R. J., & Slaby, A. E. (1984). *Clinical social work in health care: New biopsychosocial approaches.* New York: Praeger.

Wallack, L. (1994, Winter). Media advocacy: A strategy for empowering people and communities. *Journal of Public Health Policy,* 421–436.

Wallack, L., Dorfman, L., Jernigan, D., & Themba, M. (1993). *Media advocacy and public health: Power of prevention.* Newbury Park, CA: Sage.

Walley, A. Y., & Roll, F. J. (2007). Principles of caring for alcohol and drug users. In T. E. King, Jr., & M. B. Wheeler (Eds.), *Medical management of vulnerable and underserved patients: Principles, practice, and populations* (pp. 341–350). New York: McGraw-Hill.

Warren, R. (1977). *Social change and human purpose.* Chicago: Rand McNally.

Washington, K. T., Bickel-Swenson, D., & Stephens, N. (2008). Barriers to hospice use among African Americans: A systematic review. *Health & Social Work, 33*(4), 267–274.

Watkins, E. L. (1985). The conceptual base for public health social work. In A. Gitterman, R. B. Black, & F. Stein (Eds.), *Public health social work in maternal and child health* (Report of the Working Conference of the Public Health Social Work Advisory Committee for the Bureau of Health Care Delivery and Assistance). New York: Columbia University School of Social Work.

Watters, F. (1961). Group Health Association Inc. Washington, DC. *Group Practice, 10,* 661–674.

Wax, J. (1982, August). *Workshop on social work power and conflict negotiation.* Sponsored by Mid-Northern Ohio Society of Hospital Social Work Directors, Akron, OH.

Weick, A. (1986). The philosophical context of a health model of social work. *Social Casework, 67,* 551–559.

Weil, M. O., & Gamble, D. N. (1995). Community practice models. In R. L. Edwards (Ed.), *Encyclopedia of social work* (19th ed.). Washington, DC: National Association of Social Workers.

Weiner, J. (1994). Financing long-term care: A proposal by the American College of Physicians and the American Geriatrics Society. *Journal of the American Medical Association, 271,* 1525–1529.

Weiner, J. M., & Illson, L. H. (1994). Health care reform in the 1990s: Where does long-term care fit in? *The Gerontologist, 34,* 402–408.

Weiss, J. (1995). Genetic technology, ethics, and the family. In J. B. Rauch (Ed.), *Community-based, family-centered services in a changing health care environment.* Arlington, VA: National Maternal and Child Health Clearinghouse.

Weissensee, M. G., Kjervik, D. K., & Anderson, J. B. (1995). A tool to assess the cognitively impaired elderly. *Journal of Case Management, 4*(1), 29–33.

Weissert, W. G., & Hedrick, S. C. (1994). Lessons learned from research on effects of community-based long-term care. *Journal of the American Geriatric Society, 42,* 348–353.

Weissman, A. (1976). Industrial social services: Linkage technology. *Social Casework, 57,* 50–54.

Wells, S. J. (2008). Child abuse and neglect. In T. Mizrahi & L. E. Davis (Eds.), Encyclopedia of social work (20th ed.). Washington, DC: National Association of Social Workers and Oxford University Press. Retrieved from http://www.oxford-naswsocialwork.com

White, M., Gundrum, G., Shearer, S., & Simmons, W. J. (1994). A role for case managers in the physician office. *Journal of Case Management, 3*(2), 62–68.

White, S. W. (1993, Winter). Mental illness and national policy. *National Forum,* 2–3.

Wickizer, T. M., Von Korff, M., Cheadle, A., Maeser, J., Wagner, E. H., Pearson, D., et al. (1993). Activating communities for health promotion: A process evaluation method. *American Journal of Public Health, 83,* 561–567.

Wildon, V. R. (1994). Go beyond "home" to a hometown. *Journal of Long-Term Care Administration, 22*(2), 9.

Willer, B., & Intagliata, J. (1982). Comparison of family care and group homes as alternatives to institutions. *American Journal of Mental Deficiency, 86,* 588–595.

Wilkinson, R., & Marmot, M. (Eds.). (2003). *Social determinants of health: The solid facts* (2nd ed.). Copenhagen, Denmark: World Health Organization.

Williams, J. K. (1993). Case management: Opportunities for service providers. *Home Health Care Services Quarterly, 14,* 5–40.

Williams, S. J. (1991). An overview and management introduction. In A. Ross, S. J. Williams, & E. L. Schafer (Eds.), *Ambulatory care management.* Albany, NY: Delmar.

Williams, T. F. (1990). Foreword. In C. Zuckerman, N. N. Dubler, & B. Collopy (Eds.), *Home health care options: A guide for older persons and concerned families* (pp. ix–xii). New York: Plenum.

Wilson, D. (1979). The Iowa experimental swing-bed program. In M. M. Melum (Ed.), *The changing role of the hospital: Options for the future.* Chicago: American Hospital Association.

Wilson, K. B. (2007). Historical evolution of assisted living in the United States, 1979 to the present. *The Gerontologist, 47*(Special Issue III), 8–22.

Winkler, M. E. (1980). Saving face in the status race. *Health & Social Work, 5*(2), 27–33.

Winton, M. A., & Mara, B. A. (2001). *Child abuse and neglect: Multidisciplinary approaches.* Boston: Allyn & Bacon.

Witmer, J. M., & Sweeney, T. J. (1992). A holistic model for wellness and prevention over the life span. *Journal of Counseling & Development, 71*, 140–148.

Wolf, R. S. (2000). *Elder abuse in the family: An interdisciplinary model for research.* New York: Springer.

Wolf, R. S., & Pillemaer, K. (1994). What's new in elder abuse programming? Four bright ideas. *The Gerontologist, 34*, 126–129.

Wolfred, T. R. (1991). Ending the HIV epidemic: A call for community action. In S. Petrow, P. Frank, & T. R. Wolfred (Eds.), *Ending the HIV epidemic: Community strategies prevention and health promotion* (pp. 132–139). Santa Cruz, CA: Network.

Wood, B. (1994, November–December). 18 steps toward image enhancement. *Nursing Homes*, 13.

Wood, K. M., & Geismar, L. L. (1989). *Families at risk: Treating the multiproblem family.* New York: Human Science Press.

World Health Organization. (1958). Constitution of the World Health Organization. In *The first ten years of the World Health Organization* (pp. 459–472). Geneva: Author.

World Health Organization. (1986). The Ottawa charter for health promotion. *Health Promotion, J*, iii–v.

World Health Organization. (1989). *WHO AIDS series 5: Guide to planning health promotion for AIDS prevention and control.* Geneva: Author.

World Health Organization. (2011). *WHO definition of palliative care.* Retrieved from http://www.who.int/cancer/palliative/definition/en/

World trends & forecasts: The Internet will put hard-to-reach medical specialists in the palm of your hand (or in your chest). (2009). *The Futurist, 43*(4), 13.

World trends & forecasts: More doctors and hospitals will make use of wireless technologies. (2004, November–December). *The Futurist, 38,* 16.

World trends & forecasts: Your doctor will give you constant online checkups. (2009). *The Futurist, 43*(4), 13.

Wortman, C. B., & Lehman, D. R. (1985). Reactions to victims of life crises: Support attempts that fail. In I. G. Sarason & B. R. Sarason (Eds.), *Social support: Theory, research, and applications* (pp. 463–489). Dordrect, Netherlands: Martinus Nijhoff.

Wright, F. D., Beck, A. T., Newman, C. F., & Liese, B. S. (1993). Cognitive therapy of substance abuse: Theoretical rationale. *NIDA Research Monograph, 137*, 123–146.

Yanni, F. F. (1979). Hospital-sponsored primary care. In M. M. Melum (Ed.), *The changing role of the hospital: Options for the future.* Chicago: American Hospital Association.

Yoel, W. C., & Clair, J. M. (1994). Never enough time: How medical residents manage a scarce resource. *Journal of Contemporary Ethnography, 23*(2), 185–204.

Young, G. P., & Sklar, D. (1995). Health care reform and emergency medicine. *Annals of Emergency Medicine, 25*(5), 666–674.

Zakaria, F. (2010). Restoring the American dream. *Time, 176*(18), 30–35.

Zarit, S. H., & Zarit, J. M. (1982). Families under stress: Interventions for caregivers of senile dementia patients. *Psychotherapy: Theory, Research and Practice, 19*, 461–471.

Zastrow, C. (1985). *The practice of social work.* Belmont, CA: Dorsey.

Zavodnick, L., Katz, G., Markezin, E., & Mitchell, A. (1982). Management and organization of ambulatory care in MIS. In G. Katz, A. Mitchell, & E. Markezin (Eds.), *Ambulatory care and regionalization in multi-institutional health system.* Gaithersburg, MD: Aspen.

Zilberfein, F., & Hurwitz, E. (2004). Clinical social work practice in the end of life. In J. Berzoff & P. R. Silverman (Eds.), *Living with dying* (pp. 297–317). New York: Columbia University Press.

Zimmerman, J., & Dabelko, H. I. (2007). Collaborative models of patient care: New opportunities for hospital social workers. *Social Work in Health Care, 44*(4), 33–47.

Zimmerman, S., & Sloan, P. D. (2007). Definition and classification of assisted living. *The Gerontologist, 47*(Special Issue III), 33–39.

INDEX

Dhooper, S. S., 29, 76, 100, 110, 111, 115, 119, 127, 153, 165, 174, 178, 180, 198, 214, 226, 227, 243, 252, 268,
Diabetes, 31
Diagnosis-related groups (DRGs), 6, 41, 57, 88, 118, 133, 134, 145
Diagnostic devices, medical, 15–16
Diagnostic technologies, medical, 15
Dillard, J. M., 281
Dillon, C., 260
Disabilities, persons with
   chronic illness in, 39–40
   future needs of nonelderly, 104–105
   hospital response to needs of, 122–123
   working with, 140–141 (table)
Discharge planning, 131–136
   complexity of, 135–136, 145
   ethical considerations in, 144–146
   for AIDS patients, 142–143
   for elderly patients, 139–140
Disease prevention
   defining, 182
   See also Illness prevention/health promotion
Disease treatment era, 61
Dispensaries, 51–52, 56
Diversity, of patient population, 86–87
Dluhy, M. J., 273, 274, 275
Dobbins, N. J., 146 (note 1)
Donnelly, A. C., 205
Do-not-resuscitate orders (DNRs), 254
Dorfman, L., 198
Dower, P., 193, 196
Downsizing, 6
Drubach, D. A., 33
Drug-resistant diseases, 32–33
Drugs/diets, for prevention and treatment, 14
Dubowitz, H., 154
Dunn, C., 169, 170
Dziegielewski, S. F., 145

Ecological model, 24, 170, 184, 204–205, 209
Edlis, N., 143
Education
   medical, 21
   principles of health, 199 (table)
Educator/community activator role, 161, 187, 193–200, 199 (figure)
Edutainment, 198

Effectiveness/efficiency, enhancing social worker, 259–285
   coalition building, 272–275
   community work, 275–279
   conflict resolution, 269–272
   culturally sensitive practice, 279–281
   dealing with managed care, 281–284
   research skills, 266–269
   self-empowerment, 264–266
   strategies for, 259 (table)
   stress management, 259–261
   time management, 261–263
   worker-focused strategies, 259–269
Egan, J. J., 114, 177
Ehrlich, P., 156
Eisdorfer, C., 86, 89
Elder, J. P., 193, 196
Elder abuse, 104, 143–144
   persistence of, 38–39
   social work role, 156–157
   types of, 147 (note 3)
Elderly persons
   caseworker/counselor role *with,* 137–140
   chronic illness in, 39–40
   depression among, 10, 104, 138, 207, 221, 225, 226, 253
   functional assessment of, 138–139
   future needs of, 103–104
   hospital response to needs of, 122
   illness prevention/health promotion among, 207–208
   increase in, 9–10
   See also Elder abuse
Eliot, M. M., 183
Ell, K., 175
Elwyn, G., 249
Emergency care centers, 59–61
Emergency Medical Services Systems Act, 60
Emerson, H., 95, 185
Emic, 280
Empowerment, 139, 194–195
Enabling, 194
End-of-life care. *See* Hospice care
Enter-education, 198
Environmental analysis, 193
Epstein, J., 268
Erdmann, E., 6–7
Erickson, G., 6